Refractive
Surgery
Nightmares

Conquering Refractive Surgery Catastrophes

Refractive Surgery Nightmares

Conquering Refractive Surgery Catastrophes

EDITED BY

PROFESSOR AMAR AGARWAL, MS, FRCS, FRCOPHTH

DR. AGARWAL'S EYE HOSPITAL
RAMACHANDRA MEDICAL COLLEGE
CHENNAI, INDIA

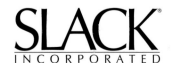

SLACK®
INCORPORATED

Delivering the best in health care information and education worldwide

www.slackbooks.com

ISBN: 978-1-55642-788-6

Published by: SLACK Incorporated
                  6900 Grove Road
                  Thorofare, NJ 08086 USA
                  Telephone: 856-848-1000
                  Fax: 856-853-5991
                  www.slackbooks.com

Contact SLACK Incorporated for more information about other books in this field or about the availability of our books from distributors outside the United States.

Library of Congress Cataloging-in-Publication Data

Refractive surgery nightmares : conquering refractive surgery catastrophes / edited by Amar Agarwal.
    p. ; cm.
  Includes bibliographical references and index.
  ISBN-13: 978-1-55642-788-6 (hardcover : alk. paper)
  ISBN-10: 1-55642-788-3 (hardcover : alk. paper)
  1. Refractive keratoplasty--Complications.   I. Agarwal, Amar.
  [DNLM: 1. Refractive Errors--surgery. 2. Postoperative Complica-
tions.   WW 340 R3325 2007]
  RE336.R4444 2007
  617.7'19059--dc22
                                    2006033366

Printed in the United States of America.

Last digit is print number: 10   9   8   7   6   5   4   3   2   1

DEDICATION

This book is dedicated to one of the finest human beings ophthalmology has produced:
Luther L. Fry

CONTENTS

Dedication v
Acknowledgments xi
About the Editor.. xiii
Contributing Authors xv
Preface xix
Foreword — Professor Thomas Neuhann xxi

SECTION I: PREOPERATIVE EXAMINATIONS PREVENTING NIGHTMARES

Chapter 1: Understanding the Orbscan to Prevent Nightmares 3
            Athiya Agarwal, MD, DO

Chapter 2: Anterior Keratoconus 11
            Sunita Agarwal, MS, DO

Chapter 3: Posterior Corneal Changes in Refractive Surgery 17
            *Smita Narasimhan, MBBS, FRSH, FERC
            and Amar Agarwal, MS, FRCS, FRCOphth*

Chapter 4: New Techniques for Exploring the Eye's Anterior Segment:
            Carl Zeiss Meditec Visante OCT................................. 25
            Georges Baïkoff, MD

Chapter 5: Pupil Size and Refractive Surgery................................. 35
            Francesco Carones, MD

SECTION II: SURFACE ABLATIONS: PRK, LASEK, EPI-LASIK, PTK

Chapter 6: Corneal Haze.. 43
            *Noel Alpins, FRACO, FRCOphth, FACS
            and George Stamatelatos, BScOptom*

Chapter 7: Photorefractive Keratectomy Complications 55
            Samuel Boyd, MD and Raymond Stein, MD, FRCSC

Chapter 8: LASEK Complications... 67
            Massimo Camellin, MD

Chapter 9: Epi-LASIK... 81
            *Vikentia J. Katsanevaki, MD, PhD; Maria I. Kalyvianaki, MD;
            Dimitra S. Kavroulaki, MD; and Ioannis G. Pallikaris, MD, PhD*

Chapter 10: The Use of Mitomycin-C in Laser Refractive Surgery.................... 89
            Francesco Carones, MD

Chapter 11: Nightmares With Phototherapeutic Keratecomy 97
            Jes Mortensen, MD

SECTION III: LASIK AND WAVEFRONT-GUIDED LASIK

Chapter 12: Flap Complications... 105
            *Melania Cigales, MD; Jairo Hoyos-Chacón, MD;
            and Jairo E. Hoyos, MD, PhD*

Chapter 13: Decentered Ablation...119
 Helen Boerman, OD; Tracy Swartz, OD, MS, FAAO;
 and Ming Wang, MD, PhD

Chapter 14: Post-LASIK Iatrogenic Ectasia 131
 Amar Agarwal, MS, FRCS, FRCOphth;
 Soosan Jacob, MS, FRCS, FERC, Dip NB;
 and Vladimir Pfeifer, MD

Chapter 15: Sands of Sahara or Diffuse Lamellar Keratitis: The Refractive
 Emergency 143
 Alexander Hatsis, MD, FACS

Chapter 16: Post-LASIK Infections 155
 Soosan Jacob, MS, FRCS, FERC, Dip NB;
 Amar Agarwal, MS, FRCS, FRCOphth;
 and Nibaran Gangopadhyay, MS

Chapter 17: Epithelial Ingrowth...163
 Amar Agarwal, MS, FRCS, FRCOphth
 and Soosan Jacob, MS, FRCS, FERC, Dip NB

Chapter 18: Dealing With Irregular Astigmatism: State of the Art 171
 Jorge L. Alió, MD, PhD and José I. Belda, MD, PhD

Chapter 19: Glare and Halos After Refractive Surgery 185
 Guillermo Simón-Castellví, MD; Sarabel Simón-Castellví, MD;
 José María Simón-Castellví, MD; Cristina Simón-Castellví, MD;
 and José María Simón-Tor, MD

Chapter 20: Complications Creating LASIK Flaps With the Intralase
 Femtosecond Laser..197
 William W. Culbertson, MD

Chapter 21: LASIK Over- and Undercorrections 203
 Luis Escaf Jaraba, MD; Alejandro Tello, MD; and
 Victor Rojas Hernandez, MD

Chapter 22: Topographic and Wavefront Aberrometry Disasters...................213
 Tracy Swartz, OD, MS, FAAO and Ming Wang, MD, PhD

Chapter 23: Customized LASIK After Previous Refractive Surgery................229
 Roberto Pinelli, MD; Patrizia Portesi, OT; and Cristian Bacchi, OD

Section IV: Lens-Based Refractive Surgery

Chapter 24: Accurate Biometry and Intraocular Lens Power Calculations 237
 Noel Alpins, FRACS, FRCOphth, FACS and
 Gemma Walsh, B Optom

Chapter 25: MIRLEX...245
 Amar Agarwal, MS, FRCS, FRCOphth; Mahipal S. Sachdev, MD;
 and Clement K. Chan, MD, FACS

Chapter 26: Refractive Shift After Pediatric Cataract Surgery 265
 Rupal H. Trivedi, MD, MSCR and M. Edward Wilson, Jr, MD

Chapter 27: Vitreoretinal Complications Associated With Refractive Surgery 275
  Clement K. Chan, MD, FACS; Steven G. Lin, MD;
  and Astha S. D. Nuthi, DO

Chapter 28: Nightmares With Presbyopic Correcting Implants 293
  Robert Jay Weinstock, MD

Chapter 29: Toxic Anterior Segment Syndrome 307
  Simon P. Holland, MB, FRCSC; Douglas W. Morck, DVM, PhD;
  Gina Chavez, BSc; Yumi G. Ohashi, BSc; and Tracy L. Lee, BSc

Chapter 30: Phakic Intraocular Lens Complications 315
  Benjamin F. Boyd, MD, FACS; Samuel Boyd, MD;
  Soosan Jacob, MS, FRCS, FERC, Dip NB;
  and Amar Agarwal, MS, FRCS, FRCOphth

SECTION V: MISCELLANEOUS

Chapter 31: Conductive Keratoplasty and Potential Complications 331
  Roberto Pinelli, MD

Chapter 32: Corneal Surgery for the Correction of Irregular Astigmatism After
  Corneal Refractive Surgery...339
  Jose L. Güell, MD; Javier A. Gaytan Melicoff, MD;
  Felicidad Manero Vidal, MD; Merce Morral MD;
  and Oscar Gris, MD

Chapter 33: Intracorneal Rings: KeraRings and Intacs..345
  Jaime R. Martiz, MD; Carlos Manrique De Lara, MD, FACS;
  and Ramon Naranjo Tackman, MD

Chapter 34: Refractive Surgery and Intraocular Pressure 351
  Soosan Jacob, MS, FRCS, FERC, Dip NB
  and Amar Agarwal, MS, FRCS, FRCOphth

Chapter 35: Dry Eye and Refractive Surgery...361
  Ahmad M. Fahmy, OD and David R. Hardten, MD

Chapter 36: Postrefractive Surgical Fitting of Contact Lenses.......................................373
  Kenneth Daniels, OD, FAAO

Index *383*

ENCLOSED VIDEO CD-ROM

Video 1: Battle of the Bulge: Post-LASIK Iatrogenic Keratectasia.............................7:43
  Soosan Jacob, MS, FRCS, FERC, Dip NB; Amar Agarwal, MS, FRCS, MS;
  Smita Narasimhan, MBBS, FRSH, FERC; Ashkok Kumar, DO, FERC;
  Nibaran Gangopadhyay, MS; Vladimir Pfeifer, MD; Athiya Agarwal, MD, DO;
  Sunita Agarwal, MS, DO; and Mr. Balasubramanian

Video 2: Flap Wars..7:46
  Soosan Jacob, MS, FRCS, FERC, Dip NB; Amar Agarwal, MS, FRCS, MS;
  Himanshu Shukla, MD; Athiya Agarwal, MD, DO; Sunita Agarwal, MS, DO;
  Jerry Tan, MD; Ming Wang, MD, PhD; Tracy Swartz, OD, MS, FAAO;
  Vladimir Pfeifer, MD; Jairo E. Hoyos, MD, PhD; Melania Cigales, MD;
  Jairo Hoyos-Chacón, MD; Nibaran Gangopadhyay, MS; T. Agarwal, MD;
  and Mr. Balasubramanian

Video 3: Perfecting Your Curves: Mastering Bimanual Phacoemulsification............7:46
Soundari S., MD; Amar Agarwal, MS, FRCS, MS;
Soosan Jacob, MS, FRCS, FERC, Dip NB; Ashkok Kumar, DO, FERC;
Nibaran Gangopadhyay, MS; Athiya Agarwal, MD, DO;
Sunita Agarwal, MS, DO; and Mr. Balasubramanian

Video 4: Pearls & Implantation Technique for the Foldable Iris
Fixated Phakic IOL...6:32
H. Burkhard Dick, MD and Mana Tehrani, MD

Video 5: Hyperopic Shift After Phacoemulsification
With Previous Radial Keratotomy..6:02
Virgilio Centurión, MD

Video 6: Cataract After Radial Keratotomy 4:47
Virgilio Centurión, MD

ACKNOWLEDGMENTS

No book can be completed without HIM and all the acknowledgment in the world is just not enough for HIM.

ABOUT THE EDITOR

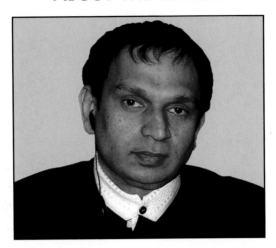

Amar Agarwal, MS, FRCS, FRCOphth is the pioneer of the phakonit procedure, which is phako with needle incision technology. This technique became popularized as bimanual phaco, microincision cataract surgery (MICS) or microphaco. He is the first to remove cataracts through a 0.7-mm tip with the technique called microphakonit. He has also discovered no anesthesia cataract surgery and FAVIT, a new technique to remove dropped nuclei. The use of an air pump, which was the simple idea of using an aquarium fish pump to increase the fluid into the eye in bimanual phaco and co-axial phaco, has helped prevent surge. This built the basis of various techniques of forced infusion for small incision cataract surgery. Dr. Aga was also the first to use trypan blue for staining epiretinal membranes and publishing the details in his four volume *Textbook of Ophthalmology*. He has also discovered a new refractive error called Aberropia. He is the first to do a combined surgery of microphakonit (700-micron cataract surgery) with a 25-gauge vitrectomy in the same patient thus having the smallest incisions possible for cataract and vitrectomy. He is also the first surgeon to implant a new mirror telescopic IOL (LMI) for patients suffering from age-related macular degeneration.

Dr. Agarwal has received many awards for his work in ophthalmology most significant being the Barraquer Award and the Kelman Award. He has also written more than 33 books that have been published in various languages including English, Spanish, and Polish. In his center, he also trains doctors from all over the world on phaco, bimanual phaco, LASIK, and the retina. Dr. Agarwal was recently appointed as Professor of Ophthalmology at Ramachandra Medical College in Chennai, India.

Contributing Authors

Athiya Agarwal, MD, DO
Dr. Agarwal's Group Of Eye Hospitals and
   Eye Research Centre
Chennai, India

Sunita Agarwal, MS, DO
Dr. Agarwal's Group Of Eye Hospitals and
   Eye Research Centre
Bangalore, India

Jorge L. Alio, MD, PhD
Instituto Oftalmológico De Alicante
Refractive Surgery and Cornea Department
Miguel Hernández University, Medical School
Alicante, Spain

Noel Alpins, FRACO, FRCOphth, FACS
University of Melbourne
Melbourne, Australia

Cristian Bacchi, OD
Instituto Laser Microchirurgia Oculare
Brescia, Italy

Georges Baïkoff, MD
Clinc Monticelli
Marseille, France

José I. Belda, MD, PhD
Vissum Corporation—Instituto Oftalmológico
   de Alicante
Department of Ophthalmology
Universidad Miguel Hernández
Alicante, Spain

Helen Boerman, OD
Wang Vision Institute
Nashville, TN

Benjamin F. Boyd, MD, FACS
Consultant Editor
Highlights of Ophthalmology
Panama, Republic of Panama

Samuel L. Boyd, MD
Editor In Chief And Executive Vice President
Highlights of Ophthalmology
Director, Laser Section and Associate Director
Retina and Vitreous Department
Clinica Boyd—Ophthalmology Center
Panama, Republic of Panama

Massimo Camellin, MD
Health Director
Sekal Microchirurgia Rovigo
Rovigo, Italy

Francesco Carones, MD
Carones Ophthalmology Center
Milano, Italy

Virgilio Centurión, MD
Instituto de Moléstias Oculares
Sao Paulo, Brazil

Clement K. Chan, MD, FACS
Medical Director
Southern California Desert Retina Consultants,
   MC and Inland Retina Consultants
Palm Springs, California
Associate Clinical Professor
Department of Ophthalmology
Loma Linda University
Loma Linda, California

Gina Chavez, BSc
University of British Columbia
Canada

Melania Cigales, MD
Ophthalmologist
Instituto Oftalmológico Hoyos
Sabadell, Barcelona, Spain

William W. Culbertson, MD
Professor of Opthalmology, Lou Higgins
   Distinguished Chair
University of Miami Miller School of
   Medicine
Director of Refractive Surgery Center
Miami, Florida

Kenneth Daniels, OD, FAAO
Adjunct Assistant Clinical Professor
Pennsylvania College of Optometry
Center for International Studies
Hopewell—Lambertville Eye Associates
Hopewell, NJ
Affiliated with the Wills—Princeton Eye Group
Laser Surgery Center
Princeton, NJ

Carlos Manrique De Lara, MD, FACS
Manrique Custom Vision Centers
Medical Director
Professor of Ophthalmology at University of
  Texas, Health Science Center
San Antonio, Texas

H. Burkhard Dick, MD
Professor and Chairman, Director
Center for Vision Science
Ruhr University
Bochum, Germany

Ahmad M. Fahmy, OD
Minnesota Eye Consultants
University of Minnesota
Minneapolis, Minnesota
Regions Medical Center
St. Paul, Minnesota

Nibaran Gangopadhyay, MS
Director, Eye Care
Techno India
Kolkata, India

Oscar Gris, MD
Instituto de Microcirugia Ocular
Barcelona, Spain

Jose L. Güell, MD
Associate Professor of Ophthalmology
Autonoma University of Barcelona
Director of Cornea and Refractive Surgery
  Unit
Instituto de Microcirugia Ocular
Barcelona, Spain

David R. Hardten, MD
Minnesota Eye Consultants
University of Minnesota
Minneapolis, Minnesota
Regions Medical Center
St. Paul, Minnesota

Alexander Hatsis, MD, FACS
Director of Refractive Surgery
Assistant Clinical Professor of
  Ophthalmology
State University of New York
Stony Brook, New York

Victor Rojas Hernández, MD
Ophthalmologist
Anterior Segment Fellowship Clínica
Oftalmológica del Caribe
Barranquilla, Colombia

Simon P. Holland, MB, FRCSC
The Eye Care Centre
Vancouver, British Columbia
Canada

Jairo E. Hoyos, MD, PhD
Chairman of Ophthalmology
Instituto Oftalmológico Hoyos
KM Study Group President
Sabadell, Barcelona, Spain

Jairo Hoyos-Chacón, MD
Ophthalmologist
Instituto Oftalmológico Hoyos
Sabadell, Barcelona, Spain

Soosan Jacob, MS, FRCS, FERC, Dip NB
Dr. Agarwal's Group Of Eye Hospitals and
  Eye Research Centre
Chennai, India

Luis Escaf Jaraba, MD
Ophthalmologist
Subspecialist Anterior Segment
Medical Director Clínica Oftalmológica del
  Caribe
Chairman Fellowship and Residency Programs
Universidad de San Martín
Barranquilla, Colombia

Maria I. Kalyvianaki, MD
Vardinogiannion Eye Institute
University of Crete, Greece

Vikentia J. Katsanevaki, MD, PhD
Vardinogiannion Eye Institute
University Of Crete, Greece

Dimitra S. Kavroulaki, MD
Vardinogiannion Eye Institute
University of Crete
Greece

Tracy L. Lee, BSc
University of British Columbia
Vancouver, British Columbia
Canada

Steven G. Lin, MD
Southern California Desert Retina Consultants,
   MC and Inland Retina Consultants
Palm Springs, California

Jaime R. Martiz, MD
Clinical Director, Refractive Surgery
Consultant, President
Woodlands Custom Vision
Woodlands, Texas

Javier A. Gaytan Melicoff, MD
Cirujano Oftalmólogo
Especialista en Córnea y Cirugía Refractiva
FHNSL México/IMO
Barcelona, Spain

Douglas W Morck, DVM, PhD
University of Calgary
Calgary, Alberta
Canada

Merçe Morral, MD
Instituto de Microcirugia Ocular
Barcelona, Spain

Jes Mortensen, MD
University Hospital of Örebro
Örebro, Sweden

Smita Narasimhan, MBBS, FRSH, FERC
Dr. Agarwal's Group Of Eye Hospitals and
   Eye Research Centre
Chennai, India

Astha S.D. Nuthi, DO
Southern California Desert Retina Consultants,
   MC and Inland Retina Consultants
Palm Springs, California

Yumi G. Ohashi, BSc
University of British Columbia
Vancouver, British Columbia
Canada

Ioannis G. Pallikaris, MD, PhD
Vardinogiannion Eye Institute
University of Crete
Greece

Vladimir Pfeifer, MD
University Eye Clinic
Klinicni Center Ljubljana
Slovenija

Roberto Pinelli, MD
Scientific Director
Instituto Laser Microchirurgia Oculare
Brescia, Italy

Patrizia Portesi, OT
Instituto Laser Microchirurgia Oculare
Brescia, Italy

Mahipal S. Sachdev, MD
Centre for Sight
New Delhi, India

Cristina Simón-Castellví, MD
Simon Eye Clinic
Barcelona, Spain

Guillermo Simón-Castellví, MD
Chief Anterior Segment Surgeon
Simon Eye Clinic
Department of Ophthalmology
University of Barcelona
Barcelona, Spain

Sarabel Simón-Castellví, MD
Chief Posterior Segment Surgeon
Simon Eye Clinic
Barcelona, Spain

José María Simón-Castellví, MD
Anterior Segment Consultant
Emergency Room
Simon Eye Clinic
Barcelona, Spain

José María Simón-Tor, MD
Chairman
Glaucoma Senior Consultant
Simon Eye Clinic
Barcelona, Spain

George Stamatelatos, BScOptom
New Vision Clinics
Melbourne, Australia

Raymond Stein, MD, FRCSC
Medical Director, Bochner Eye Institute
Chief of Ophthalmology
Scarborough Hospital
Toronto, Canada

Tracy Swartz, OD, MS, FAAO
Wang Vision Institute
Nashville, Tennessee

Ramon Naranjo Tackman, MD
Hospital para evitar la Ceguera
Chief of Cornea Department
Mexico City, Mexico

Jerry Tan, MD
Jerry Tan Eye Surgery
Camden Medical Centre
Singapore

Mana Tehrani, MD
Center for Vision Science
Ruhr University
Bochum, Germany

Alejandro Tello, MD
Ophthalmologist
Subspecialist Anterior Segment
Fundación Oftalmológica Vejarano
Clinical Professor of Ophthalmology
Universidad del Cauca
Research Department Director, Fundación
  Oftalmológica Vejarano
Popayán, Colombia.
Member of Editorial Board
Highlights of Ophthalmology
Panamá City, Panamá.

Rupal H. Trivedi, MD, MSCR
Miles Center for Pediatric Ophthalmology
Storm Eye Institute, Department of
  Ophthalmology
Medical University of South Carolina
Charleston, South Carolina

Felicidad Manero Vidal, MD
Oftalmologa
Especialista en Enfermedades Externas
Instituto de Microcirugia Ocular de
  Barcelona
Barcelona, Spain

Gemma Walsh, B. Optom
New Vision Clinics
Melbourne, Australia

Ming Wang, MD, PhD
Wang Vision Institute
Nashville, Tennessee

Robert Jay Weinstock, MD
Cataract and Refractive Surgeon
The Eye Institute of West Florida
Largo, Florida

M. Edward Wilson, Jr, MD
Miles Center for Pediatric Ophthalmology
Storm Eye Institute
Department of Ophthalmology
Medical University of South Carolina
Charleston, South Carolina

PREFACE

Nightmares give all of us sleepless nights. Whenever we have nightmares in refractive surgery, it is even more disastrous as we are treating patients mainly for a cosmetic reason. Keeping this in mind, this book has been written so that you can learn from the problems we have experienced so you do not do the same thing. The aim of this book remains "to keep it simple" in order to enable the refractive surgeon to effectively diagnose and treat the various complications that can be associated with refractive surgery.

One day, I was watching the news on CNN. The news reader announced that a person had climbed Mount Everest. I told myself "so what? Many people climb Mount Everest." The next sentence the news reader announced was that the person who climbed Mount Everest had no legs. This got me thinking—a person with no legs climbing Mount Everest. Normal bodied people are not able to do even simple things sometimes. The question then that came to my mind is where is the battle ? Does one believe the battle is in the legs? No. THE BATTLE IS IN THE BRAIN.

Many eye surgeons from all over the world ask me how to improve their surgical skills. Just like the person who climbed Mount Everest, whenever we do surgery, the battle is in our brain. When we conquer that battle, we will become better. This does not mean that we will not have nightmares in surgery. Yes, we will, but it will make us better prepared to deal with them. I hope that with this book, I have done my bit in preparing you to deal with these nightmares in refractive surgery. Nobody expects you to become the best refractive surgeon in the world, but you would expect yourself to become a bit better today than what you were yesterday. If you achieve that, you are a winner all the way.

I would like to thank my consultant, Dr. Soosan Jacob; my secretary, Mr. Kumarguru; and each and every contributing author who I keep troubling when writing my books. I would also like to thank John Bond, Jenniffer Briggs, Robert Smentek, Michelle Gatt, and the rest of the SLACK Incorporated team for helping me in every stage of this book. I do not know what I have done in my Karma to get such great human beings as friends.

I would like to end this preface with a lovely quotation from Professor Muthu:

"There are two ways to spread knowledge;
Be the candle or the mirror that reflects it.
Where I cannot be the candle,
I want to be, at least, the mirror."

Amar Agarwal, MS, FRCS, FRCOphth
Dr. Agarwal's Group of Eye Hospitals
Chennai, India

FOREWORD

Never before has the introduction of a new therapeutic modality in ophthalmology been associated with a hype comparable with that raised by refractive surgery. Glossy paper marketing brochures scream out the definitive relief of all burden and nuisance with glasses and contact lenses: freedom, beauty, a new life altogether—all seemingly without problems or risks. How could one promise a guarantee? Because this surgery is performed only by internationally reknown, experienced, or outright world-famous surgeons.

As splendid and fascinating as the possibilities of modern refractive surgery truly are in the vast majority of cases, there is also a dark side of the moon. Dr. Amar Agarwal and his outstanding international team of authors have the great merit of pointing out the dark side that so often is kept quiet with embarassment. Yes, it is in fact a nightmare when—culpably or not—a healthy, well-seeing eye with optical correction does not come out of refractive surgery as a well-seeing eye, but rather as an eye with a serious medical problem that no longer performs well, even with optical correction.

The book goes beyond just exploring the dark side of the moon. It compiles the enormous combined experience of the authors in this field to show ways to avoid such nightmares in the first place and, once confronted with an undesired outcome, how to recognize them and their cause, deal with them, and repair them to the best end result possible.

Dr. Agarwal and his team of true heavyweight champions in this specialty are not only to be greatly respected and commended for sharing with us their vast experience, but also for their honesty in letting us know that even they, with all their knowledge, responsibility, and experience, have had nightmares. That does not make the nightmares less frightening, but it teaches medical professionals modesty and responsibility in our promises to our patients, forces us to take every preventive measure and care to avoid complications, and gives us a perspective of treatment when they ocurr (and if it were only, to know, who to refer a patient to). The lesson in this book is loud and clear: good refractive surgeons do not negate complications. They inform their patients properly, avoid risks to the best contemporary standard, and, if a complication occurs, assume responsibility and care for the best available treatment.

A copy of this book belongs in the reference library of every refractive surgery center—and, so to speak, under the pillow of every refractive surgeon.

Professor Thomas Neuhann
Germany

I

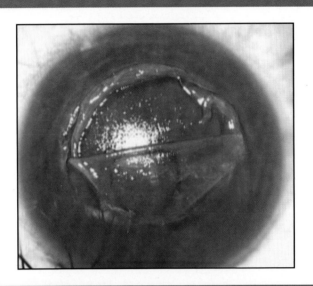

Preoperative Examinations Preventing Nightmares

Chapter 1

UNDERSTANDING THE ORBSCAN TO PREVENT NIGHTMARES

Athiya Agarwal, MD, DO

INTRODUCTION

Keratometry and corneal topography with placido disc systems were originally invented to measure anterior corneal curvature. Computer analysis of more complete data acquired by the latter has, in recent years, been increasingly more valuable in the practice of refractive surgery. The problem with the placido disc systems is that one cannot perform a slit scan topography of the cornea. This has been solved by an instrument called the Orbscan (Bausch & Lomb, Rochester, NY), which combines both slit scan and placido images to give a very good composite picture for topographic analysis. Orbscan[1-3] analysis can help diagnose primary posterior corneal elevation and other conditions and, thus, prevents one from having nightmare occurrences in refractive surgery.

PARAXIAL OPTICS

Spectacle correction of sight is designed to only eliminate defocus errors and astigmatism. These are the only optical aberrations that can be handled by the simplest theory of imaging, known as paraxial optics that excludes all light rays finitely distant from a central ray or power axis. Ignoring the majority of rays entering the pupil, paraxial optics only examine a narrow thread-like region surrounding the power axis. The shape of any smoothly rounded surface within this narrow region is always circular in cross-section. Thus from the paraxial viewpoint, surface shape is toric at most; only its radius may vary with meridional angle. Because a toric optical surface has sufficient flexibility to null defocus and astigmatism, only paraxial optics are needed to specify corrective lenses for normal eyes. Paraxial optics are used in keratometers and two-dimensional (2-D) topographic machines.

RAYTRACE OR GEOMETRIC OPTICS

The initial objective of refractive surgery was to build the necessary paraxial correction into the cornea. When outcomes are less than perfect, it is because defocus correction is inadequate. Typically, other aberrations (astigmatism, spherical aberration, coma, etc) are introduced during surgery. These may be caused by decentered ablation, asymmetric healing, biomechanical response, poor surgical planning, and inadequate or misinformation. To assess the aberrations in the retinal image, all the light rays entering the pupil must properly be taken into account using raytrace (or geometric) optics. Paraxial optics and their hypothetical toric surfaces must be abandoned as inadequate, which eliminates the need to measure surface curvature. Raytrace optics does not require surface curvature, but depends on elevation and especially surface slope. The Orbscan uses raytrace or geometric optics.

ELEVATION

Orbscan measures elevation, which is especially important because it is the only complete scalar measure of surface shape. Both slope and curvature can be mathematically derived from a single elevation map, but the converse is not necessarily true. As both slope and curvature have different values in different directions, neither can be completely represented by a single map of the surface. Thus, when characterizing the surface of nonspherical test objects used to verify instrument accuracy, elevation is always the gold standard.

Curvature maps in corneal topography (usually misnamed as power or dioptric maps) only display curvature measured in radial directions from the map center. Such a presentation is not shift-invariant, which means its values and topography change as the center of the map is shifted. In contrast, elevation is shift-invariant. An object shifted with respect to the map center is just shifted in its elevation map. In a meridional curvature view, it is also described. This makes elevation maps more intuitively understood, making diagnosis easier.

To summarize:
- Curvature is not relevant in raytrace optics.
- Elevation is complete and can be used to derive surface curvature and slope.
- Elevation is the standard measure of surface shape.
- Elevation is easy to understand.

The problem we face is that there is a cost in converting elevation to curvature (or slope) and visa versa. To go from elevation to curvature requires mathematical differentiation, which accentuates the high spatial frequency components of the elevation function. As a result, random measurement error or noise in an elevation measurement is significantly multiplied in the curvature result. The inverse operation, mathematical integration used to convert curvature to elevation, accentuates low-frequency error. The Orbscan helps in good mathematical integration, making it easy for the ophthalmologist to understand because the machine does all the conversion.

ORBSCAN I AND II

Previously, Orbscan I was used, which only had a slit scan topographic system. Then the placido disc was added in Orbscan I. Hence Orbscan II came into the picture.

SPECULAR VERSUS BACK-SCATTERED REFLECTION

The keratometer eliminates the anterior curvature of the precorneal tear film. It is an estimate because the keratometer only acquires data within a narrow 3-mm diameter annulus. It measures the anterior tear film because it is based on specular reflection (Figure 1-1), which occurs primarily at the air-tear interface. As the keratometer has very limited data coverage, abnormal corneas can produce misleading or incorrect results.

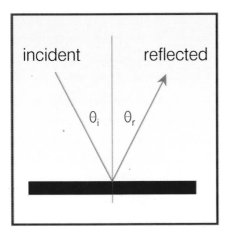

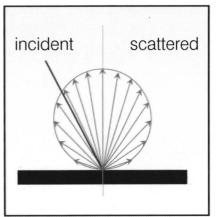

Figure 1-1. Specular reflection. This is used in keratometers. This is angle dependent.

Figure 1-2. Back-scatter reflection. This is used in Orbscan. This is omnidirectional.

Orbscan can calculate a variety of different surface curvatures, and on a typical eye, these are all different. The various curvatures equal only on a properly aligned and perfectly spherical surface. The tabulated simulated keratometer (SimK) values (magnitudes and associated meridians) are the only ones designed to give keratometer- like measurements. Therefore, it only makes sense to compare keratometry reading with SimK values.

Orbscan uses slit-beams and back-scattered light (Figure 1-2) to triangulate surface shape. The derived mathematical surface is then raytraced using a basic keratometer model to produce SimK values. Due to the difficulty of calculating curvature from triangulated data, the repeatability of Orbscan I SimK values is usually not as good as a clinical keratometer. But when several readings of the same eye are averaged, no discernible systematic error is found.

If one reading is taken and a comparison is made, the difference may be significant enough to make you believe the instrument is not working properly. So when the placido illuminator was added to Orbscan II to increase its anterior curvature accuracy, it also provided reflected data similar to that obtained with a keratometer. These reflective data are now used in SimK analyses, resulting in repeatabilities similar to keratometers and other placido-based corneal topography instruments.

Keratometry measures the tear film, while slit-scan triangulation, as embodied in Orbscan, sees through the tear- film and measures the corneal surface directly. Thus, an abnormal tear film can produce significant differences in keratometry but not with the Orbscan II.

Curvature measures the geometric bending of a surface, and its natural unit is reciprocal length, like inverse millimeters (1/mm). When keratometry was invented, this unfamiliar unit was replaced by a dioptric interpretation, making keratometry values equivalent on average (ie, over the original population) to the paraxial back-vertex power of the cornea. As it has become increasingly more important to distinguish optical properties from geometric properties, it is now more proper to evaluate keratometry in keratometric diopters. The keratometric diopter is strictly defined as a geometric unit of curvature with no optical significance. One inverse millimeter equals 337.5 keratometric diopters.

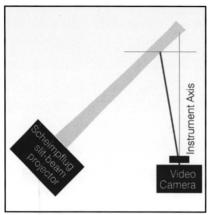

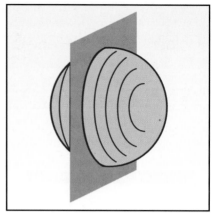

Figure 1-3. Beam and camera calibration in the Orbscan.

Figure 1-4. Ocular surface slicing by the Orbscan slit.

IMAGING IN THE ORBSCAN

In the Orbscan, the calibrated slit, which falls on the cornea, gives topographical information that is captured and analyzed by the video camera (Figure 1-3). Both slit-beam surfaces are determined in camera object space. Object space luminance is determined for each pixel value and framegrabber setting. Forty slit images are acquired in two 0.7-second periods. During acquisition, involuntary saccades typically move the eye by 50 μm. Eye movement is measured from anterior reflections of stationary slit-beam and other light sources. Eye tracking data permit saccadic movements to be subtracted from the final topographic surface. Each of the 40 slit images triangulates one slice of ocular surface (Figure 1-4). Before an interpolating surface is constructed, each slice is registered in accordance with measured eye movement. Distance between data slices averages 250 μm in the coarse scan mode (40 slits limbus to limbus). So Orbscan exam consists of a set of mathematical topographic surfaces (x, y), for the anterior and posterior cornea, anterior iris and lens and backscattering coefficient of layers between the topographic surfaces (and over the pupil).

MAP COLORS CONVENTIONS

Color contour maps have become a standard method for displaying 2-D data in corneal and anterior segment topography. Although there are no universally standardized colors, the spectral direction (from blue to red) is always organized in definite and intuitive ways.
- Blue = low, level, flat, deep, thick, or aberrated
- Red = high, steep, sharp, shallow, thin, or focused

ANALYSIS OF THE NORMAL EYE BY THE ORBSCAN MAP

The general quad map in the Orbscan of a normal eye (Figure 1-5) shows 4 pictures. The upper left is the anterior float, which is the topography of the anterior surface of the cornea. The upper right shows the posterior float, which is the topography of the posterior surface of the cornea. The lower left map shows the keratometric pattern and the lower right map shows the pachymetry (thickness of the cornea). The Orbscan is a three-dimensional (3-D)

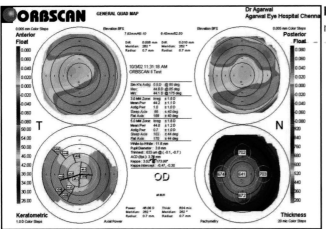

Figure 1-5. General quad map of a normal eye.

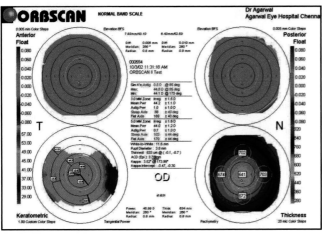

Figure 1-6. Normal band scale filter on a normal eye.

slit scan topographic machine. If we were doing topography with a machine that does not have slit scan imaging facilities, we would not be able to see the topography of the posterior surface of the cornea. Now, if the patient had an abnormality in the posterior surface of the cornea (eg, as in primary posterior corneal elevation), this would not be diagnosed. Then, if we perform LASIK on such a patient, we would create an iatrogenic keratectasia. The Orbscan helps us to detect the abnormalities on the posterior surface of the cornea.

Another facility, which we can move onto once we have the general quad map, is to put on the normal band scale filter (Figure 1-6). If we are in suspicion of any abnormality in the general quad map, then we put on the normal band scale filter. This highlights the abnormal areas in the cornea in orange to red colors. The normal areas are all shown in green. This is very helpful with generalized screening in preoperative examination of a LASIK patient.

CLINICAL APPLICATIONS

Let us now illustrate this better in a case of a primary posterior corneal elevation. If we see the general quad map of a primary posterior corneal elevation (Figure 1-7), we will see the upper left map is normal. The upper right map shows abnormality highlighted in red. This indicates the abnormality in the posterior surface of the cornea. The lower left keratometric map is normal and if we see the lower right map, which is the pachymetry map, one will see

Figure 1-7. General quad map of a primary posterior corneal elevation. Notice the upper right map has an abnormality whereas the upper left map is normal. This shows the anterior surface of the cornea is normal and the problem is in the posterior surface of the cornea.

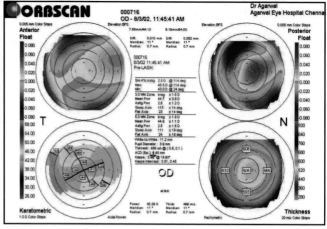

Figure 1-8. Quad map of a primary posterior corneal elevation with the normal band scale filter on. This shows the abnormal areas in red and the normal areas in green. Notice the abnormality in the upper right map.

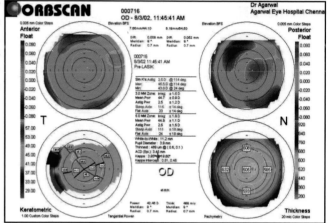

a slightly thin cornea of 505 μm, but still one cannot diagnose the primary posterior corneal elevation only from this reading. Thus we can understand that if not for the upper right map, which denotes the posterior surface of the cornea, one would miss this condition. Only the Orbscan can diagnose this.

Now, we can put on the normal band scale filter (Figure 1-8), and it will highlight the abnormal areas in red. Notice in Figure 1-8 the upper right map shows a lot of abnormality denoting the primary posterior corneal elevation. One can also take the 3-D map of the posterior surface of the cornea (Figure 1-9) and notice the amount of elevation in respect to the normal reference sphere shown as a black grid. In a case of keratoconus (Figure 1-10), all 4 maps show an abnormality, which confirms the diagnosis.

If we take a LASIK patient's topography, we can compare the patient's pre- and post-LASIK (Figure 1-11) pictures. This helps to understand the pattern and amount of ablation done on the cornea. The picture on the upper right is the preop topographic picture and the one on the lower right is the post-LASIK picture. The main picture on the left shows the difference between the pre- and post-LASIK topographic patterns. One can detect from this any decentered ablations or any other complication of LASIK surgery.

Corneal topography is extremely important in cataract surgery. The smaller the size of the incision, the less the astigmatism, and earlier stability of the astigmatism will occur. One can reduce or increase the patient's astigmatism after cataract surgery. The simple rule to follow is that where you make an incision, the area will flatten and where you apply sutures, the area

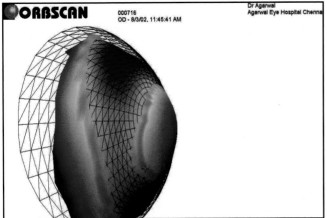

Figure 1-9. 3-D map of primary posterior corneal elevation. This shows a marked elevation in respect to a normal reference sphere highlighted as a black grid. Notice the red color protrusion on the black grid. This picture is of the posterior surface of the cornea.

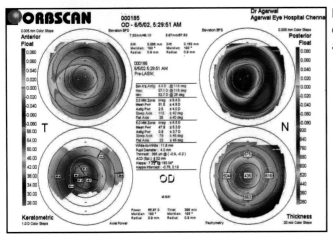

Figure 1-10. General quad map of a keratoconus patient showing abnormality in all 4 maps.

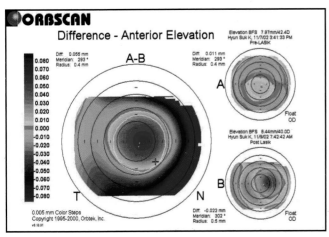

Figure 1-11. Difference of pre- and post-LASIK.

will steepen. One can use the Orbscan to analyze the topography before and after cataract surgery. For instance, in an extracapsular cataract extraction one can check to see where the astigmatism is highest and remove those sutures. In a phaco procedure, the astigmatism will be lower, and in Phakonit where the incision is sub-1.5 mm, or in microphakonit (700 microncataract surgery), the astigmatism will be the least.

We can use the Orbscan to determine the anterior chamber depth and also analyze where one should place the incision when one is performing astigmatic keratotomy. The Orbscan can also help in a good fit of a contact lens with a fluorescein pattern.

Summary

The Orbscan has changed the world of topography because it gives us an understanding of a slit scan 3-D picture. One can use this in understanding various conditions.

KEY POINTS

1. Orbscan measures elevation. Elevation is especially important because it is the only complete scalar measure of surface shape.
2. Curvature maps in corneal topography (usually misnamed as power or dioptric maps) only display curvature measured in radial directions from the map center. Such a presentation is not shift-invariant, which means its values and topography change as the center of the map is shifted. In contrast, elevation is shift-invariant. An object shifted with respect to the map center is just shifted in its elevation map.
3. Orbscan can calculate a variety of different surface curvatures, and on a typical eye, these are all different. Only on a properly aligned and perfectly spherical surface are the various curvatures equal.
4. In the Orbscan, the calibrated slit, which falls on the cornea, gives a topographical information, which is captured and analyzed by the video camera.
5. The general quad map in the Orbscan of a normal eye shows 4 pictures. The upper left is the anterior float, which is the topography of the anterior surface of the cornea. The upper right shows the posterior float, which is the topography of the posterior surface of the cornea. The lower left map shows the keratometric pattern and the lower right map shows the pachymetry (thickness of the cornea).

References

1. Agarwal S, Agarwal A, Agarwal A. *Textbook of Corneal Topography.* New Delhi, India: Jaypee; 2006.
2. Agarwal S, Agarwal A, Agarwal A. *Step by Step on Corneal Topography.* New Delhi, India: Jaypee; 2005.
3. Agarwal S, Agarwal A, Agarwal A. *Step by Step on Corneal Topography.* 2nd ed. New Delhi, India: Jaypee; 2006.

Chapter 2

ANTERIOR KERATOCONUS

Sunita Agarwal, MS, DO

INTRODUCTION

Keratoconus is characterized by noninflammatory stromal thinning and anterior protrusion of the cornea. Keratoconus is a slowly progressive condition, often presenting in a patient's teens or early 20s with decreased vision or visual distortion. Family history of keratoconus is seen occasionally. Patients with this disorder are poor candidates for refractive surgery because of the possibility of exacerbating keratectasia.[1] The development of corneal ectasia is a well-recognized complication of LASIK and attributed to unrecognized preoperative forme fruste keratoconus.

ORBSCAN

The Orbscan (Bausch & Lomb, Rochester, NY) corneal topography system uses a scanning optical slit scan that is fundamentally different than the corneal topography that analyzes the reflected images from the anterior corneal surface. The high-resolution video camera captures 40 light slits at a 45-degree angle projected through the cornea similarly as seen during slit lamp examination. It has an acquisition time of 4 seconds.[2] The diagnosis of keratoconus is a clinical one and early diagnosis can be difficult on clinical examination alone. Orbscan has become a useful tool for evaluating the disease, and with the advent of its use, morphology and any subtle changes in the topography can be detected in early keratoconus. We always use the Orbscan system to evaluate our potential LASIK candidates preoperatively to rule out anterior keratoconus.

TECHNIQUE

All eyes to undergo LASIK are examined by Orbscan. Eyes are screened using quad maps with the normal band (NB) filter turned on. Four maps included:
1. Anterior corneal elevation: NB = ± 25 μ of best-fit sphere
2. Posterior corneal elevation: NB = ± 25 μ of best-fit sphere

Figure 2-1. Showing general quad map of an eye with keratoconus.

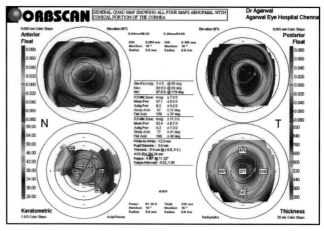

3. Keratometric mean curvature: NB = 40 to 48 D, K

4. Corneal thickness: (pachymetry): NB = 500 to 600 µm

Map features within NB are colored green. This effectively filters out variation falling within normal band. When abnormalities are seen on the NB quad map screening, a standard scale quad map is examined. For those cases with anterior keratoconus, we also generate three-dimensional (3-D) views of anterior and posterior corneal elevation. The following parameters are considered to detect anterior keratoconus: (a) radii of anterior and posterior curvature of the cornea, (b) posterior best-fit sphere, (c) difference between the thickest corneal pachymetry value in a 7-mm zone and thinnest pachymetry value of the cornea, (d) NB scale map, (e) elevation on the anterior float of the cornea, (f) elevation on the posterior float of the cornea, and (g) location of the cone on the cornea.

ANTERIOR KERATOCONUS

On Orbscan analysis in patients with anterior keratoconus, the average ratio of radius of the anterior curvature to the posterior curvature of cornea is 1.25 (range 1.21 to 1.38), average posterior best-fit sphere is –56.98 Dsph (range –52.1 to –64.5 Dsph), average difference in pachymetry value between thinnest point on the cornea and thickest point in a 7-mm zone on the cornea is 172.7 µm (range 117 to 282 µm), and average elevation of anterior corneal float is 55.25 µm (range 25 to 103 µm), average elevation of posterior corneal float is 113.6 µm (range 41 to 167 µm). Figures 2-1 to 2-6 show the various topographic features of an eye with anterior keratoconus. In Figure 2-1 (general quad map), the upper left corner map is the anterior float, the upper right corner map is the posterior float, the lower left corner is the keratometric map, while the lower right is the pachymetry map showing a difference of 282 µm between the thickest pachymetry value in a 7-mm zone of cornea (597 µm) and thinnest pachymetry value (315 µm). In Figure 2-2, normal band scale map of anterior surface shows significant elevation on the anterior and posterior float with abnormal keratometric and pachymetry maps. Figure 2-3 is a 3-D representation of the anterior float with reference sphere of 64 µm. Figure 2-4 show 3-D representation of posterior float with a reference sphere. Figure 2-5 shows an amount of elevation (color coded) of the anterior corneal surface in microns (64 µm). Figure 2-6 shows the amount of elevation (color coded) of the posterior corneal surface in microns (167 µm).

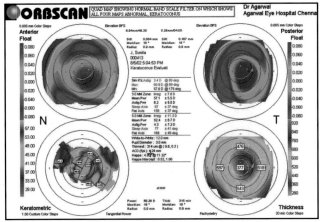

Figure 2-2. Showing quad map with normal band scale filter on in the same eye as in Figure 2-1.

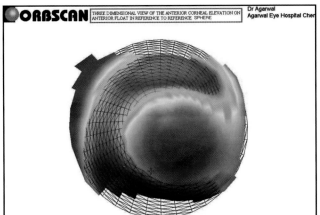

Figure 2-3. Showing 3-D anterior float.

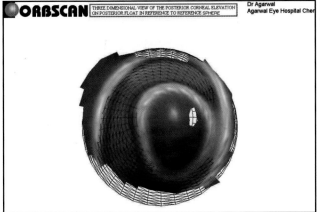

Figure 2-4. Showing 3-D posterior float.

DISCUSSION

Topography is valuable for preoperative ophthalmic examination of LASIK candidates. Three-dimensional imaging allows surgeons to look at corneal thickness, as well as the corneal anterior and posterior surface, and it can predict the shape of the cornea after LASIK surgery. Topographic analysis using a 3-D slit scan system allows us to predict which candidates

Figure 2-5. Showing 3-D anterior corneal elevation measured in microns.

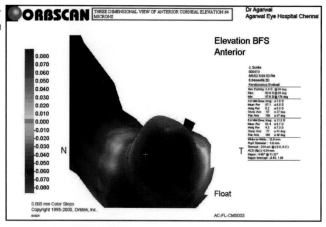

Figure 2-6. Showing 3-D posterior corneal elevation measured in microns.

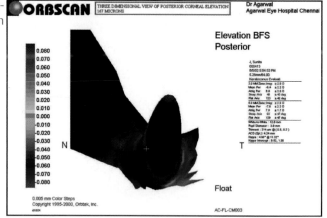

would do well with LASIK and also confers the ability to screen for subtle configurations that may be contraindications to LASIK.[3] It is known that corneal ectasias and keratoconus have posterior corneal elevation as the earliest manifestation. In addition, Wang et al have shown that the posterior corneal elevation increases after LASIK, and the increase is correlated with residual corneal bed thickness.[4] We found that patients with positive keratoconus have higher posterior and anterior elevation on Orbscan II topography.

Elevation is not measured directly by placido-based topographers, but certain assumptions allow the construction of elevation maps. Elevation of a point on the corneal surface displays the height of the point on the corneal surface relative to a spherical reference surface. Reference surface is chosen to be a sphere. Best mathematical approximation of the actual corneal surface called best-fit sphere is calculated. Posterior corneal surface topographic changes after LASIK are known. Increased negative keratometric diopters and oblate asphericity of the posterior corneal curvature (PCC) are common after LASIK and lead to mild keratectasia.[5,6] Lamellar refractive surgery reduces the biomechanical strength of the cornea that may lead to mechanical instability and keratectasia. Iatrogenic keratectasia represents a complication after LASIK that may limit the range of myopic correction.[7] Corneal ectasia has also been reported after LASIK in cases of forme fruste keratoconus.[8] Posterior corneal bulge may be correlated with residual corneal bed thickness. The risk of keratectasia may be increased if the residual corneal bed is thinner than 250 μm.[9] Age, attempted correction, and the optical zone diameter are other parameters that have to be considered to avoid post-LASIK ectasia.[10,11]

CONCLUSION

The Orbscan provides reliable, reproducible data of the anterior corneal surface; posterior corneal surface, keratometry, and pachymetry values with 3-D presentations; and all LASIK candidates must be evaluated by this method preoperatively to detect an "early keratoconus." We suggest that Orbscan II is an important preoperative investigative tool to decide the suitable candidate for LASIK and, thus, avoid any complication of LASIK surgery and helping the patient out by contact lens or keratoplasty. The following parameters must be analyzed in all LASIK candidates to rule out keratoconus (a) ratio of radii of anterior to posterior curvature of cornea: >1.21 and <1.27, (b) posterior best-fit sphere: ≥52.0 Dsph, (c) difference between thickest corneal pachymetry value at 7 mm zone and thinnest pachymetry value: >100 μm, and (d) posterior corneal elevation >50 μm.

KEY POINTS

1. The development of corneal ectasia is a well-recognized complication of LASIK and attributed to unrecognized preoperative forme fruste keratoconus.
2. Three-dimensional imaging allows surgeons to look at corneal thickness as well as the corneal anterior and posterior surface and can predict the shape of the cornea after LASIK surgery.
3. It is known that corneal ectasias and keratoconus have posterior corneal elevation as the earliest manifestation.
4. Elevation of a point on the corneal surface displays the height of the point on the corneal surface relative to a spherical reference surface.
5. Lamellar refractive surgery reduces the biomechanical strength of the cornea that may lead to mechanical instability and keratectasia.

REFERENCES

1. Seiler T, Quurke AW. Iatrogenic keratectasia after LASIK in a case of forme fruste keratoconus. *J Cataract Refract Surg.* 1998;24(7):1007-1009.
2. Fedor P, Kaufman S. Corneal topography and imaging. *eMedicine Journal.* 2001;2(6).
3. McDermott GK. Topography's benefits for LASIK. *Review of Ophthalmology.* 2002; 9:02.
4. Wang Z, Chen J, Yang B. Posterior corneal surface topographic changes after laser in situ keratomileusis are related to residual corneal bed thickness. *Ophthalmology.* 1999;106:406-409; discussion 409-410.
5. Seitz B, Torres F, Langenbucher A, et al. Posterior corneal curvature changes after myopic laser in situ keratomileusis. *Ophthalmology.* 2001;108(4):666-672.
6. Geggel HS, Talley AR. Delayed onset keratectasia following laser in situ keratomileusis. *J Cataract Refract Surg.* 1999;25(4):582-586.
7. Seiler T, Koufala K, Richter G. Iatrogenic keratectasia after laser in situ keratomileusis. *J Refract Surg.* 1998;14(3):312-317.
8. Seiler T, Quurke A W. Iatrogenic keratectasia after laser in situ keratomileusis in a case of forme fruste keratoconus. *J Refract Surg.* 1998;24(7):1007-1009.
9. Wang Z, Chen J, Yang B. Posterior corneal surface topographic changes after laser in situ keratomileusis are related to residual corneal bed thickness. *Ophthalmology.* 1999;106(2):406-409.
10. Pallikaris I G, Kymionis G D. Astyrakakis N I. Corneal ectasia induced by laser in situ keratomileusis. *J Cataract Refract Surg.* 2001;27(11):1796-1802.
11. Argento C, Cosentino MJ, Tytium A, et al. Corneal ectasia after laser in situ keratomileusis. *J Cataract Refract Surg.* 2001;27(9):1440-1810.

POSTERIOR CORNEAL CHANGES IN REFRACTIVE SURGERY

Smita Narasimhan, MBBS, FRSH, FERC and
Amar Agarwal, MS, FRCS, FRCOphth

INTRODUCTION

The development of corneal ectasia is a well-recognized complication of LASIK and among other contributory factors, unrecognized preoperative forme fruste keratoconus is also an important one. Patients with this disorder are poor candidates for refractive surgery because of the possibility of exacerbating keratectasia. It is known that posterior corneal elevation is an early presenting sign in keratoconus, and, hence, it is imperative to evaluate posterior corneal curvature (PCC) in every LASIK candidate.

TOPOGRAPHY

Topography is valuable for preoperative ophthalmic examination of LASIK candidates. Three-dimensional (3-D) imaging allows surgeons (see Chapter 1) to look at corneal thickness, as well as the corneal anterior and posterior surface, and it can also predict the shape of the cornea after LASIK surgery. Topographic analysis using a 3-D slit scan system allows us to predict which candidates would do well with LASIK and also confers the ability to screen for subtle configurations that may be contraindications to LASIK.

ORBSCAN

The Orbscan (Bausch & Lomb, Rochester, NY) corneal topography system uses a scanning optical slit scan that makes it fundamentally different from the corneal topography that analyzes the reflected images from the anterior corneal surface. The high-resolution video camera captures 40 light slits at 45 degree-angles projected through the cornea similarly as seen during slit lamp examination. The slits are projected on the anterior segment of the eye: the anterior cornea, the posterior cornea, the anterior iris, and anterior lens. The data collected from these 4 surfaces are used to create a topographic map. Each surface point from the diffusely reflected slit beams that overlap in the central 5-mm zone is independently triangulated to x, y, and z coordinates, providing 3-D data.

This technique provides more information about the anterior segment of the eye, such as anterior and posterior corneal curvature, elevation maps of the anterior and posterior corneal surface, and corneal thickness. It has an acquisition time of 4 seconds,[1] which improves the diagnostic accuracy. It also has passive eye-tracker from frame to frame and 43 frames are taken to ensure accuracy. It is easy to interpret and has good repeatability.

PRIMARY POSTERIOR CORNEAL ELEVATION

The diagnosis of frank keratoconus is a clinical one.[1-18] Early diagnosis of forme fruste keratoconus can be difficult on clinical examination alone. Orbscan has become a useful tool for evaluating the disease, and with its advent, abnormalities in posterior corneal surface topography have been identified in keratoconus. Posterior corneal surface data are problematic because they are not direct measures and there is little published information on normal values for each age group. In a patient with increased posterior corneal elevation in the absence of other changes, it is unknown whether this finding represents a manifestation of early keratoconus. The decision to proceed with refractive surgery is therefore more difficult.

Posterior Corneal Topography

One should always use the Orbscan system to evaluate potential LASIK candidates preoperatively to rule out primary posterior corneal elevations. Eyes are screened using quad maps with the normal band (NB) filter turned on. Four maps include anterior corneal elevation: NB = ±25 µm of best-fit sphere, posterior corneal elevation: NB = ±25 µm of best-fit sphere, keratometric mean curvature: NB = 40 to 48 D, and Corneal thickness (pachymetry): NB = 500 to 600 µm. Map features within NB are colored green. This effectively filters out variations falling within the NB. When abnormalities are seen on normal band quad map screening, a standard scale quad map should be examined. For those cases with posterior corneal elevation, 3-D views of posterior corneal elevation can also be generated. In all eyes with posterior corneal elevation, the following parameters are generated: (a) radii of anterior and posterior curvature of the cornea, (b) posterior best-fit sphere, and (c) difference between the corneal pachymetry value in a 7-mm zone and thinnest pachymetry value of the cornea.

Pre-Existing Posterior Corneal Abnormalities

Figures 3-1 through 3-6 show the various topographic features of an eye with primary posterior corneal elevation detected during pre-LASIK assessment. In Figure 3-1 (general quad map), the upper left corner map is the anterior float, the upper right corner map is posterior float, the lower left corner is keratometric map, while the lower right is the pachymetry map showing a difference of 100 µm between the thickest pachymetry value in a 7-mm zone of cornea and thinnest pachymetry value. In Figure 3-2, normal band scale map of anterior surface shows "with-the-rule astigmatism" in an otherwise normal anterior surface (shown in green), the posterior float shows significant elevation inferotemporally. In Figure 3-2, only the abnormal areas are shown in red for ease in detection. Figure 3-3 is a 3-D representation of the maps in Figure 3-2. Figure 3-4 shows 3-D representation of anterior corneal surface with reference sphere. Figure 3-5 shows 3-D representation of posterior corneal surface showing a significant posterior corneal elevation. Figure 3-6 shows the amount of elevation (color coded) of the posterior corneal surface in microns (50 µm).

In light of the fact that keratoconus may have posterior corneal elevation as the earliest manifestation, preoperative analysis of posterior corneal curvature to detect a posterior corneal bulge is important to avoid post-LASIK keratectasia. The rate of progression of posterior

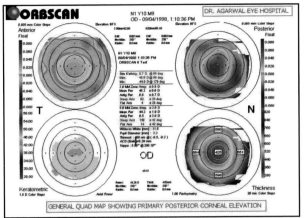

Figure 3-1. Showing general quad map of an eye with primary posterior corneal elevation. Notice the red areas seen in the top right picture showing the primary posterior corneal elevation. Notice the upper left topo picture showing the anterior float is normal.

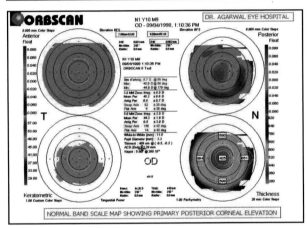

Figure 3-2. Showing quad map with NB scale filter on in the same eye as in Figure 3-1.

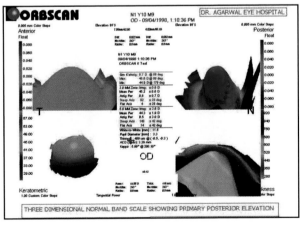

Figure 3-3. Showing 3-D NB scale map. In the top right, note the red areas that show the elevation on the posterior cornea. The anterior cornea is normal.

corneal elevation to frank keratoconus is unknown. It is also difficult to specify the exact amount of posterior corneal elevation beyond which it may be unsafe to carry out LASIK. Atypical elevation in the posterior corneal map more than 45 μm should alert us against a post-LASIK surprise. Orbscan provides reliable, reproducible data of the posterior corneal surface, and all LASIK candidates must be evaluated by this method preoperatively to detect an "early keratoconus."

Figure 3-4. Showing 3-D anterior float. Notice it is normal.

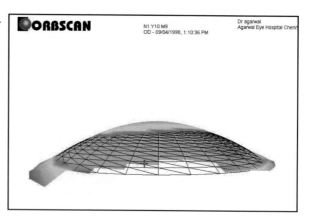

Figure 3-5. Showing 3-D posterior float. Notice in this there is marked elevation as seen in the red areas.

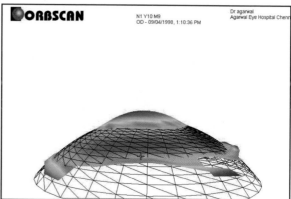

Figure 3-6. Shows 3-D posterior corneal elevation measured in microns.

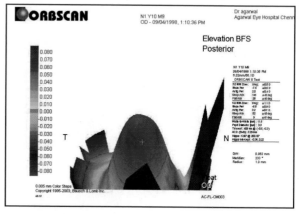

Elevation is not measured directly by placido-based topographers, but certain assumptions allow the construction of elevation maps. Elevation of a point on the corneal surface displays the height of the point on the corneal surface relative to a spherical reference surface. Reference surface is chosen to be a sphere. Best mathematical approximation of the actual corneal surface called best-fit sphere is calculated. One of the criteria for defining forme fruste keratoconus is a posterior best-fit sphere of >55.0 D.

Ratio of radii of anterior to posterior curvature of cornea ≥ 1.21 and ≤ 1.27 has been considered as a keratoconus suspect. Average pachymetry difference between the thickest and thinnest points on the cornea in the 7-mm zone should normally be less than 100 µm.

Criteria to Diagnose Primary Posterior Corneal Elevation

- Ratio of the radii of anterior and posterior curvature of the cornea should be more than 1.2. In Figure 3-2, note the radii of the anterior curvature is 7.86 mm and the radii of the posterior curvature is 6.02 mm. The ratio is 1.3.
- Posterior best-fit sphere should be more than 52 D. In Figure 3-2, note the posterior best-fit sphere is 56.10 D.
- Difference between the thickest and thinnest corneal pachymetry values in the 7-mm zone should be more than 100 μm. The thickest pachymetry value as seen in Figure 3-2 is 651 μm and the thinnest value is 409 μm. The difference is 242 μm.
- The thinnest point on the cornea should correspond with the highest point of elevation of the posterior corneal surface. The thinnest point (as in Figure 3-2's bottom right picture) is seen as a cross. This point or cursor corresponds to the same cross or cursor in Figure 3-2's top right picture and indicates the highest point of elevation on the posterior cornea.
- Elevation of the posterior corneal surface should be more than 45 μm above the posterior best-fit sphere. In Figure 3-2, you will notice it is 0.062 mm or 62 μm.

EFFECT OF POSTERIOR CORNEAL CHANGE ON INTRAOCULAR LENS CALCULATION

Intraocular lens (IOL) power calculation in post-LASIK eyes is different because of the inaccuracy of keratometry, change in anterior and posterior corneal curvatures, altered relation between the two, and change in the standardized index of refraction of the cornea. Irregular astigmatism induced by the procedure, decentered ablations, and central islands also add to the problem.

Routine keratometry is not accurate in these patients. Corneal refractive surgery changes the asphericity of the cornea and also produces a wide range of powers in the central 5-mm zone of the cornea. LASIK makes the cornea of a myope more oblate so that keratometry values may be taken from the more peripheral steeper area of the cornea, which results in calculation of a lower-than-required IOL power resulting in a hyperopic "surprise." Hyperopic LASIK makes the cornea more prolate, thus resulting in a myopic "surprise" postcataract surgery.

Post-PRK or LASIK, the relation between the anterior and posterior corneal surface changes. The relative thickness of the various corneal layers, each having a different refractive index, also changes, and there is a change in the curvature of the posterior corneal surface. All these result in the standardized refractive index of 1.3375 no longer being accurate in these eyes.

At present, there is no keratometry that can accurately measure the anterior and posterior curvatures of the cornea. The Orbscan also makes mathematical assumptions of the posterior surface rather than direct measurements. This is important in the LASIK patient because the procedure alters the relation between the anterior and posterior surfaces of the cornea as well as changes the curvature of the posterior cornea.

Thus, direct measurements such as manual and automated keratometry and topography are inherently inaccurate in these patients. The corneal power is, therefore, calculated by the calculation method, the contact lens over-refraction method, and by the computerized videokeratography (CVK) method. The flattest K reading obtained by any method is taken for IOL power calculation (the steepest K is taken for hyperopes who had undergone LASIK). One can still aim for 1.00 D of myopia rather than emmetropia to allow for any error, which is almost always in the hyperopic direction in case of pre-LASIK myopes. Also, a third- or fourth-generation IOL calculating formula should be used for such patients.

KEY POINTS

1. It is known that posterior corneal elevation is an early presenting sign in keratoconus and hence it is imperative to evaluate posterior corneal curvature (PCC) in every LASIK candidate.

2. One should always use the Orbscan system to evaluate potential LASIK candidates preoperatively to rule out primary posterior corneal elevations.

3. Ratio of the radii of anterior and posterior curvature of the cornea should be more than 1.2.

4. The thinnest point on the cornea should correspond with the highest point of elevation of the posterior corneal surface.

5. Difference between the thickest and thinnest corneal pachymetry value in the 7-mm zone should be more than 100 μm.

REFERENCES

1. Fedor P, Kaufman S Corneal topography and imaging. *eMedicine Journal*. 2001;2(6).

2. Seiler T, Koufala K, Richter G. Iatrogenic keratectasia after laser in situ keratomileusis. *J Refract Surg*. 1998;14(3):312-317.

3. Seiler T, Quurke AW. Iatrogenic keratectasia after laser in situ keratomileusis in a case of Forme Fruste keratoconus. *J Refract Surg*. 1998;24(7):1007-1009.

4. Probst LE, Machat JJ. Mathematics of laser in situ keratomileusis for high myopia. *J Cataract Refract Surg*. 1998;24.

5. McDonnell PJ. Excimer laser corneal surgery: new strategies and old enemies {review}. *Invest Ophthalmol Vis Sci*. 1995;36:4-8.

6. Seitz B, Torres F, Langenbucher A, et al. Posterior corneal curvature changes after myopic laser in situ keratomileusis. *Ophthalmology*. 2001;108(4):666-672.

7. Geggel HS, Talley AR. Delayed onset keratectasia following laser in situ keratomileusis. *J Cataract Refract Surg*. 1999;25(4):582-586.

8. Wang Z, Chen J, Yang B. Posterior corneal surface topographic changes after laser in situ keratomileusis are related to residual corneal bed thickness. *Ophthalmology*. 1999;106(2):406-409.

9. Pallikaris IG, Kymionis GD, Astyrakakis NI. Corneal ectasia induced by laser in situ keratomileusis. *J Cataract Refract Surg*. 2001;27(11):1796-1802.

10. Argento C, Cosentino MJ, Tytium A, et al. Corneal ectasia after laser in situ keratomileusis. *J Cataract Refract Surg*. 2001;27(9):1440-1448.

11. Binder PS, Moore M, Lambert RW, et al. Comparison of two microkeratome systems. *J Refract Surg*. 1997;13;142-153.

12. Hofmann RF, Bechara SJ. An independent evaluation of second generation suction microkeratomes. *Refract Corneal Surg*. 1992;8:348-354.

13. Schuler A, Jessen K, Hoffmann F. Accuracy of the microkeratome keratectomies in pig eyes. *Invest Ophthalmol Vis Sci*. 1990;31:2022-2030.

14. Behrens A, Seitz B, Langenbucher A, et al. Evaluation of corneal flap dimensions and cut quality using a manually guided microkeratome [published erratum appears in J Refract Surg 1999;15:400]. *J Refract Surg*. 1999;15:118-123.

15. Behrens A, Seitz B, Langenbucher A, et al. Evaluation of corneal flap dimensions and cut quality using the automated corneal shaper microkeratome. *J Refract Surg.* 2000;16:83-89.

16. Behrens A, Langenbucher A, Kus MM, et al. Experimental evaluation of two current generation automated microkeratomes: the Hansatome and the Supratome. *Am J Ophthalmol.* 2000;129:59-67.

17. Jacobs BJ, Deutsch TA, Rubenstein JB. Reproducibility of corneal flap thickness in LASIK. *Ophthalmic Surg Lasers.* 1999;30:350-353.

18. McDermott GK. Topography's benefits for LASIK. *Review of Ophthalmology.* 2002;9:02.

Chapter 4

New Techniques for Exploring the Eye's Anterior Segment: Carl Zeiss Meditec Visante OCT

Georges Baïkoff, MD

Introduction

Until recently, most efforts made in ocular imaging concerned posterior segment exploration. One of the most important events was the commercialization of the Carl Zeiss Meditec Stratus (Dublin, Calif) (OCT 3—820 nm wavelength), which made it possible to visualize different layers of the retina with a great deal of precision (resolution: 3 to 4 µm). Efforts are being made to develop more and more precise scanning of the neuro-sensorial layers with three-dimensional (3-D) visualization (Carmen Puliafito, Innovators Lecture, ASCRS, Washington, 2005).

Because the anterior segment could be directly observed with the slit-lamp, extensive research was not a priority. In daily practice, ultrasonic evaluations of corneal pachymetry and anterior chamber depth along the optical axis of the eye were considered sufficient. With the development of sophisticated surgical techniques, it became essential to obtain elaborate static and dynamic measurements of the anterior segment in order to meet modern safety requirements. Here, one can briefly refer to x-ray imaging of the eye (conventional x-ray, IRM, TDM), as its usage in daily practice has little chance of undergoing further development.

The choice now lies between optical and ultrasonic exploration of the anterior segment. Slit-lamp images are simply frontal images with a subjective estimation of a few external measurements of the eye.

Development of the Scheimpflug technique with oblique images resulted in a new capability to evaluate the distances in the eye's anterior segment along different optical sections. The major drawbacks of this technology are difficult mathematical reconstruction as well as scleral overexposure when taking photos. In particular, the whole of the angle area is masked by this overexposure and the fine structures are indiscernible (scleral spur, irido-corneal sinus).

The idea of using infrared wavelengths in optical coherence is expanding rapidly (IOLMaster, Visante OCT [Carl Zeiss Meditec, Dublin, Calif]).[1-2] About 10 years ago, Izatt and colleagues[3] suggested using the OCT for anterior segment imaging. Reflection of the infrared light rays is captured and analyzed by an optical sensor and appropriate software readjusts the dimensions of the images by erasing distortion errors due to different

Figure 4-1. Visante OCT.

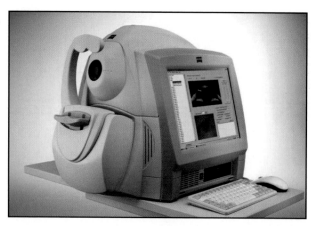

corneal optical transmission differences. Measuring software capable of evaluating the distance between 2 points, curvature radius, and angles is also integrated.

Ultrasonic exploration of the anterior segment appears to have reached its limits, whether in UBM or ultra high-frequency ultrasound equipment (Artemis [Arcscan, St. Petersberg, Fla]). Today, resolution is identical to 1310 nm wavelength anterior segment OCT available on the market (15 to 20 μm for axial resolution, 50 to 100 μm for transverse resolution). Manipulation is fairly complex and even if some ultrasonic measurements are used as references to calibrate a certain number of instruments, there is no certainty concerning the exact in vivo or ultrasonic measurements. However, the error can be considered relative as long as the reference scale remains constant with each device/technology.

THE ANTERIOR CHAMBER OPTICAL COHERENCE TOMOGRAPHY: VISANTE OCT DEVELOPED BY CARL ZEISS MEDITEC

The equipment[4-16] uses a 1310-nm wavelength, but in its present form the infrared light is blocked by pigments. However, the nonpigmented opaque structures are permeable and images can be obtained through a cloudy or white cornea or through the conjunctiva and the sclera. Axial resolution is 18 μm and transverse resolution 50 μm. The procedure is noncontact and very easy. Because of its simplicity, a technician can be rapidly trained to carry out the examinations. It is possible to choose the axis to be explored or carry out an automatic 360-degree exploration along the 4 meridians.

There is an optical target that can be focused or defocused with positive or negative lenses. Natural accommodation can be stimulated and anterior segment modifications during accommodation can be explored in vivo. Image reconstruction software has been criticized but in our experience, we were able to show that the sections obtained were perfectly reproducible. We believe that this notion of reproducibility is very important. There may be a few errors regarding the precision of the readings, but as long as the reference scale remains constant and the areas explored can easily be found during successive examinations, these errors can be considered as relative (Figures 4-1 and 4-2).

STATIC MEASUREMENT OF THE ANTERIOR SEGMENT

With the Visante OCT prototype at our disposal, we were able to explore hundreds of eyes and evaluate the different measurements of the anterior segment. We were able to show a

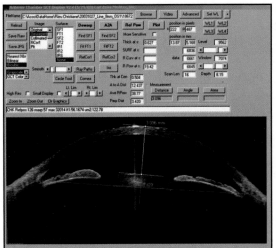

Figure 4-2. Prototype of the image exploitation software.

new notion; in most cases, the anterior chamber was not a circle. We were able to prove in vivo that in 75% of cases, the internal vertical diameter of the anterior chamber was larger than the internal horizontal diameter by at least 100 μm. Using the Artemis instrument (ultra high-frequency ultrasound) on cadaver eyes, this notion had already been put forward by Liliana Werner. This discovery has essential implications when an anterior chamber phakic or pseudophakic angle-supported implant is scheduled. The measurement obtained with the Visante OCT is much more precise than the white-to-white evaluation used until now, and it is more precise and much easier to acquire than the anterior segment images obtained with the classic B-scan instruments, even the most recent ones. What is more, with ultrasonic scanning devices, the water bath placed before the patient's cornea makes the examination difficult and because there is no fixation point, it is not possible to visualize the optical axis. The optical axis, which is a fixed reference point, allows one to know with certainty the position of the examined optical section. Thus with the Artemis, there is lack of reproducibility.

DYNAMIC EVALUATION OF THE ANTERIOR SEGMENT

Figures 4-3A and B are images of the eye of a 10-year-old with 10.00 D of accommodation. The images speak for themselves. Distortion of the anterior surface of the crystalline lens, myosis, and modifications to the anterior chamber depth during accommodation can be observed. This shows that in young subjects the anterior segment of the eye is very dynamic; for 1.00 D accommodation, there is approximately a 30-μm forward thrust of the crystalline lens' anterior pole. Therefore, it is normal to observe a 100- to 200-μm variation of the anterior chamber in a young subject (candidate for a phakic implant).

With aging, there is a reduction in the crystalline lens' flexibility and fewer modifications to the anterior segment during accommodation. However, the anterior chamber becomes flatter as the crystalline lens' anterior pole moves forward by about 20 μm per year. Specific software could perhaps be used to simulate the notion of aging of the anterior segment and, thus, help to explain that as the crystalline lens thickens with time, contact between the crystalline lens and all models of phakic implants is probable, regardless of their type of fixation in the anterior segment.

Figure 4-3. Dynamic image of accommodation of the anterior segment in a 10-year-old child (10.00 D accommodation).

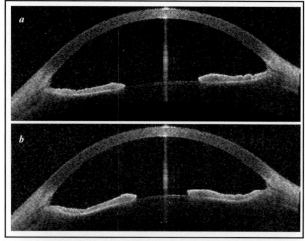

Figure 4-4. Piggyback IOLs. (A) Perfect aspect and interface's optical void. (B) Aspect of an interlenticular proliferation.

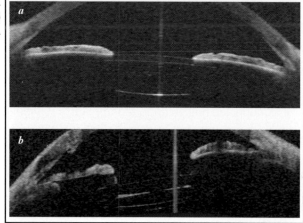

Evaluation of the Crystalline Lens With the Anterior Chamber Optical Coherence Tomography

By focusing behind the iris, it is possible to observe the entire thickness of the crystalline lens.

Pseudophakic Artificial Crystalline Lens

Figure 4-4 shows 2 examples of a piggyback implant. Figure 4-4A shows perfectly well-adapted piggyback IOLs with the main lens behind and the secondary lens in front. The interface between the 2 lenses is virtual but perfectly visible on the images. In this case, there was no proliferation of unwanted deposits on the interface. In Figure 4-4B, penetrating keratoplasty was carried out on a corneal pseudophakic edema. With the slit-lamp, an after-cataract was diagnosed postoperatively. In fact, following an examination with the OCT, we noticed a proliferation of newly formed tissues between the 2 piggyback implants. We changed our diagnosis of after-cataract to intralenticular proliferation.

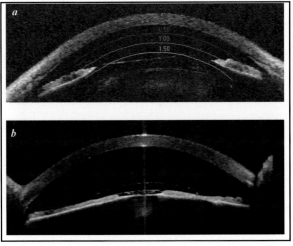

Figure 4-5. Phakic implants. (A) Posterior chamber ICL Implant. Note the edges of the optic are inside the 1.5-mm endothelial safety zone. (B) Artisan hyperopic implant with pigment dispersion in the pupil area. Note the flattening of the iris and the pigment cysts in the pupil area behind the implant.

PHAKIC IMPLANTS

Inserting a phakic implant (Artisan, Verysise) should not be done without a thorough preoperative evaluation and postoperative follow-up. Until recently, measuring the depth of the anterior chamber and checAking the endothelium cell count with a specular microscope were considered sufficient. With the development of techniques such as the OCT, surgical indications can be streamlined and a regular check-up of the anterior chamber following such an intervention is mandatory. Figure 4-5A, shows a posterior chamber implantable contact lens (ICL) inserted in a patient over the age of 45 having developed cataract and severe optical problems. Although the ICL has been placed in the posterior chamber, on the endothelial safety scale we note that the edges of the optic are approximately 1 mm from the endothelium. This distance is insufficient as it has been proved that a minimum safety distance of 1.5 mm was necessary between the edges of the lens' optic and the endothelium.

In Figure 4-5B, a pigment dispersion syndrome was observed following insertion of an Artisan hyperopic implant. Compared with a normal anterior segment, we observed that the iris was very thin and that pigment cysts had developed on the pupil between the implant and the patient's anterior capsule. We also demonstrated that a convex iris, which is a contraindication for Artisan implants, can be evaluated in a very precise way using the crystalline lens rise method (distance from the crystalline lens anterior pole to the internal diameter of the irido-corneal angle).[6,14] When the crystalline lens rise is above 600 µm, the risk of developing pigment dispersion syndrome with a drop in visual acuity is probable in 70% of cases.

THE CORNEA

For the moment, with the prototype used, corneal imaging is essentially qualitative. Although resolution is not sufficient enough to determine intracorneal disorders or specify different types of dystrophies, in Figure 4-6, 3 obvious pathologies are visible. Figure 4-6A—Terrien's degeneration with peripheral thinning, Figure 4-6B—old central descemetocele, Figure 4-6C—keratoglobus with considerable thinning of the entire cornea. In Figure 4-7, we are able to show the presence and the position of intracorneal rings used to treat myopia, and in Figure 4-8, a LASIK flap is perfectly visible with a nylon suture (marked by the arrow) to secure a "free cap."

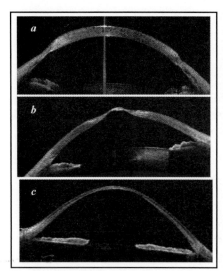

Figure 4-6. Different aspects of corneal pathologies. (A) Terrien's degeneration. (B) Descemetocele. (C)
Keratoglobus.

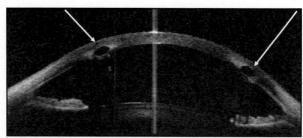

Figure 4-7. Intracorneal rings to treat myopia.

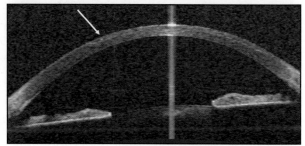

Figure 4-8. Aspect of a LASIK freecap. View of a 10-0
nylon suture.

Today, the anterior segment can be explored behind a cloudy and edematous cornea. Figures 4-9A and 4-9B are excellent examples of the performance of the Visante OCT. Figure 4-9A represents a postaphakic corneal dystrophy clearly showing anterior synechiae with vitreous strands around the iris. Because the eye is aphakic, it is easy for the surgeon to know what surgery is needed. Figure 4-9B shows a corneal edema following an endothelial graft. It was not possible to explain, with just a slit-lamp examination, why the cornea remained cloudy after surgery. However, using the OCT during a simple postop visit, we were able to observe 2 corneal stromas without adherence. In this case, the endothelio-descemetic graft was a failure because the initial corneal oedema not only remained but worsened. A normal penetrating keratoplasty was carried out later with satisfactory results.

GLAUCOMA

Visualizing angle structures as well as exploring the sclera and conjunctiva are possible with the anterior segment OCT. Figure 4-10A shows excessive scleral filtration with persistent hypotonia following surgery. Intraocular pressure was brought back to normal by scleral flap enhancement and resulted in subconjunctival filtration (Figure 4-10B). The risk of angle closure (Figure 4-11) is easy to evaluate and can be objectively and precisely measured.

CONCLUSIONS AND THE FUTURE OF ANTERIOR SEGMENT OPTICAL COHERENCE TOMOGRAPHY EXPLORATION

The main thing to remember is how simple this equipment is to use. Once the patient has fixed the target, manipulation is as easy as a corneal topography. There is no contact, the images are taken very quickly, and the technician decides which axis he or she wishes to explore.

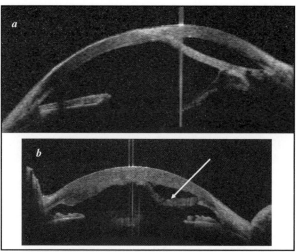

Figure 4-9. Different aspects of the anterior segment behind a corneal oedema. (A) Vitreous strands and anterior synechiae. (B) Failed descemetic graft.

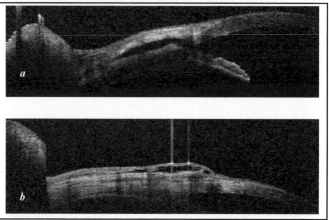

Figure 4-10. Postoperative trabeculectomy. (A) Excessive Scleral Filtration with hypotonia. (B) Conjunctival Filtration following scleral flap enhancement.

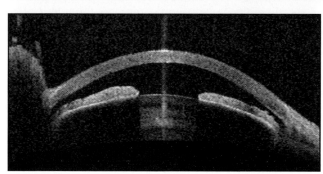

Figure 4-11. Aspect of angle-closure glaucoma.

Resolution is similar to the ultra high-frequency scanner, but the zones explored are easier to find because the fixation point is on the optical axis.

The irido-corneal angle is perfectly visible. To evaluate the measurements or to check the evolution of an anterior segment, either the irido-corneal angle sinus or the scleral spur area can be used as a reference point because both remain constants of the anterior chamber anatomy during its dynamic or senile modifications.

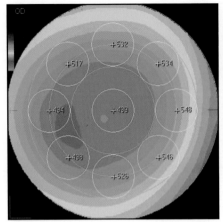

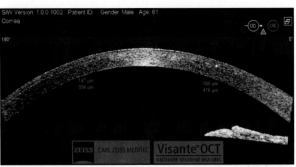

Figure 4-13. Measurement of LASIK flap thickness with corneal software.

Figure 4-12. Pachymetry map.

As it is possible to measure multiple meridians, 3-D reconstruction of the anterior segment could perhaps be the next step.

A 10-mm diameter pachymetric mapping of the cornea is already possible (Figure 4-12). Another objective for the near future would be to estimate the quality of a LASIK flap over a certain length of time (Figure 4-13).

Finally, in the laboratory, with a more appropriate wavelength and/or a modification of the power of the light ray, it has been possible to obtain images close to histology. On pseudophakic cadaver eyes, Linnola et al[17] were able to show cell proliferation on the posterior capsule. The images obtained with the high-resolution OCT that they used are very similar to a pathological study done on these same eyes.

The technological evolution of the Visante OCT for exploring the anterior segment is something to anticipate. Hopefully, in the near future, these improvements will be similar to those of OCT for exploring the posterior pole: more precise images, resolution of a few microns, and 3-D reconstruction of the structures under study. It is quite certain that this imaging system will, in daily practice, shortly replace ultrasound equipment for anterior segment exploration.

KEY POINTS

1. Until recently, most efforts made in ocular imaging concerned posterior segment exploration. One of the most important events was the commercialization of the Carl Zeiss Meditec Stratus (OCT 3—820 nm wavelength) which made it possible to visualize different layers of the retina with a great deal of precision (resolution: 3 to 4 µm).

2. The equipment uses a 1310-nm wavelength, but in its present form, the infrared light is blocked by pigments. However, the nonpigmented opaque structures are permeable and images can be obtained through a cloudy or white cornea, through the conjunctiva and the sclera.

3. There is an optical target that can be focused or defocused with positive or negative lenses. Natural accommodation can be stimulated and anterior segment modifications during accommodation can be explored in vivo.

4. Visualizing angle structures as well as exploring the sclera and conjunctiva is possible with the anterior segment OCT.

5. There is no contact, the images are taken very quickly, and the technician decides which axis he or she wishes to explore. Resolution is similar to the ultra high-frequency scanner but the zones explored are easier to find because the fixation point is on the optical axis.

REFERENCES

1. Huang D, Swanson EA, Lin CP, et al. Optical coherence tomography. *Science*. 1991;254:1178-1181.

2. Puliafito C, Hee MR, Schuman JS, et al. *Optical Coherence Tomography of Ocular Diseases*. Thorofare, NJ, SLACK Incorporated: 1996.

3. Izatt JA, Hee MR, Swanson EA, et al. Micrometer-scale resolution imaging of the anterior eye in vivo with optical coherence tomography. *Arch Ophthalmology*. 1994;112:1584-1589.

4. Baikoff G, Lutun E, Ferraz C, et al. Analysis of the eye's anterior segment with an optical coherence tomography: static and dynamic study. *J Cataract Refract Surg*. 2004;30:1843-1850.

5. Baikoff G, Lutun E, Ferraz C, et al. Refractive phakic IOLs: contact of three different models with the crystalline lens, an AC OCT study case reports. *J Cataract Refract Surg*. 2004;30:2007-2012.

6. Baikoff G, Bourgeon G, Jitsuo Jodai H, et al. Pigment dispersion and artisan implants. The crystalline lens rise as a safety criterion. *J Cataract Refract Surg*. 2005;31:674-680.

7. Baikoff G, Lutun E, Ferraz C, Wie J. Anterior chamber optical coherence tomography study of human natural accommodation in a 19-year-old albino. *J Cataract Refract Surg*. 2004;30:696-701.

8. Baikoff G, Rozot P, Lutun E, Wei J. Assessment of capsular block syndrome with anterior segment optical coherence tomography. *J Cataract Refract Surg*. 2004;30:2448-2450.

9. Baikoff G, Jitsuo Jodai H, Bourgeon G. Evaluation of the measurement of the anterior chamber's internal diameter and depth: IOLMaster vs AC OCT. *J Cataract Refract Surg*. 2004 (in press).

10. Baikoff G, Lutun E, Wei J, Ferraz C. Contact entre le cristallin naturel et différents modèles d'implants phakes. Etude avec l'OCT de chambre antérieure. A propos de trois observations. *J Fr Ophtalmol*. 2005; 28(3):303-308.

11. Rozot P, Baikoff G, Lutun E, Wei J. Evaluation d'un syndrome de blocage capsulaire tardif avec l'OCT de segment antérieur. *J Fr Ophtalmol*. 2005;28(3):309-311.

12. Baikoff G, Lutun E, Wei J, Ferraz C. Etude in vivo de l'accommodation naturelle chez un sujet albinos de 19 ans avec un tomographe à cohérence optique. A propos d'un cas. *J Fr Ophtalmol*. 2005;27(5): 514-519.

13. Baikoff G, Lutun E, Ferraz C, Wei J. Analyse du segment antérieur de l'oeil avec un tomographe à cohérence optique. Etude statique et dynamique. *J Fr Ophtalmol*. 2005;28(4):343-352.

14. Baikoff G, Bourgeon G, Jitsuo Jodai H, Fontaine A, Vieira Lellis F, Trinquet L. Migrations pigmentaires après implant Artisan: importance de la flèche cristallinienne comme critère de sécurité. *J Fr Ophtalmol.* 2005;28(6):590-597.

15. Baikoff G, Jitsuo Jodai H, Bourgeon G. Evaluation de la mesure du diamètre interne et de la profondeur de la chambre antérieure: IOLMaster vs tomographe à cohérence optique de chambre antérieure. *J Fr Ophtalmol.* 2005 (à paraître)

16. Goldsmith J, Li Y, Chalita MR, et al. Anterior Chamber width measurement by high-speed optical coherence tomography. *Ophthalmology.* 2005;112:238-244.

17. Linnola R, Findl O, Hermann, et al. Intraocular lens-capsular bag imaging with ultrahigh-resolution optical coherence tomography. Pseudophakic human autopsy eyes. *J Cataract Refract Surg.* 2005;31:818-823.

Chapter 5

Pupil Size and Refractive Surgery

Francesco Carones, MD

Introduction

Although accuracy (plano refraction) and efficacy (20/16 uncorrected vision) are certainly the 2 major goals of any refractive surgical procedure, the quality of vision also plays an important role for assessing the success of the procedure. When patients consider refractive surgery, they do not only aim for 20/16 unaided vision, they also at least want the same visual performance they had before surgery with their spectacles or contact lenses in all light conditions. In other words, patients can be very happy if they can see without glasses after surgery, but even in this situation, they may be very dissatisfied if their vision significantly worsens at night or in dim illumination. To guarantee patients the best performance in regard to night vision, the relationships between pupil size and optical zone size are to be known in detail.

Pupil Size

The size of the entrance pupil we currently see and measure does not correspond to the actual anatomical pupil size because the optical properties of the cornea magnify and displace it anteriorly. However, for clinical purposes, we may consider and measure the entrance pupil. There are several methods to measure pupil size. Needless to say, the measurement of pupil size necessary for refractive surgical purposes is the scotopic one, as pupil dilation enhances visual symptoms.

- Rulers and reference diameters. This method has been almost abandoned for refractive surgery because of its unreliability and unavailability of measuring pupil sizes at different established light conditions.
- Monocular portable infrared pupillometers. These are relatively inexpensive and popular. They provide pupil size under relatively low light conditions, but they measure one eye at a time and give no information on pupil dynamics.
- Monocular infrared pupillometers associated with corneal topographers. They provide more reliable and consistent measurements than portable pupillometers, and some of them measure some pupillary dynamic changes with different light conditions.

- Binocular infrared pupillometers. Today these instruments are the most reliable ones to assess pupil size under different set light conditions. They compensate for theoretical changes in pupil size due to accommodation thanks to a simultaneous measurement for both eyes. Some of them truly provide a dynamic measurement of changes in pupil size related to illumination.

OPTICAL ZONE

The optical zone size can be defined as the diameter of induced change in refraction delivered by the surgery, which is useful for refractive and visual purposes. For example, for a laser ablation, this is the central spherical zone bringing the correction to be made (also called the optical zone). For an IOL (either phakic or pseudophakic), this is the optical plate. For an intracorneal ring segment insertion, this is the flattened area by the segments. The optical zone has to be centered over the pupillary entrance to maximize visual performance and avoid the symptoms related to decentration.[1]

A general theoretical rule assesses that the optical zone of any refractive procedure should be as large as possible to reduce halo effects and visual disturbances at night. Regarding laser refractive surgery, wide ablation zones provide additional advantages to the surgery. They induce fewer higher-order aberrations (particularly spherical aberration), and even when performing customized ablations, induce fewer aberrations. Wide ablation zones also prove to produce more stable results with less regression of the induced refractive change.[2]

This rule, however, often gets in conflict with other surgical parameters to take into account, like the residual corneal thickness after LASIK and the total volume of ablated tissue for surface ablation. It is well known that for a certain amount of correction, the larger the ablation zone, the higher the amount of tissue removed and, consequently, the deeper the ablation thickness. This would not imply problems for lower corrections, but when attempting higher corrections using large ablation zones, it may be problematic in respect to what is considered the "safety limit" for residual stromal thickness when doing LASIK (250 μm in the stromal bed), or to avoid haze formation when performing surface ablation. In these cases, it may be necessary to reduce the ablation zone to a value that respects these safety issues.[3]

A second general rule assesses that eyes with pupil diameter smaller than 6 mm are very unlikely to have visual disturbances at night, at least for low-medium corrections. Larger pupils require larger ablation zones to avoid visual disturbances, and the same is for higher attempted corrections because of the greater light-scattering they determine at the ablation edge (Figure 5-1). Unfortunately, eyes requiring larger ablation zones to minimize night-vision problems are often those where it is more difficult to have enough stroma available for the ablation (ie, higher corrections).

PHAKIC INTRAOCULAR LENSES

When the ablation zone cannot be larger than the scotopic pupillary diameter, a sort of compromise in the surgery results has to be considered and discussed with the patient. If sharp and undisturbed quality of night vision is desired, the total amount of correction can be reduced for a planned residual refractive error, but an ablation zone larger than the scotopic pupil may be used. If emmetropia is the target of the surgery, and the patient understands and accepts the fairly disturbed night vision that an ablation zone 0.5 to 1 mm smaller than the scotopic pupil may induce, a satisfactory surgery can still be attempted. But when the patient seeks both undisturbed night vision and plano refraction, a different surgical procedure such as a phakic IOL implant may be the only surgical option. For intraocular procedures like

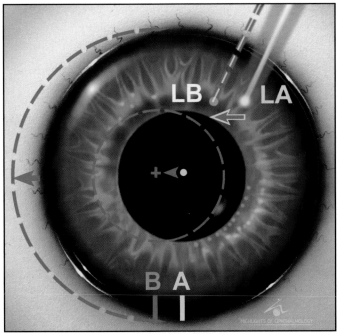

Figure 5-1. Concept of eye tracking for more accurate corneal ablations during movements of the eye. New eye tracking technology can trace eye movements by detecting displacement of the pupil. In microseconds the eye tracking computer can move the treatment spot of an Excimer laser beam appropriately to compensate for these eye movements. For example, laser beam (LA) is treating an area of the cornea when the eye is in position (A). Suddenly, during treatment, the eye moves slightly to the left to position (B). The eye tracking computer detects the movement of the pupil to the left (dotted circle) and commands the laser to track left (LB) the same amount, within microseconds. Thus the laser continues treating the same area of the cornea as desired before the eye movement takes place. Such technology aims to increase the accuracy of the desired ablation and resulting correction. (Courtesy of Benjamin F. Boyd, MD, FACS, Editor-in-Chief, *Atlas of Refractive Surgery* with permission from Highlights of Ophthalmology, English Edition, 2000.)

phakic IOL implant, there is a much smaller chance for generating visual disturbances. This is due to less light scatter generated by the edge of the optic plate, because of the lower difference in index of refraction between the aqueous humor and the IOL material, than between the air and the cornea.

GLARE AND HALOS

In conclusion, the optimal ablation zone diameter for an ideal eye would be very large, definitely larger than the scotopic pupil size. High corrections would require even larger ablations, which would require a thicker stroma. Unfortunately, the 3 key parameters—ablation zone diameter, pupil diameter, and requested correction—do not always combine together to allow it.

Night glare and halos are among the complaints more frequently reported by the patients,[4,5] particularly in treatments performed in the past or done with previous-generation excimer lasers. There are 3 main causes for night glare and halos. First, they are determined by a scattering when light rays cross the edge of the ablation. In normal light conditions, when the pupil is undilated, these scattered light rays cannot reach the visual axis thanks to the diaphragm provided by the pupil. When the pupil dilates, they may intersect the visual axis and blur vision. Second, they may be due to a severe increase in spherical aberration as a consequence of the laser ablation; the resultant multifocality may produce secondary focal images that cause the above symptoms when the pupil dilates. Finally, flap or interface problems like striae, folds, or epithelial ingrowth may induce halos and glare.

LASER ABLATION

Patients with very large scotopic pupillary diameter (8.0 mm or more) are more likely to experience night vision problems, regardless of the correction to be made. As poor candidates for refractive surgery, I usually tend to discourage them or at least I inform them about the great risk of postoperative night glare and halos. For smaller scotopic pupil sizes, I always try to set the widest available ablation zone diameter, considering the attempted correction and the residual stromal thickness. While the ablation zone should never be smaller than the scotopic pupil size, I personally recommend it to be 1.0 mm wider. When performing customized ablations, which reduce induced spherical aberration and provide a better optical quality to the ablation edges, I would not mandatorily require the additional 1.0 mm. As a general rule, even for those eyes where scotopic pupil diameter is relatively small (5.0 mm or less), I never perform treatments with ablation zone diameter smaller than 6.5 mm for myopic corrections and 6.0 mm for hyperopic corrections. In both cases, I usually add a 3.0-mm transition zone diameter for an overall ablation that is never smaller than 9.5 mm (myopia) or 9.0 mm (hyperopia). Wavefront-guided and wavefront-optimized custom ablations definitely reduce the chance of severe increase in high-order aberrations, particularly spherical aberration and, thus, they are preferred in all cases.

HIGHER POWER CORRECTION

The amount of correction to be made is a second very effective predictive factor for night vision problems: the higher, the greater. Even by using large ablation zones, corrections higher than -8.00 D (myopia) or +4.00 D (hyperopia) may induce some visual symptoms at night; usually, I do not recommend LASIK for those higher corrections in patients who perform heavy night-driving activity (eg, taxi or truck drivers).

MANAGEMENT

Once night halos occur, they are very difficult to manage. Patients usually complain about them more in the immediate postoperative period, with a reduction over time that is due both to the smoothing effect of the epithelium on the peripheral ablation edge, and to the patient's adaptation. During this period, mild miotic eye drops may help the patients in certain circumstances (eg, if patients plan to drive at night for a long period of time). Another effective solution for younger patients is to provide them with mild overcorrected minus spectacles (-0.75 D) to be used while driving at night. Through accommodation, the induced miosis reduces halos.

When symptoms persist, a customized laser retreatment seems to be the procedure of choice; the selective correction of higher-order aberrations, particularly at the ablation peripheral region, coupled with an enlargement of the ablation zone may solve the problem.[6] A second surgical option to reach similar results is the implantation of intracorneal ring segments (Figure 5-2), which helps enlarge the optical zone and restore a more prolate corneal shape.[7]

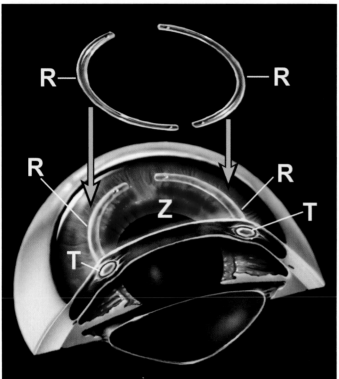

Figure 5-2. Technique for implantation of the intrastromal corneal ring. The intrastromal ring consists of 2 semicircular implants (R). They are guided into the tracts (T) on each side of the optical zone (Z). Their final position is shown in the cross-section view below. Note how the rings alter the shape of the cornea as seen in the cross-section. (Courtesy of Benjamin F. Boyd, MD, FACS, Editor-in-Chief, *Atlas of Refractive Surgery* with permission from Highlights of Ophthalmology, English Edition, 2000.)

KEY POINTS

1. To guarantee patients the best performance in night vision, the relationship between pupil size and optical zone size are to be known in detail.

2. The size of the entrance pupil we currently see and measure does not correspond to the actual anatomical pupil size, because the optical properties of the cornea magnify and displace it anteriorly, but for clinical purposes we may consider and measure the entrance pupil.

3. The optical zone size can be defined as the diameter of induced change in refraction delivered by the surgery, which is useful for refractive and visual purposes.

4. Intraocular procedures like phakic IOL implant have much less chance for generating visual disturbances. This is due to the less light scatter generated by the edge of the optic plate, due to the lower difference in index of refraction between the aqueous humor and the IOL material, than between the air and the cornea.

5. Patients with very large scotopic pupillary diameter (8.0 mm or more) are more likely to end up with night vision problems, regardless of the correction to be made.

6. Once night halos occur, they are very difficult to manage. Mild miotic eye-drops may help patients in certain circumstances. Another effective solution for younger patients is to provide them with mild overcorrected minus spectacles (-0.75 D) to be used while driving at night; through accommodation, the induced miosis reduces halos.

REFERENCES

1. Uozato H, Guyton DL. Centering corneal surgical procedures. *Am J Ophthalmol.* 1987;103:264-275.

2. Carones F, Brancato R, et al. Evaluation of three different approaches to perform excimer laser photore-fractive keratectomy for myopia. *Ophthalmic Surg Lasers.* 1996;27:458-465.

3. Joo CK, Kim TG. Corneal ectasia detected after laser in situ keratomileusis for correction of less than –12 diopters of myopia. *J Cataract Refract Surg.* 2000;26:292-295.

4. Holladay JT, Dudeja DR, et al. Functional vision and corneal changes after laser in situ keratomileusis determined by contrast sensitivity, glare testing, and corneal topography. *J Cataract Refract Surg.* 1999; 25:663-669.

5. Nixon WS. Pupil size in refractive surgery. *J Cataract Refract Surg.* 1997;23:1435-1436.

6. Alessio G, Boscia F, et al. Topography-driven excimer laser for the retreatment of decentralized myopic photorefractive keratectomy. *Ophthalmology.* 2001;108:1695-1703.

7. Fleming JF, Lovisolo CF. Intrastromal corneal ring segments in a patient with previous laser in situ ker-atomileusis. *J Refract Surg.* 2000;16:365-367.

II

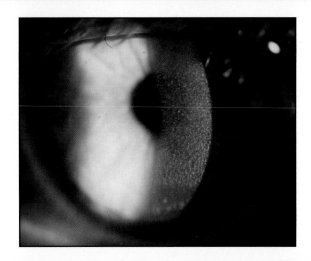

Surface Ablations: PRK, LASEK, Epi-LASIK, PTK

Chapter 6

CORNEAL HAZE

Noel Alpins, FRACO, FRCOphth, FACS and
George Stamatelatos, BScOptom

INTRODUCTION

Corneal haze presents as a superficial opacification of the normally clear cornea leading to a transient decrease in corneal transparency after excimer laser keratectomy.[1] It primarily results as part of a postoperative healing response to PRK, LASEK, or Epi-LASIK, particularly in high corrections of myopia, hyperopia, and astigmatism. Patients are not normally aware of this haze until it begins to impact their visual acuity. Haze can cause glare at night from bright lights, which may or may not interfere significantly with vision under low light conditions. Corneal haze usually reduces and disappears spontaneously within 6 to 9 months; however, it may not disappear in all cases[2] (Figure 6-1).

WHAT IS CORNEAL HAZE?

Histological and immunohistochemical studies reveal that the subepithelial haze contains newly synthesized collagen such as type III collagen, type IV collagen, fibronectin, laminin, and proteoglycans.[3-5] The first stage of wound healing in the cornea after PRK is epithelial migration along the ablated stromal bed. After re-epithelialisation, epithelial hyperplasia occurs,[6-8] which is then followed by stromal regeneration. During this phase, there is an increase in the number of stromal spindle-shaped keratocytes in the subepithelial stromal layer[9] that express smooth muscle specific alpha actin (α-SM actin) and synthesis type III collagen. Transforming growth factor $-\beta$ (TGF-β) has been proposed to be significant in inducing corneal stromal fibrosis after excimer laser keratectomy.[10] These activated stromal keratocytes (myofibroblasts) lay down an extracellular matrix.[11] From 1 month to a few months after PRK, the number of keratocytes tends to gradually diminish. The degree of corneal stromal haze after PRK correlates with the number of active fibroblasts and the amount of new extracellular matrix.[12]

The wound response following LASIK is quite different to that after PRK, LASEK, or Epi-LASIK. LASIK preserves corneal epithelium and Bowman's membrane, thereby reducing the effect of wound healing and problems associated with surface ablation.[13,14] Epithelial damage of the corneal flap due to severe dehydration or mechanical injury during LASIK

Figure 6-1. Appearance of corneal haze (grade 3.0+).

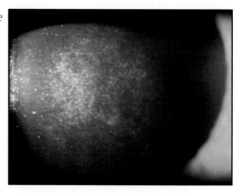

procedures can evoke excessive wound healing, leading to fibrosis or scarring. Nakamura et al hypothesized that intact epithelium is the key to the prevention of stromal haze after photoablation.[15]

ONSET OF CORNEAL HAZE

In vivo investigations of the structures responsible for corneal haze after PRK reveal a subepithelial deposition of collagen and extracellular matrix that gradually develops at the epithelial-stromal junction. This starts 1 week postoperatively, increases to a peak level between 1 and 3 months, and declines slowly thereafter.[1] However, Meyer and coauthors[16] and Lipshitz and coauthors[17] define a so-called late-onset corneal haze (LOCH) as an acute haze starting 4 to 12 months after excimer laser ablation (ie, at the time regular post-PRK haze has subsided in eyes with moderate to high myopia).[1]

CAUSES OF CORNEAL HAZE AFTER PRK

Patients with a larger attempted correction,[18-20] atopy, autoimmune conditions,[21] or high ultraviolet (UV) radiation exposure[1] may have a higher risk for corneal haze after excimer photoablation. Studies[1,16,17] have shown a correlation between post-PRK haze and UV-B exposure. These studies demonstrate that UV-B exposure after PRK exacerbates and prolongs the stromal healing response, manifested by increased keratocyte numbers and deposition of disorganized collagen in the anterior stroma.

Use of UV-protective eyewear should be encouraged during the first year after PRK especially in environments of high UV exposure (reflection from snow or water, high altitudes, or low latitudes).[1]

GRADING CORNEAL HAZE AFTER PRK

Anterior stromal haze that may be associated with photorefractive keratectomy can be classified using a grading scale as follows:
- 0 = Clear; no haze
- 0.5 = Trace corneal haze
- 1.0 = Mild corneal haze not affecting refraction
- 2.0 = Moderate corneal haze with difficult refraction
- 3.0=Corneal haze preventing refraction but anterior chamber visible
- 4.0=Severe corneal haze preventing refraction and completely obscuring iris details

PROPHYLAXIS AND TREATMENT OF CORNEAL HAZE

- Topical anti-inflammatory drugs such as 0.1% dexamethasone (Maxidex, Alcon, Ft. Worth, Tex), 0.1% fluorometholone (FML) (Allergan, Irvine, Calif) or prednisolone acetate 1% (Prednefrin Forte, Allergan) used postoperatively can prevent the development of excessive corneal haze and should be used for at least 1 month postoperatively.[22] These drugs inhibit both early and late manifestations of the inflammatory process, including fibrin deposition, fibroblast proliferation, and collagen deposition.
- Ice packs 10 minutes pre- and post-PRK together with chilled balanced salt solution (BSS) immediately after the ablation.[23]
- Severe haze affecting functional vision can be treated using phototherapeutic keratectomy (PTK) in conjunction with Mitomycin-C (MMC).

MMC is an antibiotic with antimetabolite effects (see Chapter 10) that inhibits the proliferation of keratocytes.[24] It has been used since the 1980s systemically in cancer chemotherapy[25] where its use originated, and in ophthalmology, in cases of ocular pemphygoid and following surgical treatment of glaucoma and pterygium.[26-28] MMC at a dilution of 0.02% (0.2 mg/mL) has been used in the treatment of post-PRK haze.[29] It has no effect on normal epithelial cells of the cornea provided there is no intraoperative contact of MMC with the stem cells at the limbus. There is also the prophylactic use of MMC to prevent haze applied immediately following PRK in moderate to high myopia.[30,31]

The main causes of regression and haze are overactivity and proliferation of stromal keratocytes following laser ablation.[31,32] MMC has cytotoxic effects through inhibiting DNA synthesis. MMC on the cornea can inhibit subepithelial fibrosis through preventing the proliferation of stromal keratocytes. The effects of MMC 0.02% in preventing haze have been shown by Talamo et al[29] and Xu et al[33] in experimental models. In a study by Majmudar et al, it was concluded that the application of MMC can reduce haze following PRK where prior radial keratectomy (RK) incisions existed.[34] It can also prevent the recurrence of haze after previous surgical complications such as a buttonholed LASIK flap.[35,36] The usefulness of PRK with MMC (0.2 mg/mL) for preventing haze in high myopia was reported by Carones et al.[31] Using MMC in PRK for myopia greater than -5.00 D has been shown to be safe and effective and can reduce haze formation after surgery.[32] To reduce potential toxicity, application times have reduced from the earlier standard of 2 minutes to as little as 12 seconds.[37,38]

CASE STUDY

In the case study presented below, we report our first experience in treating corneal haze post-PRK using PTK and 0.02% MMC as an adjunctive therapeutic agent. A 32-year-old male presented in 2001 inquiring about refractive laser surgery. He reported that he was a keen beach goer and spent a lot of time surfing while wearing soft disposable contact lenses for his high myopia. The preoperative parameters from the assessment are summarized in Table 6-1. A complete ocular health examination was unremarkable.

It can be seen from Figures 6-2A and 6-2B that the topographical appearance of the cornea was relatively normal. However, as the ultrasound pachymetry values were thinner than average (490 µm), the recommendation made was for PRK instead of LASIK. It was also recommended to treat one eye at a time, beginning with the nondominant left eye. This was to ensure that the patient gained functional vision and comfort before proceeding with the second eye. The patient was advised to leave his left contact lens out for 1 week preoperatively to minimize the chance of infection and allow stability of the corneal shape.

Table 6-1

Preoperative Parameters

Measurement	OD	OS
Manifest refraction	-9.50 DS/-0.50 DC Ax 170	-8.50 DS/-2.00 DC Ax 180
Cycloplegic refraction	-9.25 DS/-0.50 DC Ax 170	-8.00 DS/-2.00 DC Ax 180
BSCVA	20/20	20/20
U/S pachymetry	490 µm	490 µm
Simulated keratometry*	44.40/45.55 @ 80	45.08/46.61 @ 80

*Figures 6-2A and 6-2B

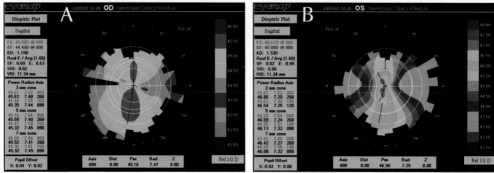

Figure 6-2. (A) Preoperative topography of the right eye. (B) Preoperative topography of the left eye.

PRK Surgery

The left eye underwent routine PRK surgery; an Amoils epithelial brush was used to remove the epithelium prior to the application of the excimer laser. The treatment programmed into the VISX STAR S2 laser (Santa Clara, Calif) was calculated using a multipass/multizone algorithm.[39] Cold BSS, Voltaren Ophtha (diclofenac sodium 5 mg/mL [Novartis, New York, NY]), and Chlorsig (chloramphenicol 5 mg/mL [Sigma Pharmaceuticals, Monticello, Iowa]) drops were subsequently used during the procedure. A bandage contact lens was applied to facilitate healing and was removed 2 days postoperatively once the epithelium had regenerated.

Postoperative topical medication was Chlorsig qid for 1 week and (once the epithelium had healed) FML (1 mg/mL) qid, tapering weekly over 1 month. Cellufresh (carmellose sodium 5 mg/mL, Allergan) lubricating drops were also used for the first month following surgery.

Postoperative Results

The results from the left surgery 6 weeks postoperatively were excellent. The patient was happy with the vision with only a minor complaint of glare at night. The results are summarized in Table 6-2. Because vision was good and there was no evidence of corneal haze at that time, arrangements were made to have PRK for the right eye. Again, the soft contact lens was removed 1 week prior to surgery. The surgical technique and postoperative topical medication were unchanged as for the left eye.

Table 6-2

Six Week Postoperative Results of Left Initial Surgery

Measurement	OS
UCVA	20/30++
Manifest refraction	Plano/-0.75 DC Ax 100
BSCVA	20/20
Slit-lamp	Clear cornea

Table 6-3

Postoperative Results of Both Eyes

Measurement	OD (Postop 4 weeks)	OS (Postop 10 weeks)
UCVA	20/20	< 20/200
Manifest refraction	+1.25 DS/-0.75 DC Ax 180	-5.00 DS
BSCVA	20/15	20/80+
Slit-lamp	Trace haze	Grade 1.5 to 2.0 haze
Simulated keratometry*	35.18/36.75 @ 90	39.20/40.89 @ 90
Intraocular pressure	12 mmHg	12 mmHg
U/S pachymetry	417 μm	518 μm

*Figure 6-3.

Four weeks after the right eye surgery, the patient reported that vision from his right eye was "good." However, he noted that the vision in his left eye (now 10 weeks postoperative) had deteriorated over the past few weeks. Indeed, this was confirmed by the reduced visual acuity measurements described in Table 6-3 and attributed to the appearance of corneal haze visible at the slit-lamp (Figure 6-3).

The development of corneal haze in high myopic PRK corrections has since been well-documented.[40,41] However, during this postoperative consultation the patient reported that he had been surfing extensively during the past month without wearing sunglasses despite being advised against this. The effect of UV radiation and the incidence of corneal haze after PRK has also been well-documented,[1,42] and it was concluded that this factor had contributed to the haze in this case.

Therapeutic Treatment of Corneal Haze

Over the course of the next 3 months, the patient's left eye was treated with topical anti-inflammatory agents in an effort to reduce the haze. Initial therapy was Maxidex (dexamethasone 1 mg/mL, Alcon) qid, later replaced with Pred Forte (prednisolone acetate 10 mg, Allergan) qid. When the haze had not resolved with topical therapy alone and the right eye began to show grade 0.5 haze, oral 25 mg cortisone was introduced bd.

Figure 6-3. Right and left eye topography at 2.5 months postoperatively.

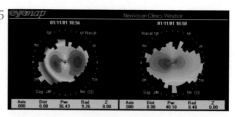

Table 6-4		
Results 6 Months Following Left Initial PRK Surgery		
Measurement	*OD (postop 4.5 months)*	*OS (postop 6 months)*
UCVA	20/120	< 20/200
Manifest refraction	-0.50 DS/-1.00 DC Ax 45	-9.75 DS
BSCVA	20/60	20/120
Slit-lamp	Grade 1.0 haze (diameter 5.0 mm)	Grade 3.0+ haze* (diameter 5.0 mm)
*Figure 6-1		

The intraocular pressure (IOP) had initially risen to 30 mmHg as a result of the topical steroid therapy. Adjunctive topical glaucoma therapy was instigated; Diamox orally (acetazolamide 250 mg, [Lederle, Madison, NJ]) with Alphagan (brimonidine tartrate 2 mg/mL, Allergan) bd and Xalatan (latanoprost; benzalkonium chloride 0.2 mg/mL [Pfizer, New York, NY) nocte were used and the IOP returned to 16 mmHg within a few days. Xalatan was therefore used in conjunction with the steroid treatment from that point, and the IOP remained well controlled.

There was no significant improvement noted in either the vision or the appearance of the corneal haze. In fact, the left eye displayed further deterioration to a grade 3 haze, as displayed in Figure 6-1. The best-corrected acuity (BSCVA) had also dropped to 20/120 in this eye. The 6-month postoperative results are summarized in Table 6-4. It should be noted that the right eye had also developed corneal haze to a lesser extent, but the unaided vision in that eye had also gradually reduced to 20/120.

Prevention of Corneal Haze Using Mitomycin-C

At this stage, the patient was restricted in his work duties because of the reduction in his vision in both eyes. He was involved in mixing paint and was required to distinguish between subtle shades of color. After extensive counseling, it was decided that surgical intervention was required.

Research through the scientific literature[31,34,43] and extensive consultation with international colleagues indicated that the use of the compound MMC could be very effective in preventing the recurrence of haze after a second surgical treatment. The risks associated with the use of MMC were researched and discussed at length with the patient.

Calculation of Residual Stromal Tissue

Once it was decided that a secondary procedure including MMC was required, the question became one of how much of the apparent myopia to treat. It cay be seen from Table 6-4

Table 6-5
Thickness of the Hyperplastic Layer of Epithelium and Haze

Calculation Of Residual Stromal Tissue For Left Eye

Preoperative corneal thickness	490 μm
Assumed epithelium thickness	60 μm
Initial treatment depth (from VISX S2 treatment printout)	120 μm
Estimated remaining stromal tissue	310 μm

Calculation of Hyperplastic Epithelial Thickness

Measured postoperative corneal thickness	518 μm
Estimated remaining stromal tissue	310 μm
Estimate of epithelium/haze thickness	208 μm

that there was almost 10.00 D of myopia present in the manifest refraction, which corrected the vision to only 20/120. Certainly, some of this myopia would be due to the presence of the haze on the cornea, but there was no way to determine how much. There may have also been some regression factors involved as evidenced by the epithelial hyperplasia.

It was decided to largely disregard the recurrence of the high myopia and to ablate the haze by phototherapeutic keratectomy (PTK). If required, a small amount of the myopia could be treated immediately following the PTK up to a maximum of 2.00 D. The haze reduction was to be monitored as the treatment progressed, and treatment ceased when the cornea appeared clear. This was done both objectively by observing the appearance of the cornea, and also by regular intraoperative pachymetry measurements to monitor the corneal thickness after epithelial removal and tissue ablation. A postoperative ultrasound pachymetry had previously been measured and found to be 518 μm. This was used to estimate the approximate thickness of the hyperplastic layer of epithelium and haze (Table 6-5).

PTK Surgical Technique Including Use of Mitomycin-C

As with the initial PRK procedure, the epithelium was removed with the Amoils epithelial brush. The PTK treatment was subsequently applied with a 6.0-mm circular ablation and a 0.3-mm transition zone. The frequency of the laser pulses was reduced to 6 Hz from the usual 10 Hz to allow the surgeon additional time to visualize the progressive removal of the haze.

After 45 pulses of PTK (11 μm) treatment, the procedure was paused for evaluation. There was still trace corneal haze remaining on objective examination under the laser microscope. It was decided to apply a minor myopic correction to further remove the haze and also to allow for any myopic regression that may have occurred. A treatment of -1.00 DS (63 pulses, 16 μm) within a 6.5-mm optic zone was applied at a rate of 6 Hz. The overall tissue removal was 27 μm.

Immediately following the myopic (second) treatment, the patient was evaluated at the slit-lamp. There was no discernible haze evident—at which point it was decided against any further treatment as this was deemed unnecessary and could result in overcorrection. The patient was taken back under the laser for the application of the MMC to prevent any

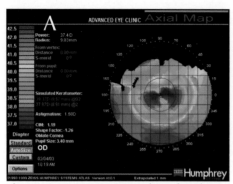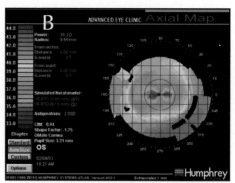

Figure 6-4. (A) Topography of right eye 6 months after secondary procedure to treat haze. (B) Topography of left eye 12 months after secondary procedure to treat haze.

future haze reformation. A Banaji shield soaked in MMC (0.02%) was applied to the cornea for 2 minutes (the recommended duration at that time). The cornea was then rinsed with 10 mL of cold BSS to flush away any remnants of MMC. As occurred after the initial surgery, a nonsteroidal anti-inflammatory drug (NSAID) was instilled, followed by a bandage contact lens and antibiotic. The contact lens was to be left in position for 2 to 3 days until corneal healing had occurred.

Postoperatively, Ciloxan (ciprofloxacin hydrochloride 3 mg/mL [Alcon]) and Predsol (minims) were prescribed qid together with Travatan (0.004% travoprost [Alcon]) nocte to keep any steroid-induced IOP rise under control.

Results Following Combined PTK/PRK With MMC

At 1 month postoperatively for treatment of haze, the results were very gratifying for both surgeon and the patient. There was a significant improvement in unaided vision, and the cornea displayed only trace haze (Figures 6-4). These results are summarized in Table 6-6.

The patient was advised to wait before considering treating the right eye for haze. This was to allow sufficient time to ensure no recurrence of corneal haze in the left had occurred and to evaluate the effectiveness of the epithelial remodelling that had occurred together with minor myopic treatment that was applied.

After 5 months (post-retreatment), it was evident that the treatment of the left eye had been successful with no noticeable haze formation and an excellent unaided vision of 20/30++. It was decided to treat the right eye in a similar fashion with a brush removal of epithelium, PTK, and minor myopic PRK.

The right eye achieved similarly excellent results as the left, and 1 month following this treatment, the patient's confidence had been restored and he had returned to full-time employment. He purchased a pair of wrap-around sunglasses that he could use during surfing and proceeded cautiously in regard to UV exposure, which included the use of a wide-brimmed hat outdoors.

Outcomes

The final review was conducted 12 months after the left eye was retreated and 7 months after the right eye was retreated. At this visit, the patient was praising the results; he was extremely pleased with his vision and level of comfort after such a frustrating but worthwhile waiting period in view of the complexity and risks of the treatment. The vision was a stable

Table 6-6
One Month Postoperative Results
Following Treatment of Left Corneal Haze

Measurement	OS
UCVA	20/30
Manifest refraction	+0.50 DS/-1.50 DC Ax 165
BSCVA	20/30
Slit-lamp	Trace haze

Table 6-7		
Results Following Treatment of Corneal Haze to Both Eyes		
Measurement	*OD (postop 7 months)*	*OS (postop 12 months)*
UCVA	20/30++	20/30-
Manifest refraction	Plano / -0.75 DC Ax 45	+1.25 DS/-1.25 DC Ax 165
BSCVA	20/30++	20/20
Slit-lamp	Trace haze	Trace haze[†]
Simulated keratometry*	37.87/39.37 @ 92	36.87/38.87 @ 92
*Figure 6-4; [†]Figure 6-5		

20/30 in each eye and 20/30++ binocularly, and the appearance of the cornea was relatively clear. These results are displayed in Table 6-7.

SUMMARY

This case demonstrates the dangers of excess exposure to UV light after PRK and the effectiveness of MMC in reducing the recurrence of corneal haze following laser vision correction with PRK. It also demonstrates how the treatment of corneal epithelial remodelling plus the corneal haze without including any significant refractive treatment may contribute to reducing any residual refractive error due to haze and epithelial remodelling. In this case, the patient apparently regressed to almost 10.00 D of myopia, though this was largely excluded in the surgical treatment plan. It was expected that the myopia would resolve by the removal of the epithelial hyperplasia and haze, as indeed was the case. If not, then subsequent refractive treatment could have been applied.

Since this initial use of MMC in the clinic 5 years ago, it has been included in all primary myopic PRK treatments where the spherical equivalent is above -4.50 DS. The 0.02% solution of MMC is still used, though the duration of application has been shortened from 2 minutes to 30 seconds for primary treatments. For PRK retreatments of low refractive magnitudes after LASIK or RK, only 15 seconds application is utilized. No similar episodes have occurred over this time with PRK treatments performed with this effective adjunctive treatment.

Acknowledgments

We would like to thank our colleagues Dr. Parag Majmudar and Dr. Francesco Carones for their advice in the management of this complex case. MMC is now a routine prophylactic part of our care with PRK and high myopia in primary treatments and in retreatments over LASIK flaps.

KEY POINTS

1. Corneal haze presents as a superficial opacification of the normally clear cornea leading to a transient decrease in corneal transparency after excimer laser keratectomy.

2. It is primarily caused as part of a postoperative healing response to PRK, LASEK, or Epi-LASIK, particularly in high corrections of myopia, hyperopia, and astigmatism.

3. Histological and immunohistochemical studies reveal that the subepithelial haze contains newly synthesized collagen such as type III collagen, type IV collagen, fibronectin, laminin, and proteoglycans

4. Patients with a larger attempted correction, atopy, autoimmune conditions, or high UV radiation exposure may have a higher risk for corneal haze after excimer photoablation.

5. Corneal haze usually reduces and disappears spontaneously within 6 to 9 months; however, it may not disappear in all cases.

References

1. Stojanovic A, Nitter TA. Correlation between ultraviolet radiation level and the incidence of late-onset corneal haze after photorefractive keratectomy. *J Cataract Refract Surg.* 2001;27:404-410.

2. Hefetz L, Nemet P. Corneal haziness. *Br J Ophthalmol.* 1997;81:637-638.

3. Goodman GL, Trokel SL, Stark WJ, et al. Corneal healing following laser refractive keratectomy. *Arch Ophthalmol.* 1989;107:1799-1803.

4. Balestrazzi E, De Molfetta V, Spadea L, et al. Histological, immunohistochemical and ultrastructural findings in human corneas after photorefractive keratectomy. *J Refract Surg.* 1955;11:181-187.

5. Hanna KD, Pouliquen Y, Waring GO, et al. Corneal stromal wound healing in rabbits after 193 nm excimer laser ablation. *Arch Ophthalmol.* 1989;107:895-901.

6. Taylor DM, L'Esperance FA Jr, Del Pero RA, et al. Human excimer laser lamellar keratectomy. A clinical study. *Ophthalmology.*1989;96:654-664.

7. McDonald MB, Frantz JM, Klyce SD, et al. One-year refractive results of central photorefractive keratectomy for myopia in the nonhuman primate cornea. *Arch Ophthalmol.* 1990;108:40-47.

8. Del Pero RA, Gigstad JE, Roberts AD, et al. A refractive and histopathologic study of excimer laser keratectomy in primates. *Am J Ophthalmol.* 1990;109:419-429.

9. Moller-Pedersen T, Cavanagh HD, Petroll WM, et al. Neutralizing antibody to TGF-beta modulates stromal fibrosis but not regression of photoablative effect following PRK. *Curr Eye Res.* 1998;17:736-747.

10. Kaji Y, Soya K, Amano S, Oshika T, Yamashita H. Relation between corneal haze and transforming growth factor-β1 after photorefractive keratectomy and laser in situ keratomileusis. *J Cataract Refract Surg.* 2001;27:1840-1846.

11. Darby I, Skalli O, Gabbiani G. Alpha-smooth muscle actin is transiently expressed by myofibroblasts during experimental wound healing. *Lab Invest.* 1990;63:21-29.

12. Fantes FE, Hanna KD, Waring GO, et al. Wound healing after excimer laser keratomileusis (photorefractive keratectomy) in monkeys. *Arch Ophthalmol.* 1990;108:665-675.

13. Pallikaris IG, Siganos DS. Excimer laser insitu keratomileusis and photorefractive keratectomy for correction of high myopia. *J Refract Corneal Surg*. 1994;10:498-510.

14. Park CK, Kim JH. Comparison of wound healing after photorefractive keratectomy and laser in situ keratomileusis in rabbits. *J Cataract Refract Surg*. 1999;25:842-850.

15. Kunihiko Nakamura, Daijiro Kurosaka, Hiroko Bissen-Miyajima, Kazuo Tsubota. Intact corneal epithelium is essential for the prevention of stromal haze after laser assisted in situ keratomileusis. *Br J Ophthalmol*. 2001;85:209-213.

16. Meyer JC, Stulting RD, Thompson KP, Durrie DS. Late onset of corneal scar after excimer laser photorefractive keratectomy. *Am J Ophthalmol*. 1996;121:529-539.

17. Lipshitz I, Loewenstein A, Varssano D, Lazar M. Late onset corneal haze after photorefractive keratectomy for moderate and high myopia. *Ophthalmology*. 1997;104:369-373.

18. Pietila J, Makinen P, Pajari S, et al. Photorefractive keratectomy for -1.25 to -25.00 diopters of myopia. *J Refract Surg*. 1998;14:615-622.

19. Gabrieli CB, Pacella E, Abdolrahimzadeh S, et al. Excimer laser photorefractive keratectomy for high myopia and myopic astigmatism. *Ophthalmic Surg Lasers*. 1999;30:442-448.

20. Corbett MC, Prydal JI, Verma S, et al. An in vivo investigation of the structures responsible for corneal haze after PRK, and their effect on visual function. *Ophthalmology*. 1996;103:1366-1380.

21. Cua IY, Pepose JS. Late corneal scarring after photorefractive keratectomy concurrent with the development of systemic lupus erythematosus. *J Refract Surg*. 2002;18:750-752.

22. Vetrugno M, Maino A, Quaranta GM, Cardia L. The effect of early steroid treatment after PRK on clinical and refractive outcomes. *Acta Ophthalmologica Scandinavica*. 2001;79:23.

23. Kitazawa Y, Maekawa E, Sasaki S, Tokoro T, Mochizuki M, Ito S. Cooling effect on excimer laser photorefractive keratectomy. *J Cataract Refract Surg*. 1999;25:1349-1355.

24. Katzung BG. *Clinical Pharmacology*. San Mateo, Calif: Appleton and Lange; 1988.

25. Soloway MS, Treatment of superficial bladder cancer with intravesical mitomycin C: analysis of immediate and long-term response in 70 patients. *J Urol*. 1985;134(6):1107-1109.

26. Donnenfeld ED, Perry HD, Wallerstein A, et al. Subconjunctival mitomycin C for the treatment of ocular cicatricial pemphigoid. *Ophthalmology*. 1999; 106(1):72-78.

27. Kitazawa Y, Kawase K, Matsushita H, Minobe M. Trabeculectomy with mitomycin. A comparative study with fluorouracil. *Arch Ophthalmol*. 1991;109(12):1693-1698.

28. Hayasaka S, Noda S, Yamamoto Y, Setogawa T. Postoperative instillation of low dose mitomycin C in the treatment of primary pterygium. *Am J Ophthal*. 1988;106:715-718.

29. Talamo JH, Gollamudi S, Green WR, De La Cruz Z, Filatov V, Stark WJ. Modulation of corneal wound healing after excimer laser keratomileusis using topical mitomycin-C and steroids. *Arch Ophthalmol*. 1991;109:1141–1146.

30. McCarty CA, Aldred GF, Taylor HR. Comparison of results of excimer laser correction of all degrees of myopia at 12 months postoperatively. The Melbourne Excimer Laser Group. *Am J Ophthalmol*. 1996; 121:372–383.

31. Carones F, Vigo L, Scandola E, Vacchini L. Evaluation of the prophylactic use of mitomycin-C to inhibit haze formation after photorefractive keratectomy. *J Cataract Refract Surg*. 2002;28:2088–2095.

32. Hashemi H, Taheri SMR, Fotouhi A, Kheiltash. Evaluation of the prophylactic use of mitomycin–C to inhibit haze formation after photorefractive keratectomy in high myopia: a prospective clinical study. *BMC Ophthalmol*. 2004;4:12.

33. Xu H, Liu S, Xia X, Huang P, Wang P, Wu X. Mitomycin-C reduces haze formation in rabbits after excimer laser photorefractive keratectomy. *J Refract Surg*. 2001;17:342–349.

34. Majmudar PA, Forstot SL, Nirankari VS, et al. Topical mitomycin-C for subepithelial fbrosis after refractive corneal surgery. *Ophthalmology*. 2000;107:89-94.

35. Lane HA, Swale JA, Majmudar PA. Prophylactic use of mitomycin-C in the management of buttonholed LASIK flap. *J Cataract Refract Surg*. 2003;29:390–392.

36. Weisenthal RW, Salz J, Sugar A, et al. Photorefractive keratectomy for treatment of flap complications in laser in situ keratomileusis. *Cornea*. 2003;22:399–404.

37. Majmudar, PA. Mitomycin C and PRK haze. *Cataract and Refractive Surgery Today*. 2001.

38. Majmudar PA, Estates H. How to make the most of mitomycin-C. *Review of Ophthalomolgy.* 2004; 11:7.

39. Alpins NA, Taylor HR, Kent DG, et al. Three multizone photorefractive keratectomy algorithms for myopia. *J Refract Surg.* 1997;13:535-544.

40. Kuo IC, Lee SM, Hwang DG. Late-onset corneal haze and myopic regression after photorefractive keratectomy (PRK). *Cornea.* 2004;23(4):350-355.

41. Kaji Y, Yamashita H, Oshika T. Corneal wound healing after excimer laser keratectomy. *Semin Ophthalmol.* 2003;18(1):11-26. Review.

42. Lipshitz I, Loewenstein A, Varssano D, Lazar M. Late onset corneal haze after photorefractive keratectomy for moderate and high myopia. *Ophthalmology.* 1997;104:369-373; discussion by JH Talamo, 373-374.

43. Majmudar PA, Epstein RJ. Mitomycin-C treatment for post-PRK corneal haze. *Video Journal of Cataract and Refractive Surgery.* 2001.

Chapter 7

PHOTOREFRACTIVE KERATECTOMY COMPLICATIONS

Samuel Boyd, MD and Raymond Stein, MD, FRCSC

Photorefractive keratectomy (PRK) was the first laser vision correction procedure adopted by ophthalmologists and patients around the globe. Today laser in situ keratomileusis (LASIK) is the predominant refractive procedure. However, there is renewed enthusiasm for PRK because of its safety profile and superior outcomes in the correction of higher-order aberrations. PRK plays a role in refractive surgery when patients are reluctant to undergo incisional surgery, when ophthalmologists have a preference for PRK or are in their learning curve with laser vision correction, or if there is a contraindication to LASIK. There are certain conditions in which a patient may be a better candidate for PRK than LASIK. These relative LASIK contraindications include:

- Epithelial anterior basement membrane dystrophy because of the risk of epithelial ingrowth.
- Keratoconus because of the risk of corneal ectasia.
- Difficulty in achieving satisfactory suction for the microkeratome cut.
- Corneal thinning in which less than 250 μm of tissue would be left in the bed.

PREOPERATIVE ASSESSMENT

Refractive errors that can be treated with PRK with a satisfactory visual outcome include myopia up to −12.00 D, astigmatism up to 6.00 D, and hyperopia up to 5.00 D.[1] The best results with the lowest incidence of complications occur in the lower ranges of myopia, astigmatism, and hyperopia; the higher the refractive error, the greater the chance of regression and corneal haze. There are a number of conditions in which a patient may be a poor candidate for PRK such as progressive myopia or unstable refractive error, cataracts, collagen vascular disease, unrealistic expectations, and advanced dry eye syndrome.

During pregnancy or nursing, there may be hormonal changes that could alter the refractive error. In addition, medications (sedation, pain medications, and possibly eye drops) can be transmitted to the fetus via the mother's bloodstream or to the baby through breast milk. For these reasons, refractive surgery should not be performed on pregnant women or nursing mothers. It has been demonstrated that there is a 13.5 times higher chance of regression

Figure 7-1. Placido disk, reflected pattern, abnormal cornea. In a cornea with abnormal curvature (note high spot in corneal cross section—arrow), the reflected pattern of the placido disk shows distortion of the rings. The steeper portion of the cornea reflects the rings in a pattern in which they appear closer together (R). Familiarity with the types of reflective distortions produced by the cornea can be used to note the location of steep, flat, and asymmetric areas for the purpose of devising a proper treatment approach. (Courtesy of Benjamin F. Boyd, MD, FACS, Editor-in-Chief, *Atlas of Refractive Surgery* with permission from Highlights of Ophthalmology, English Edition, 2000.)

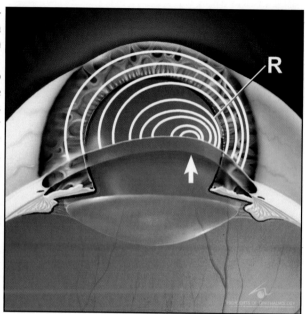

in females on oral contraceptives.[2] Patients should be counseled of this apparent increased risk.

Computerized videokeratography has become the standard of care to rule out subtle abnormalities of the cornea. Videokeratography is used to identify early keratoconus or "keratoconus suspect," corneal warpage, and asymmetric or irregular astigmatism (Figure 7-1). Each condition has a different prognosis. Patients with keratoconus have asymmetric and/or irregular astigmatism, and the standard laser ablation is not capable of correcting this abnormality. Even if the myopia were reduced, any residual irregular astigmatism would require a rigid contact lens for correction. Topographically-linked or wavefront-guided ablations have the potential to correct irregular astigmatism. The other concern of treating unrecognized keratoconus patients is the potential for litigation if keratoconus is detected postoperatively and thought to be caused by the laser procedure.

Patients with keratoconus and a relatively stable refractive error that correct to a satisfactory level with glasses are candidates for PRK but not for LASIK. Although there are higher incidences of regression and the need for an enhancement, the visual outcomes and patient satisfaction levels have been excellent.

Because patients may be given topical steroids postoperatively, it is important to rule out the presence of glaucoma or a glaucoma suspect who may be more susceptible and vulnerable to raised intraocular pressures with topical steroids. This is especially important in the higher ranges of myopia because of the greater risk of significant corneal haze that may require a course of intensive topical steroids.

Fundoscopy is a very important exam in myopic patients because there is the possibility of a retinal hole or degenerative retina (Figure 7-2). It also rules out any optic disc or macular disease as a baseline measurement. Patients with myopic degeneration and loss of best corrected visual acuity (BCVA) are at higher risk for progressive visual loss because of the natural history of their disease. A patient that loses vision postlaser vision correction will generally not accept the diagnosis of progression of myopic degeneration. Surgeons should be conservative when dealing with patients with any macular disease.

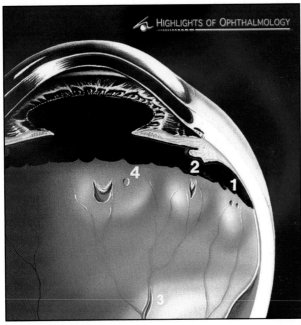

Figure 7-2. Location and types of retinal holes often missed. Identification of all retinal breaks is fundamental for a successful result. In this figure we show several locations and types of retinal holes often missed during evaluation: 1) small round holes located far peripherally near the ora serrata; 2) small horseshoe tears at the posterior edge of the vitreous base; 3) posteriorly located juxtavascular slit-like tear; 4) obscure hole easily missed during examination due to atrophy of the choroid. (Courtesy of Benjamin F. Boyd, MD, FACS, Editor-in-Chief, *Retinal and Vitreoretinal Surgery—Mastering the Latest Techniques* with permission from Highlights of Ophthalmology, English Edition, 2002.)

Advanced keratitis sicca with diffuse superficial punctate keratopathy or corneal filaments is a contraindication for PRK. Other contraindications for the excimer laser procedure include uveitis, cataract, retinopathies, and significant lagophthalmos.

Patients with active systemic connective tissue diseases (eg, systemic lupus, rheumatoid arthritis) are considered poor PRK candidates because of the potential for poor epithelial healing and the risk of a corneal melt.

Patients with a history of keloid formation of the skin are no longer considered a contraindication to PRK. There does not appear to be an increased risk of corneal haze.

Careful patient selection and review of the risk:benefit ratio of PRK are important considerations. Patient information and education are primary prerequisites for PRK or other refractive procedures. The patient should understand the excimer laser procedure and postoperative evaluation by reading information sheets and obtaining information from patient counselors, the surgeon, and other patients.

The patient should have realistic expectations. The ideal outcome would be one in which the patient can see very soon afterwards, at least as well without glasses or contact lenses as he or she had previously been able to see with the best possible glasses or contacts, and do so with no side effects. It is very important that the patient's expectations are reasonable and that he or she understands the possible ways in which his or her expectations might not be met.

PHOTOREFRACTIVE KERATECTOMY FOLLOWING OTHER SURGICAL PROCEDURES

PRK can alter the refractive error after previous eye surgery. There is an increased risk of corneal haze when PRK is performed after penetrating keratoplasty, radial keratotomy, or LASIK. The best outcomes are after cataract surgery.

Treating postradial keratotomy (RK) patients should be done with caution. Some patients after RK will complain not only of poor vision due to undercorrection, overcorrection, or induced astigmatism but also of fluctuating vision and problems with night vision. PRK enhancements will not improve night vision problems, nor can they correct vision fluctuations. The patient may blame the PRK surgeon for not correcting the pre-existing vision problems caused by the RK. Patients who have had 4-incision RK often do well with PRK enhancements. Patients with 8 or more RK incisions tend to do poorly with a high incidence of corneal haze. The etiology for this is not known and may be related to a dellen-like effect due to the corneal contour. It is not recommended to perform PRK enhancements for patients who have had RK with more than 8-incisions. If the patient had 8-incision RK and if the pre-RK refractive error was less than −6.00 D, he or she should usually do well with a PRK enhancement. However, if the refractive error was greater than −6.00 D, there is a greater incidence of central corneal haze. Longitudinal studies indicate a fairly significant hyperopic drift in RK eyes. Therefore, performing a PRK enhancement on an RK patient who is −1.00 D may not be in the patient's best interest.

Also, PRK can be used to treat anisometropia after corneal transplantation.[3]

Importance of the Postoperative Management

Excimer patients should expect vision to be blurry while the epithelium is healing.[4] They should know that symptoms like ghosting, glare, and shadows are usually transient phenomena and will disappear. Changes in vision with healing of epithelium and stroma are normal during the early postoperative course.

The combination of preoperative and postoperative NSAIDs and ice application immediately postoperatively, along with a soft contact lens has resulted in a major decrease in pain that now 90% of the patients are comfortable following PRK. The 10% that do have discomfort usually have minimal to moderate discomfort overnight that quickly resolves.

EFFECT OF POSTOPERATIVE STEROIDS

The use of topical steroids post-PRK is controversial. Studies in the low myopia range (less than 6.00 D) have shown no significant difference in refractive outcome or development of haze between eyes treated with steroids and those treated with artificial tears. Our own clinical experience, especially in the high myope, is that there is greater evidence of regression and haze when steroids are not used or when they are discontinued abruptly. It is hoped that better and more effective nonsteroidal modulating medications will be developed.

Disadvantages of this use are adverse effects, such as elevated intraocular pressure, posterior subcapsular cataracts, ptosis, and reactivation of herpes simplex keratitis.

EFFECT OF NONSTEROIDAL ANTI-INFLAMMATORIES

Anti-inflammatory nonsteroidals, like diclofenac sodium (Voltaren [Novartis, East Hanover, NJ]) and ketorolac tromethamine (Acular [Allergan, Irvine, Calif]) through inhibition of prostaglandin synthesis produce a potent analgesic effect that is very important in the early postoperative period following photorefractive surgery. The use of diclofenac has been shown to promote regression and, therefore, is occasionally used when dealing with an overcorrected PRK.

The use of nonsteroidals should be combined with a topical steroid to prevent accumulation of white blood cells in the cornea, which produce corneal infiltrates.

MANAGEMENT OF COMPLICATIONS

Clinicians must understand and recognize the potential complications of PRK.[5,6] Complications can be divided into the following categories[7]:

A. Side effects of corticosteroid use
    1. Ocular hypertension

B. Early (less than 6 weeks) complications
    1. Discomfort/pain
    2. Corneal infection/sterile infiltrates
    3. Delayed epithelial healing
    4. Pseudodendrites

C. Early and/or late complications
    1. Loss of best-corrected visual acuity
    2. Halo effect
    3. Central islands
    4. Decentration
    5. Recurrent corneal erosion
    6. Ocular hypertension

D. Late (greater than 6 weeks) complications
    1. Diffuse haze
    2. Arcuate or peripheral haze

E. Refractive complications
    1. Undercorrection
    2. Overcorrection
    3. Presbyopia
    4. Regression with or without haze

F. General awareness

Side Effects of Corticosteroid Use

OCULAR HYPERTENSION

Clinical Features

In a small percentage of patients, the postoperative use of steroids can result in increased intraocular pressure (IOP).

To reduce the incidence of such occurrence, fluorometholone and Vexol (Alcon, Ft Worth, Tex) have become a commonly used postoperative topical steroid, compared to a more penetrating steroid such as prednisolone acetate or dexamethasone.

Early Complications

DISCOMFORT/PAIN

Clinical Features

Patients may experience postoperative discomfort that is similar to that of a corneal abrasion. Ninety percent of patients report little to no discomfort after PRK and 10% of patients report discomfort or pain that usually resolves in 24 to 36 hours following the procedure.

Figure 7-3. Corneal ulcer. Acutely inflamed eye with circular infiltrate in the visual axis. To proceed with an accurate diagnosis and to find the causative agent, the cornea should be scraped over the infiltrate.

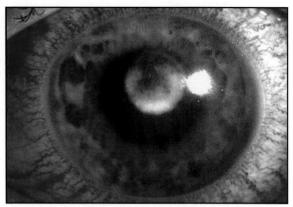

Management

The postoperative pain has been greatly reduced or eliminated by the use of NSAIDs (eg, ketorolac tromethamine 0.5% [Acular] or diclofenac sodium 0.1% [Voltaren]) during the first few days following the PRK procedure in combination with a bandage soft contact lens. Systemic medication (eg, demerol, Tylenol #3 [Ortho-McNeill, Raritan, NJ]) may be used if necessary. Cold compresses applied to the lids are often helpful. In patients with a dry eye, the wearing of a soft contact lens during the first few days after the PRK procedure can result in some irritation or discomfort. This discomfort can often be relieved by the frequent use of artificial tears. Preservative-free brands are recommended. Dry eye patients may benefit from the insertion of collagen implants or silicone punctal plugs.

CORNEAL INFECTION/STERILE INFILTRATES

Clinical Features

Occasionally, patients are asymptomatic early in the course. Pain, discharge, or redness may be present.

A corneal infection usually involves a single white infiltrate and an associated purulent discharge (Figure 7-3). Sterile infiltrates are frequently multiple in number without an associated discharge.

Management

Corneal infection and/or sterile infiltrates are rare complications and have been reported, on average, in 1 out of every 500 cases. Treat as a bacterial corneal ulcer with broad spectrum antibiotics. If the white infiltrate is small, less than 2 mm in size, consider monotherapy with a fluoroquinolone every hour during the day and taper with an improvement in the clinical course. If the infiltrate is greater or equal to 2 mm, consider treating with fortified antibiotics (eg, tobramycin 15 mg/cc and cefazolin 50 mg/cc) every 30 to 60 minutes and gradually taper).

DELAYED EPITHELIAL HEALING

Clinical Features

Persistent blurred vision occurs with an epithelial defect. The epithelial defect usually has well-defined borders. The stroma may show folds secondary to edema.

Management

If the epithelial surface is not intact by 6 days postoperatively, initiate the following steps:

- Discontinue all drops except the antibiotic. Be sure the patient is not self-medicating with topical anesthetic.
- If the soft contact lens put in place after the PRK procedure is still present, remove the lens and insert a new lens.
- If the contact lens has been removed, then you may wish to reinsert another protective contact lens.
- After the epithelium is intact, remove the protective lens and restart the topical steroid.

PSEUDODENDRITES

Clinical Features

Vision may be blurred if the pseudodendrite is in the visual axis.

Management

Pseudodendrites are not true complications, but rather a normal healing response. Do not confuse this with a herpetic lesion. A pseudodendritic pattern may be seen as the epithelial surface becomes intact in the healing process during the third and fourth days after the laser procedure. This is a normal healing pattern and will resolve within a few days. No change in the medication is required.

Early and/or Late Complications

LOSS OF BEST-CORRECTED VISUAL ACUITY

Clinical Features

The etiology of blurred vision, or loss of BCVA, can usually be detected with the standard eye examination. Occasionally, computerized videokeratography may be necessary to detect more subtle causes for loss of visual acuity.

Typical causes of loss of BCVA include:
- Epithelial irregularity
- Central islands
- Corneal haze
- Decentered ablation

Vision is typically very blurry immediately after the procedure. It generally starts to improve once the epithelium has grown back, which in most cases takes 3 to 5 days. However, vision can continue to be blurry for a number of weeks. After the epithelial defect has healed, loss of BCVA is usually secondary to an irregular epithelium, which usually smooths out over a few weeks.

Management

If epithelial irregularity with or without superficial punctate keratitis (SPK) is noted, non-preserved artificial tears should be added. Loss of acuity from other previously listed causes should be managed as outlined in this section.

HALO EFFECT

Clinical Features

Halos may be experienced in the first 4 to 6 weeks following the procedure as the epithelium heals and smooths out over the complete ablation zone.

Management

With most patients, the halo effect tends to diminish with time. In a case in which the patient is undercorrected, retreatment with a larger optical zone may alleviate the halos.

CENTRAL ISLANDS

Clinical Features

Central islands, which represent small elevated islands of tissue left centrally, may occur following PRK.[8] Central islands may cause monocular diplopia or blurred vision. The definition of a central island is a central or pericentral area of steepening that is:

- At least 1.00 D in height
- At least 1 mm in diameter
- Measured at least 1 month postoperatively

Patients may be asymptomatic or experience qualitative visual changes. The islands may be visible as a small central shadow on retinoscopy. The diagnosis can be confirmed with computerized videokeratography showing an elevation within the central or pericentral zone. The etiology is probably multifactorial.

Management

The prevention of central islands can be achieved by producing additional pulses to the central 2.5-mm area. If central islands are noted, the majority of these islands disappear after a period of months. If after 10 months there is a persistent symptomatic central island, the laser can be used to vaporize the central elevation. Computerized topography is used to determine the location, width, and steepness of the island. After mechanical epithelial removal, an ablation zone of less than 3 mm is used to flatten the island using PRK. Today, a topographically-linked or wavefront-guided ablation can be used to improve the optical quality of the cornea.

DECENTRATION

Clinical Features

Decentration can occur if the laser beam is not precisely aligned with the surgeon's eyepiece prior to the procedure. Poor patient fixation can also cause decentration. Decentration of the ablation zone can cause an increase in corneal astigmatism.[9] Eyes with higher attempted correction have a greater probability of decentration of the ablated zone because these patients have greater difficulty in maintaining fixation during treatment, due either to their greater myopia or to the longer time required for laser treatment.

Management

The use of either a topographically-based system or wavefront-guided ablation is the treatment of choice.

RECURRENT CORNEAL EROSION

Clinical Features

Patients may complain of pain, tearing, and photophobia. This is more common in the morning on awakening. The symptoms may resolve in an hour or persist for hours, if significant. An epithelial defect or erosion may be seen during the acute episode. Epithelial microcysts may be noted after the erosion has healed.

Management

Recurrent corneal erosions are more common with mechanical epithelial debridement than with laser transepithelial removal. The erosion tends to occur outside the laser area of ablation. Management is similar to that of recurrent corneal erosion with hypertonic drops and ointment. If this is not satisfactory in preventing a recurrence, a bandage soft contact lens can be used. If this is not successful, a PTK can be performed to the eroding area. The epithelium in the area is gently removed and a PTK with an optical zone of 2 to 6 mm to encompass the erosion site is selected with a depth of 5 to 8 μm.

Late Complications

DIFFUSE HAZE

Clinical Features

Corneal haze usually takes the form of a fine reticular subepithelial pattern that does not interfere with vision. Corneal clarity is graded on a scale of 0 to 4+. The haze corresponds to a corneal healing response following PRK induced by activation and migration of keratocytes (fibroblasts) and newly synthesized collagen (Figure 7-4). The haze is first noted between 2 and 4 months. The haze gradually fades by 6 to 12 months. Severe haze rarely occurs. There are some factors that may be related to increased haze: depth of ablation, laser beam homogeneity, epithelial removal method, corneal dryness during treatment, keratitis sicca, and solar exposure. Age does not seem to be an enhancing factor.

Management

If the patient has moderate or severe haze that interferes with vision, steroid drops should be increased in frequency to 5 times per day and gradually tapered over 2 to 3 months. Topical steroids are used to try to modulate the stromal wound healing response. Infrequently there may be a haze that requires a new laser treatment. It is usually best to treat the haze with a "no-touch" technique using a PTK mode. Any residual refractive error can be managed in the future with a PRK. The refractive error tends to be unreliable when there is severe corneal haze. The adjunctive use of mitomycin-C (MMC) 0.2% as a single intraoperative application for 2 minutes has been shown to decrease the incidence of recurrent haze.

If possible, it is best to wait for resolution of the haze before retreating. Patients should discontinue all drops with a stable refraction before an enhancement. If there is sufficient corneal thickness, these patients are best treated with a LASIK enhancement to minimize the wound healing response.

ARCUATE OR PERIPHERAL HAZE

Clinical Features

Haze in the peripheral area of the ablation bed can lead to a hyperopic shift and/or induced astigmatism. This peripheral haze is more commonly seen with a laser epithelial ablation that was too deep. In this case, a steep transition exists between the ablated zone and the untreated area.

Management

Peripheral haze should be managed as in the case of diffuse haze with the frequent use of steroid drops 5 times per day with a gradual tapering over 2 to 3 months. This is the only situation in which steroid drops are increased when dealing with a hyperopic refractive error.

Refractive Complications

UNDERCORRECTION

Clinical Features

The residual myopia is due to insufficient initial treatment that is more common with higher degrees of myopia. Undercorrection may result from an excessively moist cornea during the procedure.

Management

If there is an undercorrection, the patient is not satisfied with the level of vision, and is not interested in monovision, additional treatment can be performed. It is usually best to wait until the refraction is stable (3 to 6 months later).

Figure 7-4. PRK—Stromal haze formation. Some patients develop a diffuse subepithelial haze between 3 to 4 weeks following PRK. The amount of haze is not usually related to the degree of ametropia treated. It may even appear in eyes with low degrees of refractive errors. In this illustration, a grade 3 haze (H) is presented, which may significantly affect the patient's visual acuity. In most cases, the haze greatly diminishes or even disappears after 1 year. This is a major disadvantage of PRK. (Courtesy of Benjamin F. Boyd, MD, FACS, Editor-in-Chief, *Retinal and Vitreoretinal Surgery—Mastering the Latest Techniques* with permission from Highlights of Ophthalmology, English Edition, 2002.)

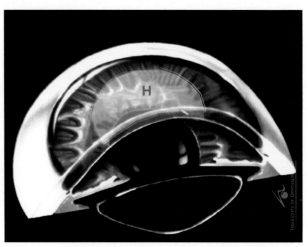

OVERCORRECTION

Clinical Features

Patients may experience blurred vision when viewing close-up objects. In some cases, particularly with those patients over 40 who are presbyopic, vision may also be blurry when viewing objects in the distance. A small amount of initial overcorrection is acceptable because some regression will often take place. Possible causes include a cornea that is too dry during the procedure and manifest preoperative refraction that did not account for accommodation.

Management

Any significant degree of hyperopia should be managed by tapering the steroid drops over 2 to 4 weeks. A more rapid withdrawal of steroids can lead to significant haze. If regression toward myopia is not satisfactory, diclofenac eye drops or a bandage contact lens can promote epithelial hyperplasia and regression. Surgical options include hyperopic PRK, conductive keratoplasty (radiofrequency), or hyperopic LASIK.

PRESBYOPIA

Clinical Features

If a patient is overcorrected, presbyopic symptoms may appear following the procedure.

Management

Reading glasses may be required, even though the patient did not require correction to read prior to the procedure.

REGRESSION WITH OR WITHOUT HAZE

Clinical Features

Regression is more likely to occur with higher degrees of myopic and/or astigmatic correction. Factors that may lead to regression include preoperative flat keratometry, small optical zones, single zone treatment, high myopia, and steep wound edges.[10,11]

Management

If regression occurs, steroid drops are either increased in frequency or restarted. If after a few months there is an improvement in the refractive error, the steroids are tapered. If the eye remains undercorrected, retreatment can be performed after the steroids have been discontinued and after the refraction becomes stable.[12]

Regression without haze can be managed with a PRK enhancement that is similar in technique to a primary procedure. If there is regression with mild haze, a transepithelial approach followed by a PRK for the residual refractive error can be performed. If there is regression with severe haze, then a "no-touch" technique using a PTK mode should be done. Any residual refractive error can be managed in the future with a PRK enhancement for myopia, astigmatism, and/or hyperopia.

SUMMARY

A thorough understanding of the preoperative assessments, techniques, and postoperative management are essential to achieve satisfactory visual outcomes. Laser safety checks are mandatory. A well-functioning excimer laser with good optics is required. The surgeon must avoid any decentration or global tilt. All aspects of the technique must be performed with attention to detail. The postoperative management requires frequent follow-up visits and psychological reinforcement of a healing process that is not instantaneous. This is evolving technology. Although the results today are impressive, the complications in the future will continue to decrease with changes in lasers, techniques, and pharmacologic management.

KEY POINTS

1. PRK plays a role in refractive surgery when patients are reluctant to undergo incisional surgery, when ophthalmologists have a preference for PRK or are in their learning curve with laser vision correction, or if there is a contraindication to LASIK.
2. There is an increased risk of corneal haze when PRK is performed after penetrating keratoplasty, radial keratotomy, or LASIK.
3. The use of topical steroids post-PRK is controversial. Disadvantages of this use are adverse effects, such as elevated intraocular pressure, posterior subcapsular cataracts, ptosis, and reactivation of herpes simplex keratitis.
4. The use of nonsteroidals should be combined with a topical steroid to prevent accumulation of white blood cells in the cornea, which produce corneal infiltrates.
5. The surgeon must avoid any decentration or global tilt.

REFERENCES

1. Stein H, Cheskes A, Stein R. *The Excimer*. 2nd ed. Thorofare, NJ: SLACK Incorporated; 1998:10-64.
2. Corbett MC, O'Brart DP, Warburton FG, Marshall J. Biologic and environmental risk factors for regression after photorefractive keratectomy, *Ophthalmology*. 1996;103(9):1381-1391.
3. Amm M, Duncker GI, Schroder E. Excimer laser correction of high astigmatism after keratoplasty. *J Cataract Refract Surg*. 1996;22(3):313-317.
4. Stein H, Stein R. *The Excimer Video Course*. St Louis, Mo: Medical Productions; 1994.
5. Boyd BF. Preoperative evaluation and considerations. *Atlas of Refractive Surgery*. Panama: Highlights of Ophthalmology; 2000:37-64.
6. Stein R. Photorefractive keratectomy. *Laser Surgery of the Eye*. Panama: Highlights of Ophthalmology; 2005:28-40.

7. Stein R, Stein H, Cheskes A. Photorefractive keratectomy. *Continuing Education Manual.* Toronto, Ont: Bochner Eye Institute; 1999.

8. Krueger RR, Saedy NF, McDonald PJ. Clinical analysis of steep central islands after excimer laser photorefractive keratectomy. *Archives of Ophthalmology.* 1996;114(4):377-381.

9. Aktunc R, Aktunc T. Centration of excimer laser photorefractive keratectomy and changes in astigmatism. *J Refract Surg.* 1996;12(2):S268-271.

10. Gauthier CA, Holden BA, Epstein D, et al. Role of epithelial hyperplasia in regression following photorefractive keratectomy. *Br J Ophthalmol.* 1996;80(6):545-548.

11. Goggin M, Foley-Nolan A, Algawa K, O'Keefe M. Regression after photorefractive keratectomy for myopia. *J Cataract Refract Surg.* 1996;22(2):194-196.

12. Matta CS, Piebenga LW, Deitz MR, Tauber J. Excimer retreatment for myopic photorefractive keratectomy failures. Six to 18 month follow-up. *Ophthalmology.* 1996;103(3):444-451.

Chapter 8

LASEK COMPLICATIONS

Massimo Camellin, MD

INTRODUCTION

Due to its main characteristics, the LASEK technique has shown very few complications, some of which are also common in PRK.[1-23] For this reason, it is important to emphasize that some LASEK surgeries may become PRK if the flap is lost during the first few postoperative hours. If the surgeon is not very skilled, he or she will believe that he or she has accomplished LASEK and will be unable to understand why his or her results are like those of a PRK. I would like to stress these considerations because during the last few years I have had to face a number of controversies in studies that say there is no difference between LASEK and PRK. PRK is not a poor technique; indeed, it works well. However, in rare cases PRK involves epithelialization delay and haze. This may occur only rarely in the experience of a refractive surgeon but when it does happen it can lead to grave complications.

Pain seems to be the most important aspect of surface techniques. The recovery time is probably like that of PRK; however, the stability of the results is largely guaranteed.

INTRAOPERATIVE COMPLICATIONS

Epithelium Management

Epithelium management is the first step toward good LASEK, but despite its relative feasibility, requires some tricks that must be taken into account in order to avoid postoperative pain and flap loss during the early hours.[1,2] The use of a toothed trephine means that every epithelium can be precut, independently of its thickness; however, when the instrument is rotated, be careful not to rotate the globe, otherwise the effect creates a circular series of notches that do not lead to the same result of increasing the alcohol flow under the epithelium itself. It is true, however, that in some cases the solution can nevertheless pass the epithelium barrier but the problem is to allow its flow, as much as possible, to detach even stubbornly attached epithelium. When one starts to rotate the trephine aid with a fixation ring, it is important to pay attention and make sure that the instrument moves at least 10 degrees in comparison to the globe. Do not exceed this safety value, because it risks the creation of a hinge that is too small, thereby increasing the risk of flap loss.

Alcohol Management

The well contains an alcohol solution, and leakage onto the conjunctiva must be avoided. An adapted well has been designed with a double edge that works better both in keeping the eye firm and at the same time containing the solution. When the correct amount of time (20 sec) has elapsed, do not take the well away before having dried the contents and rinsed it with diclofenac.

Having followed this rule, make sure that no contamination of the conjunctiva has occurred.

Unfortunately, despite best efforts, some patients move their eye during alcohol exposure and there may be some leakage onto the conjunctiva, which will immediately feel painful. At this point, abundantly rinse with diclofenac and, if exposure has been too short, apply alcohol into the well again.

Flap Tears

Starting detachment of the flap edge is the best way to begin flap making and this shows how well the flap is attached. If strong resistance is perceived, stop and reuse alcohol for 5 to 10 more seconds. This maneuver increases the alcohol flow because now there will be a real groove on the periphery of the flap and 5 to 10 seconds is enough to enormously increase the detachment. The more adherent the epithelium, the, more pressure must be applied on the spatula, which must be used vertically at its shortest side. Sometimes, tears may occur, but the worst complication is a hinge tear because of the drawback of making it difficult to recognize the right side of the flap when it has been rolled back. It is always better to manage the flap with two rounded spatulas; in this unfortunate case, the surgery can be saved by operating calmly. Having lost the hinge, one must try to increase flap stability, and this can be achieved by drying the flap for 2 minutes at the end of the procedure before fitting the contact lens.

Mitomycin-C Usage

In these cases, it is a good idea to brush the surface with mitomycin-C (MMC) 0.01% before rolling the flap back. It is usually more difficult to detach epithelium at the periphery, particularly in the upper area close to the hinge. Wide flaps are therefore more difficult to manage (ie, hyperopic treatments). When the corneal diameter is small, we must separate the epithelium close to the limbus, where it is strongly attached.

The use of MMC has been widely discussed during recent years and we have performed a study showing excellent results but a delayed recovery time and an increased corneal high-order aberration value.[3] This probably means slower epithelium regrowth; in our study, this outcome was present after a year. For this reason, we suggest using MMC only if it is necessary (ie, when the flap is unstable due to tearing or hinge problems).

An atypical use of MMC is when the patient loses the lens, and often the flap, during the first postoperative hour. The reason for this inconvenience is a dryness shown by some patients at the end of the procedure. The reason for the dryness is not clear, but probably the contemporary use of anesthetic drops, diclofenac, steroids, or maybe alcohol can temporarily reduce the secretion of the lacrimal gland. When this occurs, if the flap is lost, it seems worthwhile to pour a drop of MMC 0.01% and rinse the surface with diclofenac. In this way, we reduce the risk of PRK-type haze. The use of a single drop of MMC has never shown any complications in postoperative care.

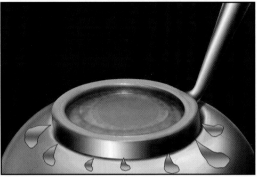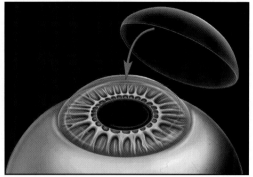

Figure 8-1. Squeezing fluid from under the flap avoids contact between nerve tips and the flap.

POSTOPERATIVE COMPLICATIONS

Pain

Pain is a debatable point in this surgery and probably it is the least comparable. Apart from some differences in pain perception from race to race, there are different results related to surgical technique (more or less correct) and the use of a good intra- and postoperative regimen.

An intraoperative regimen of drugs to be used are:
- Diclofenac (to rinse after alcohol exposure)
- Ofloxacin (this antibiotic has good penetration in the anterior chamber but is more aggressive toward epithelium than aminoglycoside; we prefer it at this stage to increase protection from infections)
- Dexamethazone + clorfenamine (This association is excellent for reducing pain and probably makes the difference between having pain or not in the postoperative period)
- Tropicamide (a light mydriatic aids in decreasing possible iris pain origin)

The postoperative regimen includes:
- Diclofenac (only when necessary)
- Gentamicin qid for 10 days
- Clobetazone bid for 30 days only after contact lens removal
- Autoserum qid for 7 days[4]
- Amino acids 7 days before surgery and 15 days after surgery[5]

If the patient refers pain on the first day, applying crushed ice several times a day is useful. There is an important surgical step in pain prevention, which is not very well understood, and that is flap squeezing. At the end of the procedure, after lens fitting, I use an applanator to squeeze all of the fluid from under the flap itself (Figures 8-1). This has the double purpose of increasing the flap stability for a vacuum mechanism and reducing nerve-end stimulus due to flap movements.

A simple example is a skin blister for tennis players. Years ago, there was only a simple cotton plaster to protect the wound, but this did not prevent pain because the nerve-ends were in contact with the blister and the cotton would often move. More recently, the Compeed (Johnson & Johnson, New Brunswick, NJ) has appeared, with the unique feature of protecting the blister with a thick and firm plastic-like strip (Figure 8-2). The working mechanism of

Figure 8-2. Compeed for protecting a blister avoids pain thanks to its thickness.

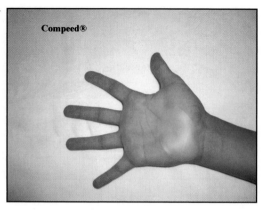

Figure 8-3. Fluid under the flap leads to pain due to stimulation of the nerves.

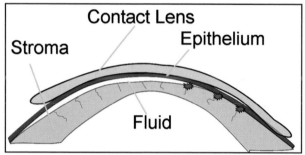

this device is simple and avoids the stimulation of the nerve fiber tips by the blister. If some fluid remains under the flap during eye movement, the contact lens may stimulate nerve ends through the flap, but if you squeeze this fluid even if the contact lens moves, it cannot move the flap, and the endings are not stimulated (Figure 8-3). There are other reasons that lead to pain, but these simple suggestions can certainly reduce the probability. In our recent analysis, strong pain was present in less than 5% of those undergoing LASEK.

Contact Lens

The contact lens itself can cause pain if it is too narrow or dirty. We are used to choosing the right basal ray according to the treatment of the patient and his or her preoperative curvature. In the past, we used lenses that were too narrow and we noticed a limbic fingerprint with vessel congestion and there were always complaints by the patients. The same happens, to a lesser degree, when the lens is dirty and this often occurs on the third day after surgery (Figure 8-4). This is probably relative, regarding materials and debris and this is not completely clear. Nevertheless, it is worthwhile to change the lens if it is too dirty, though not before the third day. The risk is to have a flap that is too weak and that can be broken by lid movements. Personally, in these cases, I fit a new lens, possibly wider for another 3 days. If the patient loses his or her lens after 2 days, this is less dangerous for haze risk because the greater cytokine release has occurred during the first 10 hours[6] and, therefore, stroma protection is useful in this period only. In these cases, I simply refit a new lens without using in any MMC.

The choice of removing the lens early is good but we should at least check the flap integrity. To achieve this certainty, there is only one way, and that is to use macromolecular fluorescein under the lens. This particular drug is used to check soft contact lenses as it only dyes the exposed stroma and not the poly-hema. In this way, we can be very sure about the

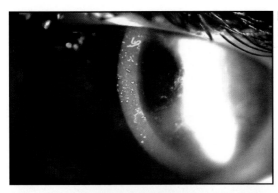

Figure 8-4. Dirty lens after 3 days following LASEK surgery.

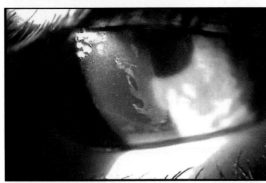

Figure 8-5. Flap tear due to early lens removal.

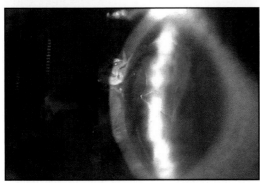

Figure 8-6. Late tear following finger injury 2 months after surgery.

quality of the flap and therefore decide to remove the lens. Nowadays, we are always used to removing the lenses after 7 days so we are sure of no tears or flap loss risk to the patient. As you can see in Figure 8-5, the flap can tear if the lens is removed too soon; this complication is caused by eyelid movements.

Flap Tear

In LASEK, more than in PRK, epithelium has good adherence only after a few months due to the poor inflammatory reaction. Unfortunately, during the first postoperative months patients can damage flap integrity with unwanted contact (Figures 8-6 and 8-7).

Septic Infiltrations

Septic infiltrations seem to affect the peripheral area of the cornea where, because it is not protected by the epithelium, the stroma is exposed. We have had a high number of peripheral

Figure 8-7. Fluorescein picture of same patient as in Figure 8-6 having late tear following finger injury 2 months after surgery.

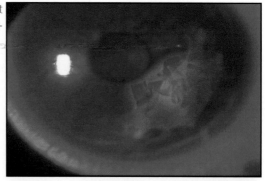

Figure 8-8. (A) Infiltration in the eye wearing hydrogel contact lens. (B) Fluorescein picture of patient having infiltration in the eye wearing hydrogel contact lens.

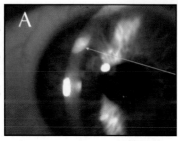
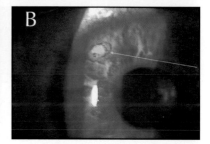

infiltrations, with hydrogel lenses, which appear characteristically rounded, small, and quite deep. (Figures 8-8A and B). Infiltrations in the eye-wearing hydrogel contact lens are possible due to the *Staphylococcal Aureo* toxin.[7] We have seen this phenomenon in 27% of these lenses, which we have since abandoned. Now, we prefer to use an alphafilcon A polymer (66% water), even if it is less permeable to oxygen. In all infiltrations, which are 0.6% of the whole statistic, we have instilled 1 drop of iodopovidon 10% with no loss of BCVA noted.

Epithelium Thinning

Epithelium thinning complications more frequently appear close to the central area. For reasons still unknown, epithelium can be slow to regrow and we suspect the reason is poor viability in the inner layers of the epithelium itself. After a LASEK procedure, epithelium is renewed and the old layer disappears in 3 or 4 days; in some cases, the viability is so good that the new one joins the old instead of slipping under it. As we know, the inner layer has the ability to regrow 8 to 10 times,[8] and wound healing in these cases follows another path. The substitution of cells belonging to the old flap is progressive but taking into account this process is physiologically slow in that it can oppose the movement of the newly born limbal cells toward the center. Fortunately, this paradox is rare, but the surgeon must immediately recognize it. It is worthwhile to suspend steroids and increase artificial tears (Figures 8-9).

Patient refraction in these cases is hyperopic and often with an irregular astigmatism, but progressively it reaches the target in 1 or 2 months without consequences. In 3 cases, this thinning has shown some negative features as in DLK. The superficial stroma was slightly whitish and the refraction was greatly hyperopic. Everything was uneventful over 3 months, but I still cannot explain the causes of this problem. The stroma progressively clarified and no line was lost (Figures 8-10).

More recently, we have had some of these cases in an operating session when I tried a new contact lens. The material was 2-hydroxyethylmetacrylate monomer 99% + methacrylic acid + ethylene glycol dimethacrylate monomer, and the suspicion is an interaction of this material with benzalconium chloride. This interaction risks toxic monomer release (which

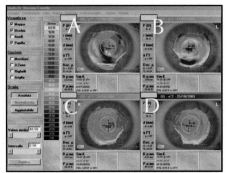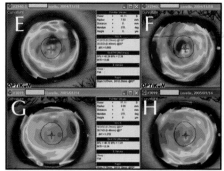

Figure 8-9. Example 1 (Left). Localized epithelial thinning, (A) right eye, (B) left eye, (C) right eye after 1 month, (D) left eye after 1 month. Complete fixing of the problem in 1 month. Example 2 (Right). Localized epithelial thinning, (E) right eye, (F) left eye, (G) right eye after 2 months, (H) left eye after 2 months. Only small defects are still present at 2 months in both eyes.

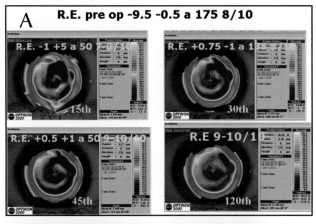

Figure 8-10. (A) Vast epithelial thinning and its healing process with time. There are still some irregularities after 4 months, but the BCVA has been recovered. (B) Corneal aspect of epithelium thinning up.

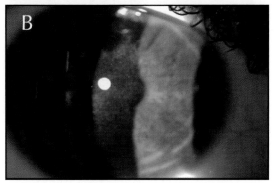

has already been reported by other authors[9]) and this can probably disturb the wound-healing process to a greater or lesser degree (Figure 8-11). Nevertheless, in all of these cases, the preoperative BCVA was achieved in 3 months, and only a slight opacity was recognized for 1 year.

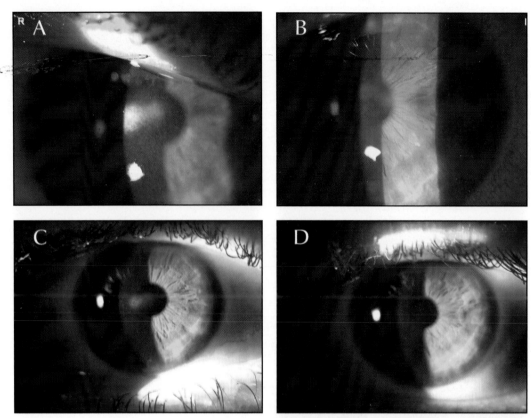

Figure 8-11. (A) Right eye central opacity diffuse in the epithelium with this monomer. (B) Left eye diffuse opacity. (C) Right eye after 2 months. (D) Left eye after 2 months. (E) Topographical aspect with disappearing of the flat area in the center of the right eye in 2 months.

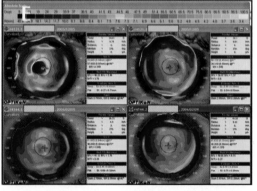

Inclusions Under the Flap

Sometimes debris or small particles of tissue can be trapped under the flap but this has not shown itself to be a real problem. During flap renewal, all these unwanted impurities are expelled and none of them can be detected within a month. Therefore, washing under the flap at the end of the procedure is not very useful.

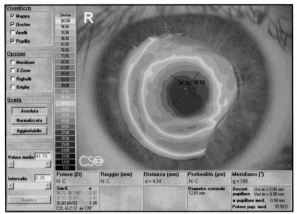

Figure 8-12. Small optical zone following myopia treatment.

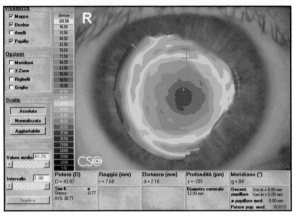

Figure 8-13. Loss of the correction with time due to a small optical zone. The optical zone progressively reduces due to stromal regrowth.

LONG-TERM COMPLICATIONS

Over- and Undercorrections

An immediate hypo- or hypercorrection is obviously due to laser failure and not to the regrowth of epithelium or stroma. If this occurs, it is worthwhile treating it within 2 months because it is easy to detach the new epithelium and correct the remaining defect. In this case, I always use MMC 0.02% for 2 minutes because the keratocytes can be very active due to reoperation and the risk of haze is significant. We always prefer to use alcohol even if it is possible to detach the epithelium without it because patients treated without it have shown more pain.

Otherwise, if the hypocorrection is delayed, it is due to an epithelial regrowth followed by a stromal one.[10,11] Usually, it is common to observe these late reactions when optical zones are small in comparison to treated myopia (Figures 8-12 and 8-13). More precisely, the reason lies in the unadapted transition zone, which is usually too steep if the optical zone is narrow. It is a paradox, but the higher the myopia we have to operate on, the wider the optical zones needed. Nonetheless, it is possible to try to reduce these regressions by using a topical steroid, but it is fundamental to check the eye pressure weekly. Often, we observe a transitory effect that disappears as we suspend the drug, but in rare cases, there is a stable reduction.

Figure 8-14. (A,B) Small optical zone following LASIK surgery for myopia. (C,D) Retreatment to wide in the optical zone. +2 sphere has been crossed with -2 sphere.

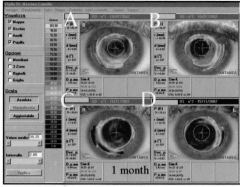

We don't like to abuse steroid usage due to the high risk of cataract.[12] The lack of Bowman's membrane increases these risks. If we have a new regression after 2 months, it is better to not insist, but to reoperate using a wider optical zone and a linked treatment if available. It is also possible to cross positive and negative spheres to increase the diameter of the treatment[13] (Figure 8-14).

If we insist on a small treatment, this will increase the difference of the curvature and after starting an overcorrection, there could be an unpredictable undercorrection. Overcorrection can derive from the wrong laser management, an error in the refraction or a variation in stromal hydration. This last phenomenon is the only one strictly related to LASEK because during flap detachment, an unskilled surgeon, by losing time, is responsible for dehydration of the stroma. It is clear that if the stroma loses water, the photoablative rate increases with the unwanted side effect of excess ablated tissue.[14] We must also consider the fact that during aging, water contained in tissue reduces and in elder patients, this can lead to overcorrection.[15] Unfortunately, we cannot determine if the patient has a high or low level of water inside the stroma. If we add MMC, and we suggest it only in selected cases, we may observe an overcorrection of about 10%.[16]

Our experience has shown an increased corneal high order aberration level,[17] which is an index of epithelium irregularity. In short, if our patient is older than 40, we suggest reducing the setting by 10% to 15%, as other authors have noted,[18] while if the surgical time has been too long, hydrating the stroma with BSS is sufficient. Both these suggestions are empirical ones and therefore may cause errors. Given that a retreatment is always possible, it is better to perform it within 3 months so as to avoid excessive adherence of epithelium and stroma.

Haze

Haze is uncommon in recent years (also in PRK[19] procedures), but it has not completely disappeared. Improvements in laser beams have greatly reduced such complications in PRK (apart from re-epithelization delay cases, in which haze is unavoidable[20]), while it is rare in LASEK. In our statistical analysis of LASEK, the epithelium was completely renewed within 4 days in 83.3% of patients and within 6 days in all. The difference with PRK is clear in that as with LASEK there is always a sheet protecting the stroma; therefore, re-epithelization time has a different meaning.

The unwanted "haze" complication has a single and certain origin called apoptosis. This is the way an injured cell dies without the negative sequel of necrosis. Stromal apoptosis means keratocytes die on a stimulus with cytokines coming from epithelial cells and stromal cells. These cytokines have different effects on wound healing both positive and negative.[21] When the stroma is exposed, the epithelium immediately produces molecules to accelerate epithelium regrowth. This is clearly a defense mechanism, but when it is too strong, it has the side effect of an increased release of cytokines that can activate keratocytes transforming them into myofibroblastes. These cells, by producing an extracellular matrix, tend to rebuild the ablated tissue. The 2 well-known consequences are a loss of correction and loss of BCVA (or at least contrast sensitivity).

Why should LASEK reduce this risk? The answer is due to the presence of a basal layer (lamina lucida) that by covering the stroma avoids contact with tear film that contains diluted cytokines.[22] The importance of the flap is greater during the first 24 hours in which cytokine release is abundant. In short, even nonviable epithelium has the role of protecting stroma from contamination and reducing the tendency of too rapid epithelium regrowth.[23] If one remembers, it is important to squeeze fluid from under the flap because we avoid nerve stimulation and reduce pain. Pain reduction also reduces epiphora and, therefore, the risk of contaminating the stroma with cytokines. The double mechanism is the protection of the stroma as a barrier and the reduction of pain, which has the positive effect of reducing apoptosis.

Therefore, LASEK has the characteristics of reducing haze and regression. It is obvious that some patients can lose their flap, which transforms their surgery into a PRK. We observed some rare cases of haze but the degree and percentage were low. In myopia patients, we observed only 0.7% of third-degree haze in one eye.

Pain When Waking Up

Pain when waking up is relatively common during the first few months after surgery and is related to dryness that every eye experiences during sleep. When a patient suddenly wakes up and opens his or her eyes, there can be some small superficial epithelial tears, so small they usually disappear in a few minutes. In our experience, only 25% of patients had this symptom during the first 6 months, while only 2% continued to refer it at 1 year. The best way to solve this problem is to instil a drop of artificial tears before sleeping and gently move the eyelids with one's hands before opening the eyes. We didn't notice any epithelial suffering in these patients during examinations.

SUMMARY

By concluding this short report, we can affirm that LASEK does not have the propensity to create grave complications. It certainly reduces PRK complications, but we wish to point out once again that LASEK is not only a surgery but also a procedure and must be followed in all its steps to obtain the excellent results we have had until now.

KEY POINTS

1. Epithelium management is the first step toward a good LASEK but, despite its relative feasibility, requires some tricks that must be taken into account in order to avoid postoperative pain and flap loss during the early hours.

2. The use of MMC shows excellent results but a delayed recovery time and an increased corneal high-order aberration value. This probably means slower epithelium regrowth. For this reason, use MMC only if it is necessary (when the flap is unstable due to tearing or hinge problems).

3. At the end of the procedure, after lens fitting, use an applanator to squeeze all fluid from under the flap itself. This has the double purpose of increasing the flap stability for a vacuum mechanism and reducing nerve-end stimulus due to flap movements.

4. The contact lens itself can cause pain if it is too narrow or too dirty.

5. Septic infiltrations seem to affect the peripheral area of the cornea, where, because it is not protected by the epithelium, the stroma is exposed.

REFERENCES

1. Camellin M. *Camellin LASEK Technique. LASEK, PRK, and Excimer Laser Stromal Surface Ablation.* New York, NY: Marcel Dekker; 2005;7:73-82.

2. Camellin M. *LASEK & Asa Storia Tecnica Risultati a Lungo Termine.* Canelli: Fabiano Editore; 2004:117.

3. Camellin M. Laser epithelial keratomileusis with mitomycin C: indications and limits. *J Refract Surg.* 2004;20:S693-S698.

4. Nizzola F, Zizzola GM, Ascari A, Torlai F. Autologous serum therapy following PRK. *J Refract Surg.* 2001;suppl:269.

5. Vinciguerra P, Camesasca FL, Ponzin D. Use of amino acids in refractive surgery. *J Refract Surg.* 2002; 18:S374-377.

6. Wilson SE, Molecular cell biology for the refractive corneal surgeon: programmed cell death and wound healing. *J Refract Surg.* 1997;13:171-175.

7. CCLRU. (Cornea and Contact Lens Research Unit—The University of New South Wales – Sidney NSW 2052 Australia) and LVPEI (LV Prasad Eye Institute—LV Prasad Marg Banjara Hills Hyderabad 500034 India). Guida alle reazioni corneali con infiltration, osservate nella pratica contattologia. Ciba Vision; 2003.

8. Pellegrini G, et al. Cultivation of human keratinocyte stem cells: current and future clinical application. *Cell Eng.* 1998;36:1-13.

9. Casini M. Sistemi chimici di disinfezione e pulizia in contattologia. *Otoforum.*1986;52-60.

10. Sandvig KU, Kravik K, Haaskjold E, Blika S. Epithelial wound healing of the rat cornea after excimer laser ablation. *Acta Ophthalmologica Scandinavica.* 1997;75:115-119.

11. Lee YC, Wang IJ, Hu FR, Y-Kao WW. Immunohistochemical study of subepithelial haze after photo-therapeutic keratectomy. *J Refract Surg.* 2001;17:334-341.

12. Maitchouk D, Smirennaia E, Kourenkov V. Corneal pharmacodynamics after photorefractive keratectomy and laser in situ keratomileusis in rabbits. *J Refract Surg.* 2002;18:S382-S384.

13. Lafond G, Solomon L, Bonnet S. Retreatment to enlarge small excimer laser optical zones using combined myopic and hyperopic ablations. *J Refract Surg.* 2004;20:46-52.

14. Rama G, Buratto L, Dal Fiume E, Merlin U. Chirurgia della Cornea. *Fogliazza Editore.* 1993;662.

15. Rao SN, Chuck RS, Chang AH, LaBree L, McDonnell PJ. Effect of age on the refractive outcome of myopic photorefractive keratectomy. *J Cataract Refract Surg.* 2000;26:543-546.

16. Carones F, Vigo L, Standola E, Vacchini L. Evaluation of the prophylactic use of mitomycin-C to inhibit haze formation after photorefractive keratectomy. *J Cataract Refract Surg.* 2002;28:2088-2095.

17. Camellin M. Surgeon: disadvantages of mitomycin in LASEK outweigh advantages. *Ocular Surgery News.* 2005;23:28-29.

18. Dutt S, Seinert RF, Raizman MB, Puliafito CA. One-year results of excimer laser photorefractive keratectomy for low to moderate myopia. *Arch Ophthalmol.* 1994;112:1427-1436.

19. Zoltan Zsolt Nagy Z, Fekete O, Suveges I. Photorefractive Keratectomy for Myopia With the Meditec MEL 70 G-Scan Flying Spot Laser. *J Refract Surg.* 2001;17:319-326.

20. Seiler T, Holschbach A, Derse M, et al. Complications of myopic photorefractive keratectomy with the excimer laser. *Ophthalmology.* 1994;101:153-160.

21. Wilson SE, Liu JJ, Mohan RR. Stromal-epithelial interactions in the cornea. *Prog Retin Eye Res.* YEAR; 18:293-309.

22. Zhao J, Nagasaki T, Maurice DM. Role of tears in keratocyte loss after epithelial removal in mouse cornea. *Invest Ophthalmol Vis Sci.* 2001;42:1743-1749.

23. Baldwin HC, Marshall J. Growth factors in corneal wound healing following refractive surgery: A review. *Acta Ophthalmologica Scandinavica.* 2002;80:238-247.

Chapter 9

Epi-LASIK

*Vikentia J. Katsanevaki, MD, PhD; Maria I. Kalyvianaki, MD;
Dimitra S. Kavroulaki, MD; and Ioannis G. Pallikaris, MD, PhD*

INTRODUCTION

Laser in situ keratomileusis (LASIK) has been widely accepted and is currently the most popular surgical approach for photorefractive correction of ametropias, providing fast visual recovery and minimal postoperative discomfort.[1,2] However, complications that have been related [3-8] to the method, such as flap-related complications, dry eye, reported postoperative mechanical instability of the cornea, and vision-threatening inflammations, have turned many surgeons back to surface ablations. Advanced surface ablations refer to photorefractive surface surgical modalities that were developed to manage the drawbacks of traditional photorefractive keratectomy (PRK)[9,10] (ie, the postoperative pain and the formation of subepithelial haze).

LASEK

Laser assisted subepithelial keratectomy (LASEK)[11] was the first procedure that involved preservation of the epithelium in order to control corneal wound healing.[1-38] The procedure involves the use of alcohol solution for the successful in toto separation of the epithelium as a sheet. The ablation takes place on the exposed stroma, and the epithelial flap is then repositioned on the top of the cornea. Although the beneficial effect of the replaced epithelial sheet (as compared to the conventional PRK method) is still under question,[26] many studies[12-22] have shown LASEK to be a safe and effective approach for the correction of myopia and myopic astigmatism, and propose LASEK to be superior to PRK. Drawbacks of LASEK that have been reported are the dose and time-dependent[25] toxic effect of alcohol on the corneal epithelium,[23,24] the interpatient variability of the ease of making epithelial flaps[26] necessitating variable application times of the alcohol solution[27] as well as the long learning curve[28] of the technique.

Figure 9-1. Electron microscopy of the basal part of the epithelial sheet. A small portion of Bowman's is included within the sheet (between arrows).

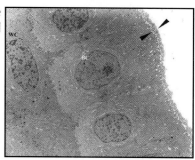

Epi-LASIK

Epi-LASIK,[29-31] as an amalgam of LASIK and surface treatment much like LASEK, also involves preservation of an intact epithelial sheet in order to control corneal wound healing. In Epi-LASIK, however, the epithelial separation is achieved by means of a customized device that can achieve the successful epithelial separation mechanically without requiring the use of alcohol. As compared to LASEK, Epi-LASIK provides a completely automated way to perform advanced surface ablation and avoids the toxic effect of alcohol on the separated epithelium.

HISTOLOGICAL FINDINGS OF MECHANICALLY SEPARATED EPITHELIAL SHEETS

During the evolution of Epi-LASIK, one of the initial goals was to determine whether mechanical separation provided any advantages as compared to alcohol-assisted, separated epithelial sheets. In a study that was conducted in the University of Crete, we cross examined epithelial sheets that were obtained either with corneal preparation with alcohol or after mechanical separation using a prototype device. We found that due to a shallower cleavage plane, the basement membrane of alcohol-assisted epithelial sheets was destroyed upon separation; a finding that was also confirmed by other investigators.[14,32] Transmission electron microscopy of mechanically separated sheets, however, showed that mechanical separation of the corneal epithelium preserved the epithelial basement membrane providing a slightly deeper cleavage plane as compared to that of alcohol[29] (Figure 9-1). As has been shown by in vitro studies,[33] the presence of an intact basement membrane is important for the control of corneal wound healing minimizing the fibrotic activation of keratocytes. Under this consideration, we assume that mechanically separated epithelial sheets are expected to be more effective in the control of postoperative inflammation and corneal wound response after PRK as compared to those separated with alcohol. Furthermore, the basement membrane is important for the viability of the epithelial sheet that is expected to act as mechanical barrier between the corneal stroma and the tear film after the surgery. Histopathological study of a small number of sheets that were harvested and examined 24 hours after the surgery[34] showed that the epithelium was morphologically close to normal at that interval. Although it is clinically evident that the replacement of the epithelial sheet does not cancel the migratory phase of epithelial healing and that it is replaced within the first days after the surgery, histopathology data provide supporting evidence that at least for the first postoperative hours the mechanically separated sheets remain viable providing a "living contact lens" to cover the ablated cornea.

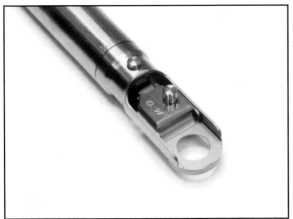

Figure 9-2. Centurion SES epikeratome for epithelial separations (Norwood Abbey, Australia).

Epi-LASIK: The Surgical Technique

The operative eye is prepared with povidone-iodine and 3 drops of topical tetracaine hydrochloride 0.5% (applied every 5 minutes before the procedure) and is covered with a sterile drape. The epithelial separations are currently performed in our center with the use of a commercially available epithelial separator (Centurion EpiEdge Epikeratome, Norwood Abbey, Australia), which is an electrically powered device (Figure 9-2) that operates under low suction similar to a conventional microkeratome. Instead of a blade, it features a disposable, oscillating polymethylmethacrylate (PMMA) separator with an advance speed of 3.5 mm/sec. The resulting separated epithelial sheet has a nasal hinge and a diameter of 9.5 to 10 mm.

Although the replacement of the epithelial sheet is not as mandatory as in the classic LASIK flap, preoperative corneal marking enables the surgeon to replace the epithelium without any stress. Before the epithelial separation, the cornea is marked with a customized marker (Epi-LASIK marker, Duckworth & Kent, Baldock, UK) that features 2 concentric circles crossed by 8 radial arms. Upon the replacement of the epithelial sheet, any deformity of the concentric cycles dictates the sheet's proper repositioning.

The manipulations on the epithelial flap can be conducted either by a moistened Merocel sponge (Medtronic, Jacksonville, Fla) or a customized spatula (Epi-LASIK spatula, Duckworth & Kent). The lift and the replacement of the separated epithelial sheet are often achieved with a single movement. Any inward or outward folds of its edges can be restored with the use of the spatula after irrigation with balanced salt solution (BSS). Once the epithelial sheet is stuck to the underlying stroma in accordance with the preoperative marks, a therapeutic contact lens is applied onto the operative eye.

Epi-LASIK: Postoperative

All eyes in our setting were operated with the Centurion SES epikeratome (Norwood Abbey) and the Wave Allegretto (Wavelight, Enlagen, Germany) laser platform. The mean time of epithelial healing in more than 500 eyes that have been operated in Crete up to date is around 5 days, ranging from 3 to 7 days. The epithelial healing is complete by day 5 in the vast majority of the operated eyes. The lenses are removed on the third day after the treatment in less than 10% of the operated eyes.

At the end of the surgery, the replaced epithelial sheet often overlays its initial gutter probably due to the intraoperative mechanical stretch on the epithelial sheet upon separation. The epithelial sheet is transparent immediately after the operation. During the healing process of the corneal surface, the borders between the newly synthesized epithelium and the remnants of the separated sheet are easily observed at slit-lamp biomicroscopy. The migrating cells gradually replace the separated epithelial sheet, which is subsequently constricted in the central area. Starting from its peripheral part around the edges on the first postoperative day, the sheet becomes hazy in its total area until about the third day after the treatment. At that time, the hazy area measures about the central 1- to 2-mm whereas a front of newly synthesized, transparent epithelium migrates from the corneal periphery toward the center of the corneal surface. After that stage, the transparency of the corneal epithelium is restored within 24 to 48 hours and the therapeutic contact lens is removed. A central healing line is often apparent after the removal of the therapeutic contact lens. The time of epithelial healing ranges from 3 to 5 days between the treated eyes.

Similarly as after LASEK,[18,19] Epi-LASIK is not a totally pain-free procedure. Postoperative pain of the treated eyes is currently assessed in our center with the use of a subjective questionnaire that patients grade pain in a scale from 0 to 4 in 2-hour intervals on the operative day and once daily in the following days. The postoperative regimens after the procedure include eye drops of diclofenac sodium 0.1% qid for 2 days and combined eye drops of tobramycin-dexamethasone qid until the removal of the therapeutic lens. After the removal of the lens, all treated eyes receive fluorometholone eye drops qid for 5 weeks in a tapered dose. Artificial tears are prescribed to be used at the patients' discretion.

In a preliminary study of 44 eyes,[29] we found that 16% of patients with treated eyes experienced a burning feeling or worse within the first 2 postoperative hours. The pain subsided within the following hours and on the first postoperative day 26% of the patients had only minor discomfort. In order to deal with this finding, we included intraoperative corneal cooling with the instillation of prefrozen BSS before the epithelial separation and after the ablation. After this alteration of the technique, in more than 200 eyes that we followed, fewer than 15% of the operated eyes had burning feeling subsiding after the first 2 hours after the treatment. The records show that less than 3% of the patients need oral analgesics or are prescribed eye drops of diluted topical anesthetic (20% tetracaine in natural tears) to control pain. By the third day after the treatment, a small minority of patients may complain of mild discomfort as new symptom. In those cases, the symptoms are mild and do not require any further medication than standard. However, even with lower pain grading, the vast majority of the patients report mild discomfort and photophobia especially the first couple of days after the treatment.

In regard to visual performance, the mean uncorrected visual acuity (UCVA) of the treated eyes corresponded well with the progress of the epithelial healing and the transparency of the replaced epithelial sheet. More particularly, UCVA is better on the first postoperative day, when the epithelial sheet is still transparent, decreases around the third postoperative day as the epithelial sheet becomes hazy, and, finally rises again when the epithelial healing is complete.

As reported in our preliminary report of 3-month results after Epi-LASIK, visual rehabilitation after the procedure is quite slow with only 48% of the eyes having unaided vision of 20/40 or better on day 1 after the procedure.[29] A larger series of 234 eyes confirmed this result, reporting 53% of eyes having 20/40 or better on day 1 increased to 78% on the day of re-epithelization. Follow-up in the same series showed that vision improved 6 months after the procedure with refractive stabilization by the third-month interval. At 1 year postop, more than 50% of the eyes gained lines of best corrected visual acuity (BCVA). The contrast sensitivity testing in 4 different spatial frequencies was equal or better than baseline at 1 year after the procedure (Katsanevaki et al, One year clinical results after epi-LASIK for myopia, data under review).

COMPLICATIONS

Using the initial version of the Centurion SES epikeratome, we recorded 7 eyes with inadvertent stromal incursion of the separator during the epithelial separation. In all cases, the incursion was very superficial and the operation was completed in accordance with the placement of the stromal crease in relation to the visual axis. In 5 eyes, the stromal penetration occurred outside the treatment zone and the operation was completed at the same session as planned, whereas in 2 eyes the irregularity implicated the treatment zone and the cases were aborted. The epithelial sheets were carefully replaced and the eyes were treated on a later date with LASIK with no further complications. The eyes were followed for 10 to 14 months. At the last follow-up visit, all eyes were within 0.5 D of the attempted correction with no loss of BCVA.

DISCUSSION

The expected beneficial effect of the replaced epithelial sheet is still controversial. Comparative clinical trials of PRK and LASEK have shown LASEK-treated eyes have lower pain scores during the first postoperative days and lower haze scores at the first postoperative month[12] and 1 year postoperatively.[13] Litwak et al[27] questioned these results and noticed greater discomfort, a longer epithelial healing period, and lower UCVA during the first 3 days in the LASEK-treated eyes. A probable reason could be the longer alcohol application used for the epithelial separation in this study. Two recent prospective, randomized studies[26,35] comparing PRK and LASEK came to no favorable outcome for the latter. Both studies included patients that had one eye treated with LASEK and the contralateral eye treated with PRK. Pirouzian et al[26] studied 30 patients and compared the subjective pain level, the rate of epithelial defect recovery, and the visual acuity in both eyes. They observed no differences between the LASEK- and the PRK-treated eyes. They noticed a different epithelial healing pattern in both groups, but the time needed for the epithelial healing was similar. They also applied the alcohol solution for 45 seconds and emphasized the unpredictability in the ease of making the epithelial flap during the LASEK procedure. Hashemi et al[35] included 42 patients in their comparative study with spherical equivalent in the range -1.00 to -6.50 D and a follow-up of 3 months. They demonstrated that LASEK was an effective, safe, and predictable technique, but found that it had no advantages over PRK regarding pain, epithelial healing time, or the refractive or visual outcome. In another study, Lee et al[36] compared epithelial healing, postoperative pain scores, and refractive results following 3 different epithelial removal techniques: conventional PRK, excimer laser (transepithelial PRK), and alcohol (LASEK). They found no significant differences in clinical outcomes, subepithelial opacity at 6 months postoperatively, and pain scores on the first 2 postoperative days. They noticed the fastest epithelial healing rate in the LASEK group. The LASEK group also demonstrated a slight undercorrection probably due to hydration of the cornea. We could assume that the different alcohol concentrations used and the variable duration of alcohol application needed for the epithelial separation result in various effects of alcohol on the epithelial sheet itself and, therefore, different results of the technique.

An issue that has arisen is whether the alcohol-assisted separated epithelial sheet is vital, in order to protect the stroma during the epithelial healing process. Some authors supported that a period longer than 20 seconds is sometimes needed for the loosening of the epithelial layer during the LASEK procedure.[17,25,27] Gabler et al[34] showed that after a 45-second exposure to alcohol solution 20% only half of the epithelial cells remained vital. Therefore, a longer exposure of the cornea to alcohol may be threatening for the viability of the epithelial flap. Hazarbassanov et al[37] used hypertonic saline solution 5% in a group of eyes and 20% alcohol solution in another group to create the epithelial flap and compared the healing time, the visual recovery, and the refractive outcome in both groups. Both techniques showed similar results, but the eyes treated with hypertonic solution had a faster epithelial healing than the alcohol treated eyes. The authors concluded that in order to avoid the toxic effect of alcohol on the epithelium and the surrounding tissues, a more epithelium-friendly method is needed. Numerous authors[16-18] agreed that epithelial separation without alcohol would be more preferable.

Our initial clinical results after Epi-LASIK for myopia have shown the efficacy, safety, and predictability of this technique. These results are comparable to many studies of LASEK-treated eyes.[12-22] Epi-LASIK is an alternative method of separating an epithelial sheet without alcohol. Except for avoiding the toxic effect of alcohol on the epithelial sheet and the corneal stroma, Epi-LASIK offers an automated way of epithelial separation with a device that resembles a microkeratome. Therefore, it may have a shorter learning curve than LASEK for an experienced LASIK surgeon. Since the initial description of Epi-LASIK by Pallikaris and the University of Crete, almost every major microkeratome manufacturing company launched an epikeratome for Epi-LASIK treatments. This response from the industry highlights the necessity within the refractive community for a method that can safely and effectively complement LASIK in the armamentarium of the refractive surgeon. Involvement of more surgeons and analysis of clinical results of larger number of eyes is expected to clarify the place of Epi-LASIK in future refractive practice.

KEY POINTS

1. Complications that have been related to LASIK, such as flap-related complications, dry eye, reported postoperative mechanical instability of the cornea, and vision-threatening inflammations, have turned many surgeons back to surface ablations.

2. Drawbacks of LASEK that have been reported are the dose and time dependent toxic effect of alcohol on the corneal epithelium , the interpatient variability of the ease of making epithelial flaps necessitating variable application times of the alcohol solution as well as the long learning curve of the technique.

3. In Epi-LASIK, however, the epithelial separation is achieved by means of a customized device that can achieve the successful epithelial separation mechanically without requiring the use of alcohol.

4. As compared to LASEK, Epi-LASIK provides a completely automated way to perform advanced surface ablation and avoids the toxic effect of alcohol on the separated epithelium.

5. Transmission electron microscopy of mechanically separated sheets show that mechanical separation of the corneal epithelium preserves the epithelial basement membrane providing with a slightly deeper cleavage plane as compared to that of alcohol.

REFERENCES

1. Pallikaris IG, Papatzanaki ME, Siganos DS, Tsilimbaris MK. A corneal flap technique for laser in situ keratomileusis. Human studies. *Arch Ophthalmol.* 1991;109(12):1699-1702.

2. Hersh PS, Brint SF, Maloney RK, et al. Photorefractive keratectomy versus laser in situ keratomileusis for moderate to high myopia; a randomized prospective study. *Ophthalmology.* 1998;105:1512-1522.

3. Pallikaris IG, Katsanevaki VJ, Panagopoulou SI. Laser in situ keratomileusis intraoperative complications using one type of microkeratome. *Ophthalmology.* 2002;109(1):57-63.

4. Carpel EF, Carlon KH, Shannon S. Folds and striae in laser in situ keratomileusis flaps. *J Refract Surg.* 1999;15(6):687-690.

5. Melki SA, Azar DT. LASIK complications: etiology, management, and prevention. *Surv Ophthalmol.* 2001;46(2):95-116.

6. Smith RJ, Maloney RK. Diffuse lamellar keratitis. A new syndrome in lamellar refractive surgery. *Ophthalmology.* 1998;105(9):1721-1726.

7. Wang MY, Maloney RK. Epithelial ingrowth after laser in situ keratomileusis. *Am J Ophthalmol.* 2000; 129(6):746-751.

8. Pallikaris IG, Kymionis GD, Astyrakakis NI. Corneal ectasia induced by laser in situ keratomileusis. *J Cataract Refract Surg.* 2001;27(11):1796-1802.

9. Seiler T, Wollensak J. Myopic photorefractive keratectomy with excimer laser; one-year follow up. *Ophthalmology.* 1991;98:1156-1163.

10. Epstein D, Fagerholm P, Hamberg-Nystroem H, Tengroth B. Twenty four-month follow up of excimer laser photorefractive keratectomy for myopia; refractive and visual outcome results. *Ophthalmology.* 1994;101:1558-1563.

11. Camellin M, Cimberle M. LASEK technique promising after 1 year of experience. *Ocular Surg News.* 2000;18(1):14-17.

12. Lee JB, Seong GJ, Lee JH, Seo KY, Lee YG, Kim EK. Comparison of laser epithelial keratomileusis and photorefractive keratectomy for low to moderate myopia. *J Cataract Refract Surg.* 2001;27(4):565-570.

13. Shah S, Sebai Sarhan AR, Doyle SJ, et al. The epithelial flap for photorefractive keratectomy. *Br J Opthalmol.* 2001;85:393-396.

14. Azar DT, Ang RT, Lee JB, et al. Laser subepithelial keratomileusis: electron microscopy and visual outcomes of photorefractive keratectomy. *Curr Opin Ophthalmol.* 2001;12(4): 323-328.

15. Camellin M. Laser epithelial keratomileusis for myopia. *J Refract Surg.* 2003;19:666-670.

16. Anderson NJ, Beran RF, Schneider TL. Epi-LASEK for the correction of myopia and myopic astigmatism. *J Cataract Refract Surg.* 2002;28:1343-1347.

17. Claringbold VT. Laser-assisted subepithelial keratectomy for the correction of myopia. *J Cataract Refract Surg.* 2002;28:18-22.

18. Shahinian L. Laser-assisted subepithelial keratectomy for low to high myopia and astigmatism. *J Cataract Refract Surg.* 2002;28:1334-1342.

19. Rouweyha RM, Chuang AZ, Mitra S, Phillips CB, Yee RW. Laser Epithelial Keratomileusis for myopia with the Autonomous Laser. *J Refract Surg.* 2002;18:217-224.

20. Taneri S, Zieske JD, Azar DT. Evolution, techniques, clinical outcomes, and pathophysiology of LASEK: review of the literature. *Surv Ophthalmol.* 2004;49:576-602.

21. Partal AE, Rojas MC, Manche EE. Analysis of the efficacy, predictability and safety of LASEK for myopia and myopic astigmatism using the Technolas 217 excimer laser. *J Cataract Refract Surg.* 2004;30:2138-2144.

22. Taneri S, Feit R, Azar DT. Safety, efficacy and stability indices of LASEK correction in moderate myopia and astigmatism. *J Cataract Refract Surg.* 2004;30:2130-2137.

23. Kamm O. The relation between structure and physiological action of the alcohols. *J Amer Pharm Assoc.* 1921;10:87-92.

24. Kim SY, Sah WJ, Lim YW, Hahn TW. Twenty percent alcohol toxicity on rabbit corneal epithelial cells: electron microscopic study. *Cornea.* 2002;21(4):388-392.

25. Chen CC, Chang JH, Lee JB, Javier J, Azar DT. Human corneal epithelial cell viability and morphology after dilute alcohol exposure. *Invest Ophthalmol Vis Sci.* 2002;43(8):2593-2602.

26. Pirouzian A, Thornton JA, Ngo S. A randomized prospective clinical trial comparing laser subepithelial keratomileusis and photorefractive keratectomy. *Arch Ophthalmol.* 2004;122:11-16.

27. Litwak S, Zadok D, Garcia-de Quevedo V, Robledo N, Chayet AS. Laser-assisted subepithelial keratectomy versus photorefractive keratectomy for the correction of myopia. A prospective comparative study. *J Cataract Refract Surg.* 2002;28:1330-1333.

28. Chalita MR, Tekwani NH, Krueger RR. Laser epithelial keratomileusis: outcome of initial cases performed by an experienced surgeon. *J Refract Surg.* 2003;19:412-415.

29. Pallikaris IG, Naoumidi II, Kalyvianaki MI, Katsanevaki VJ. Epi-LASIK: comparative histological evaluation of mechanical and alcohol-assisted epithelial separation. *J Cataract Refract Surg.* 2003;29(8):1496-1501.

30. Pallikaris IG, Katsanevaki VJ, Kalyvianaki MI, Naoumidi II. Advances in subepithelial excimer refractive surgery techniques: Epi-LASIK. *Curr Opin Ophthalmol.* 2003;14(4):207-212.

31. Pallikaris IG, Kalyvianaki MI, Katsanevaki VJ, Ginis HS. Preliminary clinical results of an alternative surface ablation procedure. *J Cataract Refract Surg.* 2005;31:879-885.

32. Espana EM, Gruetereich M, Mateo A, et al. Cleavage plane of corneal basement membrane components by ethanol exposure in laser-assisted subepithelial keratectomy. *J Cataract Refract Surg.* 2003;29:1192-1197.

33. Stramer BM, Zieske JD, Jung JC, Austin JS, Fini ME. Molecular mechanisms controlling the fibrotic repair phenotype in cornea: implications for surgical outcomes. *Invest Ophthalmol Vis Sci.* 2003;44(10):4237-4246.

34. Katsanevaki VJ, Naoumidi II, Kalyvianaki MI, Pallikaris IG. Epi-LASIK: histological findings of epithelial sheets 24 hours after the treatment. *J Refract Surg* (In press).

35. Hashemi H, Fotouni A, Foudazi H, Sadeghi N, Payvar S. Prospective, randomized, paired comparison of laser epithelial keratomileusis and photorefractive keratectomy for myopia less than -6.50 diopters. *J Refract Surg.* 2004;20:217-222.

36. Lee HK, Lee KS, Kim JK, Kim HC, Seo KR, Kim EK. Epithelial healing and clinical outcomes in excimer laser photorefractive surgery following three epithelial removal techniques: mechanical, alcohol and excimer laser. *Am J Ophthalmol.* 2005;139:56-63.

37. Hazarbassanov R, Ben-Haim O, Varssano D, et al. Alcohol- vs. hypertonic saline-assisted laser-assisted subepithelial keratectomy. *Arch Ophthalmol.* 2005;123:171-176.

38. Kim JK, Kim SS, Lee HK, Lee IS, et al. Laser in situ keratomileusis versus laser-assisted subepithelial Keratectomy for the correction of high myopia. *J Cataract Refract Surg.* 2004;30:1405-1411.

THE USE OF MITOMYCIN-C IN LASER REFRACTIVE SURGERY

Francesco Carones, MD

INTRODUCTION

In Europe, unlike the United States, excimer laser photorefractive keratectomy (PRK) has been the predominant refractive surgical procedure for years. Subepithelial fibrosis with wound healing is probably the major complication of any kind of surface ablation. Its clinical appearance at slit-lamp examination consists of an opacity, variable in density, commonly called haze. This can be very mild, thus not inducing any visual impairment. It usually tends to regress spontaneously with time. In the majority of cases, haze is simply reported by the ophthalmologist during postoperative examinations, while the patient does not convey any visual problems.

CORNEAL HAZE

Haze formation embodies the excessive wound healing response to the corneal tissue ablation and is characterized by stromal reaction, keratocyte activation, and collagen and amorphous material deposition. Certain circumstances tend to magnify both haze density and chance of appearance. Among them, the amount of intended correction is probably the most important: the higher, the worse.[1-4] But other factors, like ultraviolet (sun) exposure, delay in re-epithelialization, and irregularity of the ablation surface, are also implicated in haze formation. Dense haze may significantly impair vision by reduced best spectacle-corrected visual acuity (BSCVA), induced regression, induced irregular astigmatism, and provoked visual symptoms such as blurred vision, halos, glare, and ghost images.

Treatment of severe haze involves the use of pharmaceuticals applied topically. Corticosteroid produced some controversial results and is frequently ineffective.[5,6] The second category of drugs employed are antimetabilites, of which mitomycin-C (MMC), 5 fluorouracil, and thio-pepa[7] are those used most. Haze can be removed by a second laser ablation in a therapeutic fashion, but this approach also is often ineffective because laser ablation generated the haze in the first place and may induce haze recurrence.

Figure 10-1. This image shows the microsponge soaked with 0.02% MMC solution positioned over the corneal stroma immediately after scraping.

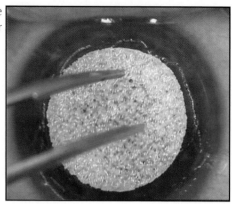

Mitomycin-C

MMC is a systemic chemotherapeutic agent. It is commonly used topically after glaucoma surgery, pterygium excision, in the treatment of conjunctival and corneal intraepithelial neoplasia, and in the treatment of ocular pemphigoid. Rationale to its use relies on its long-term, possibly permanent, cytostatic effect on tissue. More specifically, its use after PRK is intended to inhibit subepithelial fibrosis as the result of an abnormal activation or proliferation of stromal keratocytes following laser ablation.[8] This use was originally proposed by Talamo and associates on an experimental model.[9] Haze reduction following MMC administration was also documented by Xu and associates in rabbit eyes.[10] More recently, Majmudar and coworkers reported a successful series of eyes treated using a 0.02% (0.2 mg/mL) MMC solution, to remove haze after PRK and radial keratotomy.[11]

The peculiar action of MMC on the corneal tissue allows 2 possible applications in the field of laser surface ablation. It can be used therapeutically in those eyes already exposed to surface ablation that present significant haze, or it can be used in a prophylactic fashion to avoid haze formation in those treatments at risk.

Mitomycin-C For the Treatment of Haze

The rationale to this therapy is the removal of haze by any methods (excimer laser PTK, mechanical scraping), and the application of MMC to inhibit further haze formation. I have had excellent results by manual scraping. The technique is as follows.

The corneal epithelium is removed using a 20%-diluted alcohol solution, applied topically by filling the barrel of a 9.0-mm Hoffer marking trephine. The alcohol and the epithelium are gently removed with Merocel surgical microsponges (Medtronic, Jacksonville, Fla). Once the epithelium is removed, using a Desmarres sharp blade, the stromal surface is scraped quite vigorously in an attempt to remove as much newly generated tissue as possible. This process is complete when no material is visible on the sharp edge of the blade itself. At this point, the stromal surface should look not much more transparent than before scraping (slit-lamp examination is mandatory at this aim), but also much more regular and smooth. Immediately after scraping, a circular Merocel microsponge soaked with a 0.02% (0.2 mg/mL) MMC solution is placed on top of the stromal surface (Figure 10-1). This has to be left in place for 2 minutes. The surface is then irrigated copiously with 20 cc balanced salt solution (BSS) to remove all MMC particles.

Obviously, the scar can be also removed using the excimer laser in a therapeutic fashion, where the choice is based upon the surgeon's personal experience. In this case, the surgeon

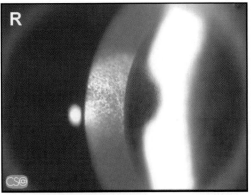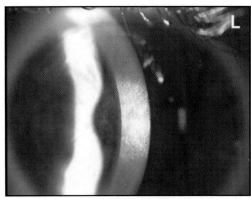

Figures 10-2. The image shows a very severe haze (grade 4) that was evident in both eyes of the same patient who was treated for −12.00 D correction by myopic PRK.

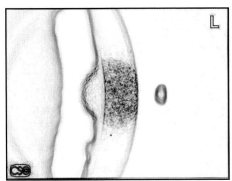

Figure 10-3. The digital image processing of the left eye image, aimed at evidencing tissue irregularity, shows the very high degree of tissue scarring.

may consider programming either a plano correction or a refractive procedure, depending on the refraction. It is important to notice that with all approaches there will be some unpredictable refractive change due to the removal of fibrotic tissue; thus, the programmed refractive change should be conservative.

Postoperatively, a bandage contact lens is applied to both eyes and left in place until re-epithelialization is complete (usually 4 days). During this period, antibiotic drops and nonsteroidal anti-inflammatory drops are applied four times per day, together with artificial tears. The patient is also prescribed oral narcotics as needed for pain. Once the bandage contact lens is removed, topical fluorometholone drops are applied three times per day for 2 weeks, and then twice a day for the other 2 weeks. Artificial tears are administered as needed thereafter.

RESULTS

The results attainable by this therapy are very successful. My personal series involves more than 80 treated eyes with a follow-up now exceeding 7 years, and the results are overlapping to those we published previously.[12]

Figures 10-2 through 10-5 show a case story of both eyes of the same patient who underwent PRK for -12.00-D correction in the year 1996 and had this therapy in 1998. The patient was in a lamellar keratoplasty waiting list at another center. In both eyes, the opacity was so dense that it interfered with iris details visualization at slit-lamp examination, and the irregularity generated by the scarring was so severe that a very high irregular astigmatism was seen with corneal topography. In both eyes, BSCVA was 20/40 (preoperative BSCVA was referred

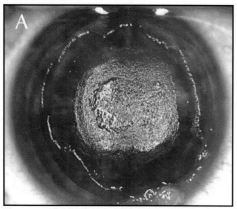 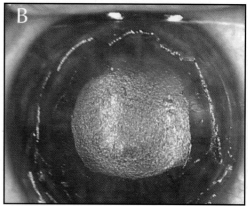

Figures 10-4. These 2 images were taken during surgery. A shows the stromal surface just before starting scraping. Note the irregularity of the surface. B shows the surface after scraping; it is much smoother than before.

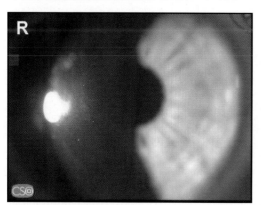 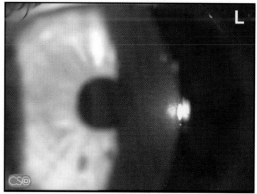

Figures 10-5. The slit-lamp examination of both eyes 7 years after treatment showed a transparent cornea with no trace of haze.

to be 20/16) with –4.75 D in RE and –4.50 D in LE, while uncorrected visual acuity (UCVA) was 20/800 in both eyes. Haze was reported to appear 1 year after surgery, immediately following a long vacation that the patient took during the summer, in a high UV exposure country. UCVA and BSCVA before haze onset were reported to be 20/16 in both eyes with plano refraction. Immediately after haze appearance, both eyes were treated for 6 months with a high-dosage topical corticosteroid eye drop therapy (dexametazone qid) that was ineffective in reducing haze and reversing myopic regression. One month after treatment, both corneas were completely transparent, with no haze at all. UCVA and BSCVA acuities were 20/20, with +0.25-D refraction in both eyes. Corneal topography revealed a quite regular surface, with no irregular astigmatism. These findings did not change over a 7-year follow-up period (see Figure 10-5). Corneal transparency was maintained; haze did not reoccur; and the UCVA and BSCVA, as well as refraction, remained stable. No long-term toxic effects, like corneal melting and endothelial changes, were noticed.

This case mimics the average results achievable when MMC is used to avoid further haze formation once the scar is removed.[13-15] Corneal transparency, once restituted, maintains over time in the vast majority of cases. Regression of the induced correction is a common finding when haze occurs. The graph presented in Figure 10-6 shows the change in refraction

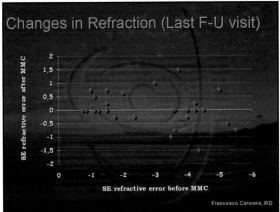

Figure 10-6. This graph shows the reduction in myopic regression and the hyperopic shift due to the therapy with MMC in eyes with haze.

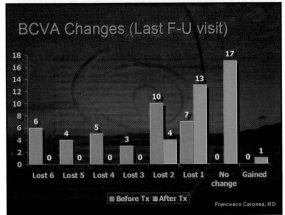

Figure 10-7. This graph shows the substantial gain in BSCA experienced by the eyes with the treatment.

toward the original achieved correction that commonly follows the therapy, thus suggesting that the surgeon should conservatively program the laser to correct any residual refractive error at the time of haze removal. Figure 10-7 presents the change in BSCVA in between, before, and after the treatment, compared to the preoperative (pre-PRK) status. The gain is significant in most of the cases and may mean avoiding more invasive procedures like penetrating keratoplasty. Recurrence of haze is quite rare and in all cases milder than the original onset. Literature assesses haze recurrence around 5% to 10% of cases; in these cases, a second approach may be advisable. Also, this therapeutic approach is more likely to be successful when applied to new scars; recent-onset haze is easier to remove, and recurrence is even less frequent.

MMC has some potential side effects and complications, as discussed in the following section. Thus, the question is at what stage this therapy should be considered. In other words, should the surgeon accept the potential, yet very rare, risk of side effects and complications and proceed with the treatment, or wait for natural haze disappearance using conventional (steroid) therapy? My personal indication to MMC therapy is in eyes in which haze compromises BSCVA and/or induces severe quality of vision disturbances, and previous steroid therapy was unsuccessful. In these cases, I like to proceed to scraping and MMC application as soon as the patient agrees.

Mitomycin-C for Prophylactic Use to Avoid Haze Formation

In all cases of surface ablation at risk of haze formation, MMC may be applied prophylactically to avoid such complications. Indications include not only high volumes of ablated tissue (high attempted corrections, generically speaking), but also surface ablation enhancements; ablation on the top of a previous LASIK flap either for enhancement purposes or to manage a flap complication[16-18] (aborted, buttonhole, irregular); and ablation over previous refractive surgery (radial keratotomy), therapeutic corneal surgery (penetrating keratoplasty), or keloid formers.

MMC is delivered in the same manner as for therapeutic purposes; after the ablation, a 0.2 mg/mL (0.02%)-soaked microsponge is positioned over the corneal stroma. The original protocol consisted of a 2-minute application time. Today, several investigators propose shorter application times according to individual nomograms based upon attempted correction and ablation depth (1 minute, 30 seconds, 12 seconds) in order to reduce the risk of potential side effects and complications. Results are reported as well for longer application times. Once the microsponge is removed, it is suggested to abundantly wash the corneal surface and the entire conjunctival sac in order to remove all MMC remnants. Postoperative care should be carried out in the same way as conventional surface ablation; there are no contraindications to the use of a bandage contact lens or to the replacement of the epithelial layer in a LASEK or Epi-LASIK fashion. Steroids and lubricants should be administered according to individual protocols and experience.

Results are astonishing.[19-22] MMC does not interfere with re-epithelialization or early wound healing. Haze rates are extremely low (when present) even for high corrections and ablation depths. Particularly, all complicated cases such as complicated LASIK flaps, RK, and PKP treatments do behave as "virgin" eyes. The accuracy of the procedure is reported as much higher than surface ablation without the use of MMC and with lower standard deviations. All published series report a marked trend to overcorrection (in the range 10% to 15%, according to the laser used and individual nomograms), thus suggesting a programmed undercorrection when using MMC.

The potential use of MMC is of particular interest for those eyes with limited stromal thickness, where LASIK is contraindicated. These eyes may benefit from the great accuracy of MMC prophylactic therapy and the application of wide ablation diameters as well.

My personal indications to the prophylactic use of MMC foresee its applications in all complicated eyes (complicated LASIK flaps, surface ablation in eyes after RK and PKP, PRK enhancements, etc). In all these cases, particular care has to be considered when removing the epithelium in order not to induce any keratocyte activation or tissue damage. My personal protocol involves the use of the routine concentration of MMC (0.2 mg/mL) for a 2-minute application. Another matter is virgin eyes. I use MMC for attempted ablation depth of 80 µm or more. I always use the same concentration (0.2 mg/mL), while the application time goes for 30 seconds for ablation depth up to 100 µm, and 1 minute for higher ablation depth.

Safety Issues

The major criticism in the use of MMC after laser refractive surgery concerns the potential side effects and complications associated with its long-term cytostatic action on tissues when applied in a topical fashion on the corneal stroma. Several authors reported corneoscleral melt after MMC application after pterygium excision.[23-24] Also, the long-term integrity of the endothelial layer is supposed to be at risk.

It is worth mentioning that all reports that refer to corneoscleral melting differ in substance from the approach used after refractive surgery. First, the concentration of MMC was reported to be higher, and for application times longer than the 2-minute maximum time. It is currently performed when MMC is applied on the corneal stroma. Second, the previous melting reports always involve the conjunctivo-scleral district, which is substantially different from the cornea as regard the tissue structure, vascularization, and origin.

It is estimated that more than 100,000 procedures have been applied with the use of MMC worldwide, and there are no reports of corneal melting or endothelium toxicity over a 8-year follow-up period. However, the use of MMC has to be very cautious, in order to reduce at minimum these potential risks. The concentration has to be 0.2 mg/mL because higher concentrations determined the previously reported complications while lower concentrations are therapeutically not effective. The application time should never exceed 2 minutes, and studies are being done to evaluate the efficacy at shorter application times. After MMC application, it is suggested to wash the corneal surface and the entire conjunctival sac quite abundantly using BSS in order to avoid the interaction of MMC both with the epithelial stem cells and the conjunctiva. The use of MMC according to these rules has been proven safe and effective.

KEY POINTS

1. Subepithelial fibrosis with wound healing is probably the major complication of any kind of surface ablation. Its clinical appearance at slit-lamp examination consists of an opacity, variable in density, commonly called haze.

2. Haze formation embodies the excessive wound healing response to the corneal tissue ablation and is characterized by stromal reaction, keratocyte activation, and collagen and amorphous material deposition.

3. Mitomycin-C (MMC) is a systemic chemotherapeutic agent. The rationale to this therapy is the removal of haze by any methods (excimer laser PTK, mechanical scraping), and the application of MMC to inhibit further haze formation.

4. Immediately after scraping, a circular Merocel microsponge soaked with a 0.02% (0.2 mg/mL) MMC solution is placed on top of the stromal surface. This has to be left in place for 2 minutes. The surface is then irrigated copiously with 20 cc BSS to remove all MMC particles.

5. In all cases of surface ablation at risk of haze formation, MMC may be applied prophylactically to avoid such complications.

REFERENCES

1. McCarthy CA, Aldred GF, Taylor HR. Comparison of results of excimer laser correction of all degrees of myopia at 12 months postoperatively. *Am J Ophthalmol.* 1996;121:372-383.

2. Krueger RR, Talamo JH, McDonald MB, et al. Clinical analysis of excimer laser photorefractive keratectomy using a multiple zone technique for severe myopia. *Am J Ophthalmol.* 1995;119:263-274.

3. Sher NA, Hardten DR, Fundingsland B, et al. 193-Nm excimer photorefractive keratectomy in high myopia. *Ophthalmology.* 1994;101:1575-1582.

4. Carson CA, Taylor HR. Excimer laser treatment for high and extreme myopia. *Arch Ophthalmol.* 1995;113:431-436.

5. Gartry D, Kerr Muir MG, Lohmann CP, Marshall J. The effect of topical corticosteroids on refractive outcome and corneal haze after photorefractive keratectomy. *Arch Ophthalmol.* 1992;110:944-952.

6. Carones F, Brancato R, Venturi E, et al. Efficacy of corticosteroids in reversing regression after myopic photorefractive keratectomy. *Refract Corneal Surg.* 1993;9(suppl):S52-56.

7. Penno EA, Braun DA, Kamal A, et al. Topical thiopepa treatment for recurrent corneal haze after photorefractive keratectomy. *J Cataract Refract Surg.* 2003;29:1537-1542.

8. Shipper I, Suppelt C, Gebbers JO. Mitomycin C reduces scar formation after excimer laser (193 nm) photorefractive keratectomy in rabbits. *Eye.* 1997;11:649-655.

9. Talamo JH, Gollamudi S, Green RW, et al. Modulation of corneal wound healing after excimer laser keratomileusis using topical mitomycin C and steroids. *Arch Ophthalmol.* 1991;109:1141-1146.

10. Xu H, Liu S, Xia X, et al. Mitomycin C reduces haze formation in rabbits after excimer laser photorefractive keratectomy. *J Refract Surg.* 2001;17:342-349.

11. Majmudar P, Forstrot L, Dennis R, et al. Topical mitomycin-C for subepithelial fibrosis after refractive corneal surgery. *Ophthalmology.* 2000;107:89-94.

12. Vigo L, Scandola E, Carones F. Scraping and mitomycin C to treat haze and regression after photorefractive keratectomy for myopia. *J Refract Surg.* 2003;19(4):449-54.

13. Porges Y, Ben-Haim O, Hirsh A, et al. Phototherapeutic keratectomy with mitomycin C for corneal haze following photorefractive keratectomy for myopia. *J Refract Surg.* 2003;19:40-3.

14. Raviv T, Majmudar PA, Dennis RF, et al. Mitomycin-C for post-PRK corneal haze. *J Cataract Refract Surg.* 2000;26:1105-6.

15. Weisenthal RW, Salz J, Sugar A, et al. Photorefractive keratectomy for treatment of flap complications in laser is situ keratomileusis. *Cornea.* 2003;22:399-404.

16. Muller LT, Candal EM, Epstein RJ, Dennis RF, Majmudar PA. Transepithelial phototherapeutic keratectomy/photorefractive keratectomy with adjunctive mitomycin-C for complicated LASIK flaps. *J Cataract Refract Surg.* 2005;31(2):291-296.

17. Carones F, Vigo L, Scandola E, Vacchini L. Evaluation of the prophylactic use of mitomycin-C to inhibit haze formation after photorefractive keratectomy. *J Cataract Refract Surg.* 2002;28(12):2088-2095.

18. Lacayo GO, Majmudar PA. How and when to use mitomycin-C in refractive surgery. *Curr Opin Ophthalmol.* 2005 Aug; 16 (4):256-259.

19. Gambato C, Ghirlando A, Moretto E, Busato F, Midena E. Mitomycin C modulation of corneal wound healing after photorefractive keratectomy in highly myopic eyes. *Ophthalmology.* 2005;112(2):208-218.

20. Hashemi H, Taheri SM, Fotouhi A, Kheiltash A. Evaluation of the prophylactic use of mitomycin-C to inhibit haze formation after photorefractive keratectomy in high myopia: a prospective clinical study. *BMC Ophthalmol.* 2004;4(1):12.

21. Rubinfeld RS, Pfister RR, Stein RM, et al. Serious complications of topical mitomycin-C after pterygium surgery. *Ophthalmology.* 1992;99:1647-1654.

22. Dougherty PJ, Hardten DR, Lindstrom RL. Corneoscleral melt after pterygium surgery using a single intraoperative application of mitomycin-C. *Cornea.* 1996;15:537-540.

Chapter 11

Nightmares With Phototherapeutic Keratectomy

Jes Mortensen, MD

Introduction

The exact edging capability (Figure 11-1) of the excimer laser is useful in treating superficial corneal opacities, corneal scars, dystrophies, and irregularities.[1-3] This part of the excimer laser use is commonly referred to as phototherapeutic keratectomy (PTK).[1-3] The VISX B 2020 laser (Santa Clara, Calif) is a broad beam laser that is able to treat PTK and myopia with or without astigmatism. The VISX Star is able to treat PTK, myopia, astigmatism, and hyperopia using a scanning mode. The Technolas 217c and 217z (Bausch & Lomb, Rochester, NY) are flying spot lasers that can treat the aforementioned and even perform custom ablation.

Phototherapeutic Keratectomy

The excimer laser treats with a cool beam. The temperature is only increased by 5°C. The ArF excimer laser emission is 193 nm. At 193 nm, a single ultraviolet (UV) photon has energy of 6.4 eV, which exceeds the covalent bond strength of many molecules. The excimer laser removes 0.22 to 0.25 μm of the corneal tissue per pulse. PTK is focused on the surface of the cornea with an excimer laser beam by which it is possible to smooth the surface and even change the curvature of the cornea and the refractive power of the cornea.

Recurrent Erosion

This was first described by Hansen in 1872. It causes sudden onset of pain in the affected eye, with photophobia and epiphora . The treatment enforces healing between the posterior layer of the epithelium and the Bowman's membrane. We ablate 5 to 8 μm of Bowman's membrane after removing the epithelium, which is often poorly adherent.

Nightmares

Do not treat too much, especially if you have an emmetropic or hyperopic patient. An 8-μm ablation could give a change in refraction of +0.50 to +0.75 D, so you might end up with unintended hyperopia and a dissatisfied patient. Videokeratography can often help you if you

Figure 11-1. Human hair cut by the excimer laser.

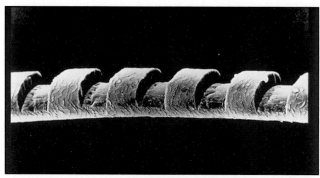

Figure 11-2. An 83-year-old woman with Groenow type I corneal dystrophy. PTK was done on the patient. Visual acuity before PTK was 20/200. Visual acuity after PTK was 20/30.

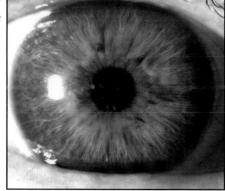

are not able to localize the erosion at the moment of healing, as it will often show irregularity of the afflicted area. If the erosions are near the visual axis, the treatment should always be properly centered to omit any irregularity of the surface that could disturb the visual acuity or visual quality of the eye. If you are used to treating transepithelially 45 to 50 μm, be sure that the epithelium is in situ.

Conclusion

The treatment is often very successful. Our experience is that the treatment is lasting, but a new erosion might appear in a new area. Complications are few. Healing may take several weeks, so an extended wear contact lens is often useful if the patient can tolerate it. Local corticosteroid is not needed during the healing.

CORNEAL DYSTROPHIES

Corneal dystrophies are often defined as primary, inherited, bilateral disorders of the cornea affecting transparency or refraction. The disorders often disturb vision. The dystrophies are often assessed anatomically into pre-Bowman's layer, Bowman's layer, anterior stromal, stromal, and endothelial dystrophies. Dystrophies are congenital and will recur, so the PTK procedure may be repeated in the future.

Figure 11-2 shows a patient with Groenow type I corneal dystrophy. The lesions are sharply demarcated and confined to the axial portion of the cornea, usually beginning in the most superficial portion of the stroma. The deposit is believed to come from the epithelium. Recurrent erosion and irregularity are often the biggest problems. The eye was treated like recurrent erosion, transepithelially using methylcellulose as a masking agent.

Nightmares

The deeper you treat, the more hyperopic shift will be induced. The visual acuity is often more affected by the irregularity of the surface than of the opacities in the corneal stroma. A hard contact lens could give important information before treating. Never make a flap to treat the remaining posterior opacities, as the materials produced after the treatment will collect at the interface. Aggressive PTK treatment can inflict haze and exaggerate the cloudiness of the corneas, adding fibrous tissue and severe irregularity and leading to the need for penetrating keratoplasty.

Conclusion

PTK treatment of different corneal dystrophies often gives very good results, especially if the problem is due to recurrent erosion and the cornea's surface irregularity is not too severe. Try to treat as little as possible to obtain the desired result because the dystrophy can often give similar problems in the future. Never try LASIK because the materials produced by the dystrophic process might collect in the interface.

CORNEAL SCARS

Evaluation is important to understand what has caused the scarring of the cornea. The evaluation is done using the slit-lamp and Videokeratography. The irregularity of the corneal surface might be a bigger cause to the visual problem than the cloudiness of the stroma. You can always try to put on a hard contact lens to evaluate if a simple smoothing of the corneal surface would be sufficient before you do a corneal transplantation.

Traumatic macular corneal opacities can be very deep and produce a major change in the refraction. First, smooth the surface and after that go for the change of refraction. Inform the patient that you may need to do more sessions. Always try to remember that what has been removed by the excimer laser will not come back.

Nightmares

Reviving an old viral herpetic keratitis could be devastating for the result. If you are uncertain as to what caused the opacity, always suspect virus and then give systemic antiviral medications to prevent a recurrence of the infection. Remember to carefully evaluate the sensitivity of the cornea. If you are treating a cornea with a diminished sensitivity, you could have a big problem. The same applies if the lacrimation is in any way adversely affected owing to reduced production or corrupted lubricating ability. Sjögren's syndrome and postherpetic scars are relatively contraindicated. Careful evaluation of the blinking ability and the state of the palpebrae is also of major importance.

Do not forget to be very conservative and do remember that the cornea heals very slowly. A 29-year-old man woke up after he had been wearing his contact lenses for at least 24 hours. He did not remember to remove the lenses, as he had been celebrating all night. Evaluation showed finger counting both eyes, the spectacles he wore showed that he was –18.00 D in both eyes. Slit-lamp microscopy showed contact lenses "glued" to the epithelium and heavy edema of both corneas (Figure 11-3). The contact lenses were removed, resulting in almost total removal of the epithelium. At first, severe infection was suspected, but this could not be confirmed. The corneas were cloudy and had severe edema. The diagnosis of severe ischemia of the corneas was proposed. The patient stayed for 3 weeks and slowly regained some vision; the epithelium healed with severe scarring and irregularity. Visual acuity as best was 20/80 in his right eye and finger counting in the left eye. The videokeratographies showed severe irregularity (Figures 11-4). I waited for 1 year and then the right eye was treated 50 μm

Figure 11-3. Cloudy cornea with severe edema.

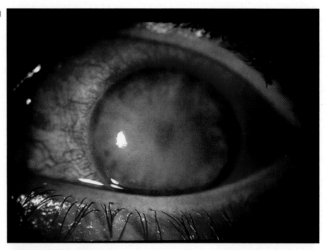

Figure 11-4. Videokeratography showing severe irregularity.

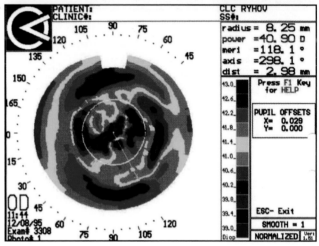

transepithelially with PTK. I tried to smooth the surface. The result was 20/40 with a contact lens. The patient was very happy after that. The patient was seen at my clinic 7 years later: VA 20/20 both eyes and Orbscan II was done (Figures 11-5 and 11-6).

Conclusion

Corneal scars are a heterogeneous group, consisting of eyes with corneal dystrophies and scars after keratitis or trauma. Try first to smoothen the surface of the cornea if you are uncertain what causes the diminished visual acuity. Treat as little as possible so the procedure can be repeated. If you are uncertain what caused the scar, consider herpetic virus. Do not treat a cornea with diminished sensitivity or very dry eyes.

MISCELLANEOUS

In the early days, we treated pterygium with PTK by smoothening the denuded area after surgical excision of the pterygium. We hoped to abolish or diminish the recurrence of the pterygium. We did not see any success in that. The only indication for PTK is if you have corneal macular opacities or irregularities of the cornea in conjunction with the pterygium.

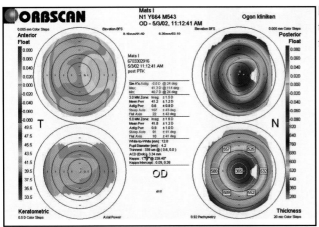

Figure 11-5. Videokeratography by the Orbscan showing regular surface.

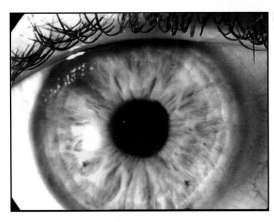

Figure 11-6. Cornea of patient seen in Figure 11-3 after 7 years.

These should be treated as earlier described. Another group that can be treated are those patients with band-shaped keratopathy. The treatments are done transepithelially followed by polishing of the surface.

Nightmares

Before treating, be sure what you want to achieve—better visual acuity and pain relief or only pain relief. Believing that every erosion of the corneal epithelium can be treated by PTK might lead to a melting of the cornea, especially in denervated corneas.

Conclusion

PTK is not superior to ethylenediaminotetraacetic acid (EDTA) in treating band-shaped keratopathy.

SUMMARY

PTK can be of great benefit for patients, minimizing the need of corneal grafting or in many cases postponing the time for grafting. Recurrent erosion that is difficult to treat can often be successfully cured with PTK. A thorough evaluation of the eye is mandatory before treating with the excimer laser. Tissue is always removed and can never be added by the laser. If you do not always bear that in mind, nightmares may haunt you.

KEY POINTS

1. The exact edging capability of the excimer laser has been found useful in treating superficial corneal opacities, corneal scars, dystrophies, and irregularities.
2. A thing you should be very careful about is not to treat too much, especially if you have an emmetropic or hyperopic patient in a case of recurrent corneal erosion.
3. Visual acuity is often more affected by the irregularity of the surface than of the opacities in the corneal stroma.
4. A hard contact lens could give important information before treating.
5. If you are uncertain as to what caused the corneal opacity, always suspect a viral infection and then give systemic antiviral medications to prevent a recurrence of the infection.

REFERENCES

1. Trokel SL, Srinivasan R, Braren B. Excimer laser surgery of the cornea. *Am J Ophthalmol.* 1983;96:710-715.
2. Mortensen J, Ohrstrom A. Excimer laser photorefractive keratectomy for treatment of keratoconus. *J Refract Corneal Surg.* 1994;10:368-372.
3. McDonnell PJ, Seiler T. Phototherapeutic keratectomy with excimer laser for Reis-Buckler´s corneal dystrophy. *J Refract Corneal Surg.* 1992;8:306-310.

III

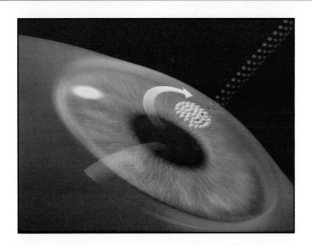

LASIK and Wavefront-Guided LASIK

Chapter 12

FLAP COMPLICATIONS

Melania Cigales, MD; Jairo Hoyos-Chacón, MD; and Jairo E. Hoyos, MD, PhD

INTRODUCTION

In the last few years, LASIK has become the most popular refractive technique. However, like all surgical procedures, LASIK is not without its possible complications. These complications can be intraoperative (arising while creating the flap with the microkeratome or during ablation with the excimer laser) or postoperative. The incidence of these complications diminishes throughout the surgeon's learning curve and with each technological development.

One of the most important steps when performing LASIK surgery is creating the corneal flap using the microkeratome. A good corneal flap needs to be smooth and even, of an appropriate thickness (including the epithelium, Bowman's membrane, and anterior stroma), and of a diameter that allows the exposure of sufficient stromal bed to perform the ablation (Figure 12-1). At times, the obtained characteristics of the flap are not those desired, and we should be very aware of the possible complications that can arise while creating the flap using the microkeratome. In this way, we will be able to prevent them or suitably resolve any complications that could occur.

FREE CAP

When in situ keratomileusis became popular at the end of the 1980s, we removed a complete corneal disc that was then sutured back onto the cornea. In 1991, Avalos and Guimaraes developed the sutureless technique for keratomileusis, using air to help dry and adhere the disc onto the stromal bed.[1] The technique continued to be developed, and in 1990 to 1991 Pallikaris et al[2] suggested creating an incomplete disc joined to the cornea by a small hinge. This was the birth of the corneal flap. Today, whenever LASIK is performed, we use the microkeratome to create a corneal flap because this is considered the safest way of preventing disc displacement and loss.

To create the flap, we must stop the motion of the microkeratome before it completes its full stroke, or alternatively use a stopper. When the corneal disc is unattached to the cornea by a hinge, then we have what is called a free cap (Figure 12-2).

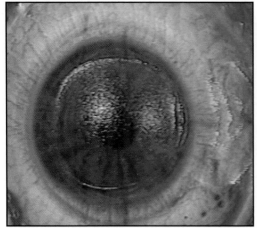

Figure 12-1. Good flap in LASIK needs to be smooth, even, and with enough diameter to perform the ablation.

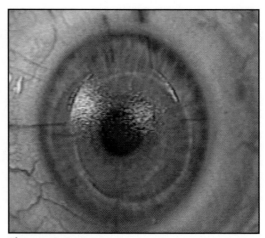

Figure 12-2. Free cap.

Figure 12-3. The automated corneal shaper (ACS) microkeratome includes calibration lenses that help calibrate the stopper depending on the diameter predicted for the flap.

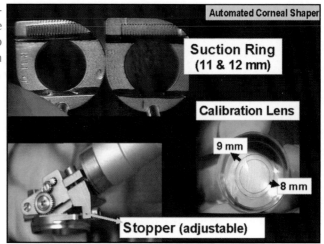

Causes

Perhaps the most frequent cause of a free cap is a very flat cornea. Patients with flat corneas and a mean keratometry of less than 41.00 D present a higher risk of a free cap occurring.[3] A flat cornea will protrude relatively less into the suction ring compared to a steep cornea, and this will give rise to a smaller diameter disc and a free cap. This problem only affects primary flat corneas since a flat cornea secondary to refractive surgery will behave exactly as the original corneal curvature. Some microkeratomes include calibration lenses that help calibrate the stopper, depending on the diameter predicted for the flap (Figures 12-3 and 12-4). Other instruments have several suction rings and stoppers that are selected according to the keratometric readings (Figure 12-5).

Management

When a free cap is obtained, we are confronted with 2 potential complications during the surgical procedure. The most serious of these is that it is often impossible to differenti-

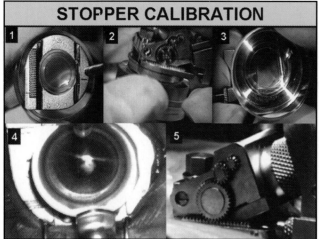

Figure 12-4. Stopper calibration with the ACS: (1) The suction ring is adapted on the calibration lens; (2) The microkeratome head is put on the suction ring; (3) The microkeratome is advanced until the edge of the blade arrives at the 8-mm or 9-mm circle of the calibration lens and the stopper is adjusted; (4) The applanation lens is used to evaluate the disc diameter before the microkeratome cut; (5) The flap is cut with the stopper previously calibrated.

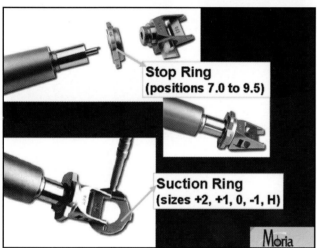

Figure 12-5. The LSK ONE microkeratome (Moria, Doylestown, Pa) has several suction rings with different sizes and a stop ring with different positions, which are selected according to the keratometric readings.

ate between the epithelial and stromal sides of the disc.[4] If the disc is replaced with the epithelial side face-down, there is a risk of epithelialization of the interface and loss of the disc. A further complication arises from the difficulty of repositioning the disc in its exact position. If the disc is rotated on the stromal bed, this commonly gives rise to astigmatism. Every LASIK surgeon must be aware of the possibility of a free cap and must be prepared for this complication by always using the epithelial reference markings.

We find it extremely useful to make 4 radial and one pararadial markings on the cornea. We use a 4-incision RK marker painted with a gentian violet labeler for the radial markings (Figure 12-6A), and then add the pararadial marking with an astigmatic marker (Figure 12-6B). We wash the cornea with balanced salt solution (BSS) to quickly remove all traces of alcohol from the gentian violet, given its toxic effect on the corneal epithelium. The pararadial marking helps us to identify the epithelial surface of the disc and the 4 radial markings serve as references to replace the disc in its original position and avoid inducing any astigmatism.

When a free cap occurs, the disc usually is inside the microkeratome and needs to be carefully retrieved with fine forceps or another instrument so as not to damage it.

Figure 12-6. Epithelial reference markings: (A) A 4-incision RK marker painted with a gentian violet labeler is used to make 4 radial markings; (B) A pararadial marking with an astigmatic marker is added.

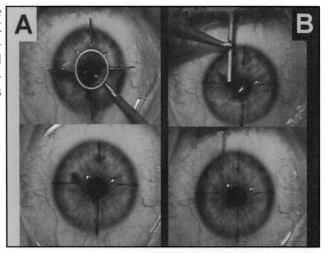

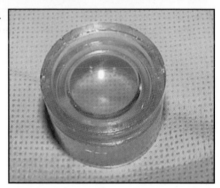

Figure 12-7. Antidesiccation chamber.

We can continue with the surgical procedure and during the ablation, the disc must be kept in the antidesiccation chamber (Figure 12-7) with the epithelial surface facing downwards. The disc must not be hydrated to avoid edema formation, although we do recommend the use of a drop of BSS on the epithelial surface for its preservation.

Once the ablation is complete, the bed is flushed and then dried with a Merocel sponge (Medtronic, Jacksonville, Fla). A drop of BSS is applied to the apex (Figure 12-8A). Using the Barraquer spatula, we recover the disc from the antidesiccation chamber and place it on the bed with the help of fine forceps (Figure 12-8B). The BSS enables us to easily mobilize the disc with the help of 2 Merocel sponges until it is aligned with the radial markings (Figure 12-8C). To finish, we dry the edges thoroughly and wait until the disc is attached to its bed (Figure 12-8D).

Complications

The most feared complication with a free cap is the loss of the disc, so certain precautions need to be taken before the patient leaves the clinic. First, lids are closed using 2 crossed adhesive strips for approximately 30 minutes after surgery. We then check the patient and if we find that the disc has moved, we reposition it and close the lid until the next day. If the disc is found to be in the right position, the patient goes home wearing only an eye shield and is instructed to follow the general directions for flaps. Due to the risk of losing the disc, we prefer to personally remove the eye shield or patch the next day so that we do not discard any dressing before making sure the disc is adhered to the cornea.

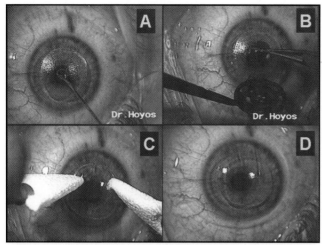

Figure 12-8. Replace the disc on the bed: (A) A drop of BSS is applied to the apex. (B) Using the Barraquer spatula, the disc is recovered from the antidesiccation chamber and placed it on the bed with the help of fine forceps. (C) With the help of 2 Merocel sponges, the disc is aligned with the radial markings. (D) The edge of the disc is dried and it is attached to its bed.

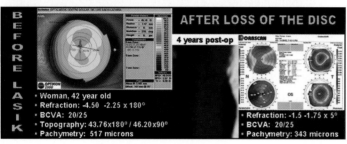

Figure 12-9. Free cap in a myopic patient. One hour after surgery the flap loss was noticed and it was treated as a PRK (occluding the eye until epithelium was achieved and using topical steroids for 6 months). The final result after flap loss was satisfactory and stable from 6 months until today (4 years), with a little irregular astigmatism and a minimum haze. (Courtesy Dr Salva and Dr. Bofill).

There have been reports of traumatic detachment of a disc despite having the security of a flap, and even cases of surgical amputation of the flap as an attempt to control an infection. In both these situations, some of the thickness of the cornea and the Bowman's membrane are lost.[5] The most simple treatment option is to wait for the re-epithelialization of the cornea and to treat the case as we would treat a PRK to avoid haze.[6] One would think that as corneal tissue was removed, the eye would finish up with tremendous hyperopia, but the results obtain do not show any hyperopic deviations and residual defects are usually slightly irregular myopic astigmatisms[6] (Figure 12-9). We should not forget that the corneal disc has two parallel sides and, therefore, has no refractive power of its own. If the final visual outcome is unsatisfactory, we should move onto undertaking a lamellar keratoplasty.

INCOMPLETE FLAP

During a keratectomy, the microkeratome can stop before completing its stroke and give rise to an incomplete flap and a corneal bed of insufficient size to perform an ablation.

Causes

Some microkeratomes have a protection mechanism (designed to impede continuous cutting and greater complications) that automatically stops if there is a loss of suction pressure while conducting the keratectomy.[7]

Figure 12-10. Buttonhole.

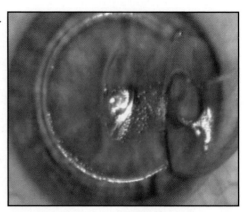

However, at times, the driving motor of the instrument may fail.[7] One of the most common reasons for an automatic microkeratome with an electric motor to breakdown is entry of the water used to help the instrument slide. For this reason, it is not indicated to sterilize the electric motor with vapor (we must use ethylene oxide). It is, therefore, recommended to have the microkeratome checked by the manufacturer on a routine basis.

In other cases, the microkeratome becomes blocked by the eyelashes or eyelids.[3] It is, thus, essential to prepare the surgical field well, covering eyelids and eyelashes with adhesive strips so that they do not interrupt the microkeratome stroke. Also, only use blepharostats that open the eye widely.

Management

The size of the exposed corneal bed can be measured with the caliper to see if it will be large enough for the ablation. We could even perform the ablation by slightly decreasing the optical zone and protect the hinge to avoid its ablation.

However, when the exposed bed is insufficient for ablation, surgery should be suspended; do not attempt to prolong the keratectomy by manual dissection because this induces irregular astigmatism that is not easily resolved.[8] A few months later, a slightly deeper keratectomy can be attempted. If we make it shallower and part of the first flap remains on the bed, during ablation, tissue might be moved and lost provoking irregular astigmatism and intense hyperopization.[9]

THIN FLAPS AND BUTTONHOLES

It is widely accepted by LASIK surgeons that the ideal flap thickness is 130 to 160 μm. This measure is determined by the plate in the microkeratome head. However, most microkeratomes generally produce thinner cuts than expected, and several pachymetric studies have indicated a high degree of variability in the thicknesses achieved.[10] Thin flaps are commonly associated with the complication of a central hole known as a buttonhole (Figure 12-10).

Causes

The most common causes of thin flaps and buttonholes are inadequate suction, poor blade quality, steep corneas, and microkeratome malfunction.[11]

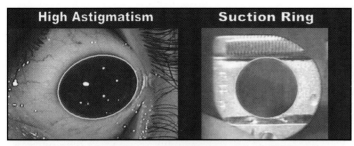

Figure 12-11. Inadequate fit of the suction ring on the eyeball is possible in the case of high astigmatism. The astigmatic eye is oval and the suction ring is round.

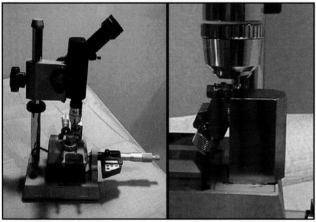

Figure 12-12. Magnum Diamond Micron-scope is useful to check and calibrate the blade's microkeratome. The microkeratome head set up with the blade and the 160-µm plate is placed under the microscope in a vertical position using a specially designed metal holder.

INADEQUATE SUCTION

The suction ring induces an ocular hypertension above the 70 to 100 mmHg required to perform the keratectomy. We use the Barraquer tonometer to monitor this pressure. As the surgeon becomes more skilled and experienced, there is a tendency to discontinue the use of the tonometer. However, it is important to remember that it is the only reliable method of detecting this complication and, if the required pressure is not reached, the keratectomy should not be performed.

Lack of pressure may be due to an inadequate fit of the suction ring on the eyeball. This commonly occurs in the case of small sunken orbits or astigmatic eyes (Figure 12-11), over which it is difficult to place the ring.[11] During the learning curve of this technique, a prolonged suction time leads to conjunctival edema that prevents the suction ring adapting to the eyeball, and requires a partial peritomy (however, now that topical anesthesia is used, it is better to postpone surgery when this situation arises, although it is rare).

POOR BLADE QUALITY OR SHARPNESS

A dull blade creates a thin and perhaps irregular cut.[12] Sometimes, remnants of Bowman's membrane can be seen on the stromal bed. Blade quality varies considerably and for this reason it is crucial to check and calibrate the blade in order to reject those with an irregular edge or a small gap (the distance between the blade and plate correlates with the thickness of the keratectomy)[11] (Figures 12-12 and 12-13).

Many surgeons reuse the same blade for 4 or 5 eyes. After each pass, the blade loses its sharpness, creating a thinner cut each time. We recommend using a new blade for each patient.

Figure 12-13. Measuring the gap (distance between the blade and plate correlates with the thickness of the keratectomy): (A) Using the microscope's controls, the vertical line on the eye-piece is aligned with the front end of the blade in the image and 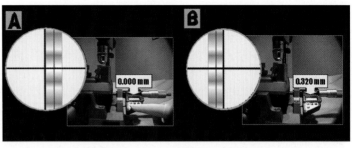 the micrometer's digital marker is set at zero; (B) Next, the same line is aligned with the end of the blade in the image and the digital micrometer indicates the measurement in microns. The image observed through the microscope is the blade and its mirror image, thus the measurement needs to be divided by 2 to give the blade gap. In the picture, the micrometer indicates 320 μm and the blade gap is, therefore, 160 μm.

Steep Corneas

Corneal curvatures greater than 46.00 D cause thin and large diameter discs and carry a risk of buttonhole due to corneal buckling during the microkeratome pass.[13] In the case of a steep cornea, we recommend the use of a 180-μm plate or a blade with a larger gap.

Microkeratome Malfunction

The microkeratome requires careful cleaning and assembly before each use to minimize any secondary complications due to malfunction. We also recommend sending the microkeratome to the manufacturer for periodic revisions and resetting. In 1993, we had 3 consecutive buttonhole cases resulting from microkeratome malfunction and the problem was corrected by simply changing the microkeratome head. A similar problem was reported by other authors.[13]

Management

We believe that whenever one of these complications occurs at the time of creating the flap (buttonhole or thin irregular cut remnants of Bowman's membrane on the stromal bed), the best solution is to interrupt the procedure and replace the flap and then attempt another keratectomy 3 or 6 months later using a thicker plate. It is not always easy to reposition these flaps because they tend to wrinkle and dislocate due to their lack of consistency. It is important to align the disc correctly and wait as long as necessary until it reattaches. The use of an eye patch is recommended. The outcome is usually favorable. There is generally no leukoma or visual loss.[13] However, if a central leukoma develops, we perform a PTK before performing a new LASIK procedure.

Some surgeons[14] prefer to use PRK in patients with previous buttonhole using mitomycin-C (MMC) to prevent corneal haze. In this way, the use of the microkeratome could be avoided.

In some cases, the flap obtained is thin but even then it is possible to perform the ablation. However, a common complication associated with these thin flaps is the formation of a flap striae (Figure 12-14). These flap striaes are not always easy to remove given their lack of consistency.

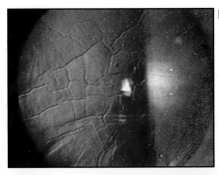

Figure 12-14. Flap folds and wrinkles.

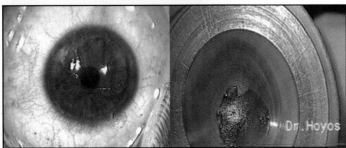

Figure 12-15. Lost suction.

Suction Loss

To perform the keratectomy, an intraocular pressure of 70 to 100 mmHg induced by the suction ring is necessary. A lack of pressure may be due to inadequate fitting of the suction ring on the eyeball. If suction is completely lost and the microkeratome continues to function, we will obtain a free, irregular, and small cut possibly affecting the pupillary area (Figure 12-15).[3] Most of the new instruments have a protection mechanism to stop cutting when there is a loss of suction. These models at most will give rise to an incomplete flap.

Management

When suction loss occurs, a free irregular cut is obtained and the best solution is to interrupt the surgery and replace the disc. We are confronted with all free cut difficulties: recognition between the epithelial and stromal sides, and the difficulty of repositioning the disc in its primary position. In this case, the irregular edge of the disc helps us, but we must be prepared for the complication by always using the epithelial reference markings.

The thin disc is usually inside the microkeratome and needs to be very carefully retrieved with fine forceps so as not to damage it. Replacing the disc on its bed is similar to the free cap management technique described above Figure 12-16. Due to the risk of losing the disc, we prefer to patch the eye until the next day. The outcome is usually favorable and we can then attempt another keratectomy 3 or 6 months later using a thicker plate.

Irregular Bed

While performing the keratectomy, the microkeratome should be guided so that it undergoes uniform movements to achieve a smooth, even corneal bed. Any malfunction of the automatic microkeratome, or slipping of the manual instrument, preventing a uniform stroke can give rise to an irregular resection leading to an uneven stromal bed (Figure 12-17).

Figure 12-16. Lost suction management: (A) Using the Barraquer spatula, the disc is recovered from the anti-desiccation chamber and placed on its bed with the help of fine forceps. (B) The interface is flushed and the disc is aligned. (C) The edge of the disc is dried until it is attached. (D) One day postop we can see the cornea dyed with fluorescein.

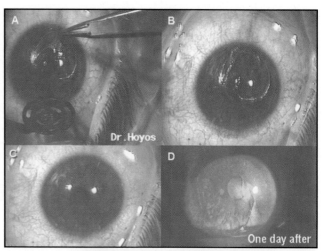

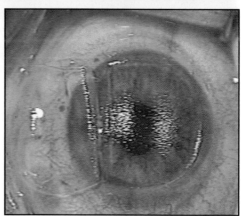

Figure 12-17. Irregular cut.

Management

If any irregularity affects the area where the ablation will be performed, surgery should be suspended to avoid an irregular astigmatism. We can attempt another keratectomy 3 or 6 months later using a thicker plate.

The irregularity is in the bed and in the stromal face of the flap as a mirror image. The ablation on an irregular bed induces a modification of the corneal bed, but the flap remains without changes. For this reason when the flap is replaced, it is not possible to match them, inducing striaes and irregular corneal surface.

EPITHELIAL DEFECTS

The epithelium of the corneal flap can become damaged during the keratectomy, causing late and painful visual recovery.

Causes

This complication is more common in diabetic or elderly patients or in those with dystrophy of the Bowman's membrane because the corneal epithelium is more fragile.[15] In this subset of patients, both eyes may show epithelial alterations. However, there are also certain

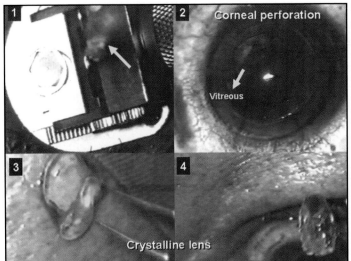

Figure 12-18. Corneal perforation with the ACS microkeratome: (1) The plate in the microkeratome head is not properly adjusted and during keratectomy the crystalline is jet-propelled (arrow); (2) The corneal perforation is associated with the loss of crystalline lens and vitreous; (3 and 4) The crystalline lens is found outside the eye in the surgical field.

intraoperative conditions that will induce damage to epithelial cells, such as excessive topical anaesthetic (which can be toxic for this delicate layer) or a keratectomy performed on a dry epithelium.[7] Anesthetics should be kept to a minimum and, if possible, should be free of preservatives. Moreover, the cornea should be moistened at the time of the keratectomy to help the microkeratome slide over the cornea and prevent abrasion of the corneal epithelium.

Management

If the corneal epithelium is damaged, we should be careful when handling the flap and should meticulously wash the interface to avoid seeding epithelial cells causing its epithelialization.[4] We prefer to reposition the altered epithelium, but if this is not possible, we carefully remove it. To avoid a painful postoperative course, it is best to include a mydriatic in the patient's normal medication and cover the eye or use a therapeutic contact lens until the cornea becomes re-epithelialized. The postoperative course of these cases is usually good, although there are reports of recurrent erosion syndromes,[16] which could be caused by a pre-existing dystrophy of the Bowman's membrane going unnoticed in the preoperative examination. A further possible cause is the transient corneal denervation that occurs after LASIK.[17]

CORNEAL PERFORATION

Corneal perforation is the most serious complication related to the use of the microkeratome and occurs when we forget to position the plate in the instrument head or when it is not properly adjusted.[18] Due to an increased intraocular pressure during keratectomy, corneal perforation is usually associated with the partial or total loss of the iris and crystalline lens and even with the loss of eye contents (Figure 12-18). To avoid this devastating complication, new microkeratome models do not have interchangeable plates; they have different heads to obtain different cutting depths.

Management

The management of this complication is complex and stressful, but we should remain calm and attempt to recompose the globe with the help of viscoelastic, followed by suturing the cornea. At a later date, select the best surgical option to restore the patient's vision.

KEY POINTS

1. A good corneal flap needs to be smooth and even, of an appropriate thickness (including the epithelium, Bowman's membrane, and anterior stroma), and of a diameter that allows the exposure of sufficient stromal bed to perform the ablation.

2. The most frequent cause of a free cap is a very flat cornea. Patients with flat corneas and a mean keratometry of less than 41.00 D present a higher risk of a free cap occurring.

3. During a keratectomy, the microkeratome can stop before completing its stroke and give rise to an incomplete flap and a corneal bed of insufficient size to perform an ablation.

4. Thin flaps are commonly associated with the complication of a central hole known as a buttonhole.

5. Any malfunction of the automatic microkeratome, or slipping of the manual instrument, preventing a uniform stroke can give rise to an irregular resection, leading to an uneven stromal bed.

REFERENCES

1. Buratto L, Brint S, Ferrari M. Keratomileusis. In: Buratto L, Brint SF, eds. *LASIK: Principles and Techniques.* Thorofare, NJ: SLACK Incorporated; 1998:9-21.

2. Pallikaris IG, Papatzanaki ME, Stathi EZ, Frenschock O, Georgiadis A. Laser in situ keratomileusis. *Laser Surg Med.* 1990;10(5):463-468.

3. Jacobs JM, Taravella MJ. Incidence of intraoperative flap complications in laser in situ keratomileusis. *J Cataract Refract Surg.* 2002;28(1):23-28.

4. Slade SG. LASIK complications and their management. In: Machat JJ, ed. *Excimer Laser Refractive Surgery.* Thorofare, NJ: SLACK Incorporated; 1996:358-400.

5. Sridhar MS, Rapuano CJ, Cohen EJ. Accidental self-removal of a flap—a rare complication of Laser in situ Keratomileusis. *Am J Ophthalmology.* 2001;132(5):780-782.

6. Eggink FA, Eggink CA, Beekhuis WH. Postoperative management and follow-up after corneal flap loss following laser in situ keratomileusis. *J Cataract Refract Surg.* 2002;28(1):175-179.

7. Buratto L, Brint S. Complications of LASIK. In: Buratto L, Brint SF, ed. *Custom LASIK: Surgical Techniques and Complications.* Thorofare, NJ: SLACK Incorporated; 2003:161-224.

8. Holland SP, Srivannaboon S, Reinstein DZ. Avoiding serious corneal complications of laser assisted in situ keratomileusis and photorefractive keratectomy. *Ophthalmology.* 2000;107(4):640-652.

9. Peters NT, Iskander NG, Gimbel HV. Minimizing the risk of recutting with a Hansatome over an existing Automated Corneal Shaper flap for hyperopic laser in situ keratomileusis enhancement. *J Cataract Refract Surg.* 2001;27(8):1328-1332.

10. Gokmen F, Jester JV, Petroll WM, McCulley JP, Cavanagh HD. In vivo confocal microscopy through-focusing to measure corneal flap thickness after laser in situ keratomileusis. *J Cataract Refract Surg.* 2002;28(6):962-970.

11. Cigales M, Hoyos JE. J. Thin flaps and buttonholes. In: Buratto L, Brint SF, ed. *Custom LASIK: Surgical Techniques and Complications*. Thorofare, NJ: SLACK Incorporated; 2003:224-225.

12. Cummings A, Lavery F. Flap complications. In: Agarwal S, Agarwal A, Pallikaris IG, et al, eds. *Refractive Surgery*. New Delhi, India: Jaypee; 2000:329-339.

13. Leung AT, Rao SK, Cheng AC, et al. Pathogenesis and management of laser in situ keratomileusis flap buttonhole. *J Cataract Refract Surg.* 2000;26(3):358-362.

14. Lane HA, Swale JA, Majmudar PA. Prophylactic use of mitomycin-C in the management of a button-holed LASIK flap. *J Cataract Refract Surg.* 2003;29(2):390-392.

15. Krüger J. Managing recurrent epithelial ingrowth. In: Buratto L, Brint SF, ed. *Custom LASIK: Surgical Techniques and Complications*. Thorofare, NJ: SLACK Incorporated; 2003:233.

16. Ti SE, Tan DT. Recurrent corneal erosion after laser in situ keratomileusis. *Cornea.* 2001;20(2):156-158.

17. Battat L, Macri A, Dursun D, Pflugfelder SC. Effects of laser in situ keratomileusis on tear production, clearance, and the ocular surface. *Ophthalmology.* 2001;108(7):1230-1235.

18. Tabbara KF, El-Sheikh HF, Vera-Cristo CL. Complications of laser in situ keratomileusis (LASIK). *Eur J Ophthalmol.* 2003;13(2):139-146.

Please see Flap Wars video on enclosed CD-ROM.

Chapter 13

DECENTERED ABLATION

Helen Boerman, OD; Tracy Swartz, OD, MS, FAAO; and Ming Wang, MD, PhD

INTRODUCTION

Significantly decentered excimer ablations result in loss of best corrected visual acuity (BCVA) due to irregular astigmatism and cause symptoms such as glare, night vision difficulty, ghosting, and diplopia. Possible causes of decentration include poor fixation due to poor patient instruction, anxiety, oversedation, blurry vision due to high refractive error, or the exposed stromal bed causing difficulty seeing the laser's target. It can also be due to improper stabilization of the patient's eye with a Thornton ring during ablation. In order to prevent decentration, careful preoperative and intraoperative instructions are key, especially with regard to the fixation target, keeping both eyes open, warning patients about sounds and smells that might startle them, and keeping the body and head still during surgery.[1,2]

DECENTERED ABLATION

To adequately define decentration of the ablation zone, a review of the differences between curvature and elevation maps is necessary. Dioptric curvature maps indicate surface shape using the axial radius of curvature, or the distance along the normal from the surface to the optic axis.[3] Once a radius is determined, it is converted to a dioptric value using a paraxial keratometry formula. This value indicates the surface refractive power when incident rays are normal to the cornea; therefore, it is valid for the corneal apex only. When this formula is applied to all corneal points, radius-based dioptric maps misrepresent corneal power. Instead, radius-based dioptric maps should be thought of as dioptric curvature maps.

In contrast, elevation maps using an appropriate reference surface can describe subtle variations in surface geometry and are valuable when true topography is required.[3] Elevation maps are incredibly useful in both diagnosing and treating decentration and in monitoring surface changes.

An example of the difference between axial and elevation maps can be seen in Figure 13-1 for a keratoconic cornea. Keratoconus presents a corneal condition resulting in progressive decentration of the corneal apex. On the axial map, keratoconus appears as an area of inferior steepening. On the elevation map, the cornea is elevated superior to the

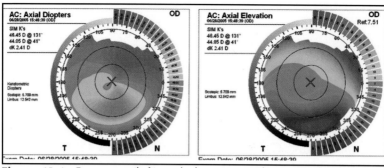

Figure 13-1. Curvature (left) and elevation (right) maps for a kerato-conic cornea are noticeably different. On the axial map, keratoconus appears as an area of inferior steepening. On the surface height map, the elevation appears superior to the area of thinning.

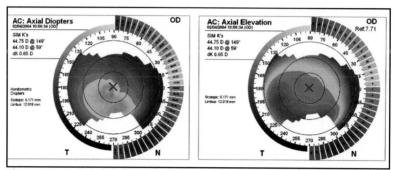

Figure 13-2. Axial (left) and elevation (right) maps for a patient with a decentered ablation. The elevation map shows an inferior decentration of the treatment zone in this patient S/P hyperopic LASIK.

area of thinning. Figure 13-2 demonstrates curvature and elevation maps for a patient with a decentered ablation. The elevation map shows a decentration of the optical zone. Note the inferior decentration of the treatment in this patient who previously underwent a myopic LASIK treatment. The key observation on curvature maps is the dioptric difference between the superior and inferior keratometric readings. The key observation on elevation maps is the misalignment of the center of ablation from the optical center.

TYPICAL CASE PRESENTATION

A patient with a decentered ablation generally presents with the following clinical signs and symptoms:

- A decentration of the ablation zone on corneal topography
- Increased higher-order aberrations as measured using wavefront aberrometry, predominantly coma
- The appearance of a tail on point spread functions (PSF)
- Reduced BCVA that improves only with gas permeable lenses
- A cylinder measurement on autorefraction and wavefront that differs from manifest refraction
- A history of reduced vision immediately following surgery that fails to improve with time

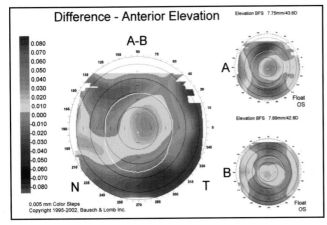

Figure 13-3. The elevation map prior to hyperopic LASIK (bottom right) and S/P hyperopic LASIK (top right), with the difference map showing the induced change (enlarged map).

TOPOGRAPHIC DECENTRATION

To evaluate decentration on corneal topography, both axial curvature and elevation maps are useful. The axial algorithm provides the refractive result of ablation (ie, the optical zone). A large corneal curvature gradient between treated and untreated cornea, such as that resulting from a highly myopic correction, creates a smaller optical zone, increasing the refractive effect of the decentration.[4]

The elevation algorithm delineates the location and size of the ablation zone. Decentration of the ablation zone can be measured by comparing the distance between the center of the flattened zone and the center of the entrance pupil on preoperative and postoperative elevation maps using a difference map (Figure 13-3).[5,6]

WAVEFRONT ABERRATIONS

Wavefront aberrometry shows increased higher-order aberrations in patients S/P LASIK, specifically those with decentered ablations. Mrochen et al[5] found that subclinical decentrations less than 1 mm significantly increase wavefront aberrations, deteriorating the optical quality of the retinal image. On average, all Zernike coefficients increased postoperatively, with coma being the predominant high-order aberration. They found that decentrations as small as 0.2 mm increased wavefront aberrations. However, decentrations less than 0.5 mm have been considered clinically insignificant.

Wavefront aberrometers typical display aberrations using several methods, including PSF and Snellen letter appearance from the patient's perspective. Patients with increased coma as a result of decentration present with wavefront maps and point spread functions similar to that in Figure 13-4A. The Snellen letter E (Figure 13-4B) for the same patient is also shown.

MANAGEMENT

Relieving patients of symptoms associated with decentration may be complex. The most frequently used method involves gas permeable lenses, which reshape the anterior cornea optically and restore visual quality. These fittings often require reverse geometry lenses or aspheric lenses to be successful. This is time-consuming, and most patients do not want to venture down the road that motivated them to pursue refractive surgery initially.

Figure 13-4. (A) A typical aberrometry map and point spread function in a patient with significant coma. (B) Snellen letter E as seen by the same patient.

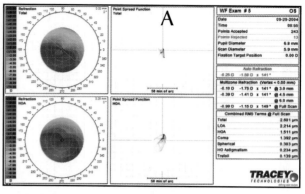

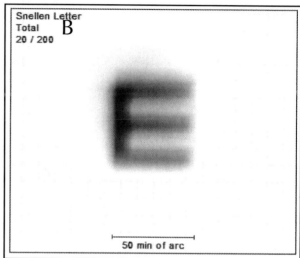

Surgical options for treatment of decentered ablations are limited. For mild degrees of decentration following photorefractive keratectomy (PRK), a small-diameter ablation (3 to 4 mm) at the edge of the original optical zone can serve to enlarge the optical zone in the pupillary axis. Another technique involves a series of 3 small-diameter ablations at the edge of the decentered ablation followed by phototherapeutic keratectomy (PTK) smoothing. A complication of this, however, is a hyperopic shift due to the removal of tissue centrally. These 2 methods are difficult S/P LASIK because the enhancement will be constrained by the size of the original bed. Ablating over the edges of the bed poses a risk for epithelial ingrowth.

Custom-Corneal Ablation Pattern (Custom–CAP) (VISX, Santa Clara, Calif) received United States Humanitarian Use Device approval for the treatment of decentrations in 2002. Elevation data are obtained using the Humphrey Atlas (Carl Zeiss Meditech, Dublin, Calif), and a software program allows simulation of surgeon-directed ablations of chosen location, shape, size, and depth to improve corneal topographic appearance. Although effective, Custom-CAP does not address the refractive error. While most surgeons consider improvement in best correction and reduction of symptoms a surgical success, many patients are frustrated by the lack of improvement or, in some cases, worsening of uncorrected vision. The use of a placido-based system for elevation data may limit its success. Wavefront-driven custom treatment may be used to correct decentrations, assuming the technology currently

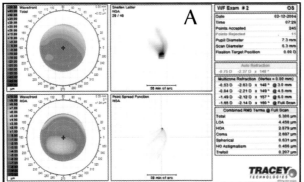

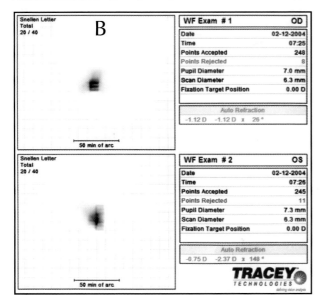

Figure 13-5. (A) The wavefront aberrometry map with PSF for the left eye S/P an initially decentered treatment with attempted correction using wavefront-guided ablation. Note the residual coma. (B) The difference in Snellen letter appearance between the eyes S/P attempted correction of the original decentration OS.

available is able to detect the irregularities reliably. Hartmann-Shack aberrometers may fail when attempting to measure eyes with considerable irregularity due to limitations of the lenslet array. While decentrations may increase higher-order aberrations, attempting to correct the aberrations may not fully correct the topographical errors. These systems assume a normal prolate cornea in treatment planning, and the refractive error corrections may be less accurate. Thus, these treatments may be less effective than topographically directed treatments.

Retreatment using conventional enhancement techniques rarely corrects the problem and typically increases the effective decentration. This occurs because the neural axes (visual axis and line of sight) and the optical axis (geometrical) are not aligned in cases of decentration. Image placement on the fovea requires the eye to rotate, making full correction of the optical problem unlikely when all measurement and planning occurs on the visual axis. Conventional technology is not able to decouple these axes, and treats solely on the visual axis information. Thus, the decentration remains, as shown in Figure 13-5, where wavefront maps and Snellen representations show significant coma.

The advancement of Scheimpflug imaging to create three-dimensional (3-D) models of corneal shape may be the missing link to accurate topographically-driven treatments. These systems measure the corneal shape directly and with greater accuracy than placido or slit

Figure 13-6. (A) A decentered ablation as seen on elevation topography. (B) The simulated elevation map after ablation to correct the decentration using the morphological axis.

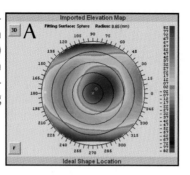
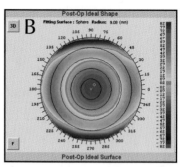

scanning methods. Combining precise topographical measurements with sophisticated software programs, such as the Corneal Integrated Planning and Treatment Algorithm (CIPTA) (Ligi, Taranto, Italy) software, may enable treatment of irregular astigmatism. CIPTA incorporates dynamic pupillometry, topography, a scanning laser, and sophisticated software for surgical planning to correct for irregularities and improve corneal asphericity. It determines the location of the morphological axis and bases treatment on this rather than the visual axis. It can incorporate the manifest refraction in planning in addition to regularizing the cornea to restore visual quality. Examples of a decentered ablation as viewed on an elevation map and postoperative simulation after corrective ablation are shown in Figure 13-6.

CASE EXAMPLES

Case I

A 47-year-old male underwent bilateral LASIK, which was complicated by severe diffuse lamellar keratitis (DLK) requiring flap relifts 5 days postoperatively. He reported blurry vision that had remained unchanged since his surgery. Upon presentation, he was wearing gas permeable lenses to correct his distorted vision, which was greater in his right eye. Manifest refraction of –1.75 +2.25 x 040 in this eye improved his unaided vision of 20/100 to 20/25, and reduced the blur by 50% subjectively. Topography revealed irregular astigmatism in both eyes, greater in the right eye due to an inferotemporal decentration of the ablation zone (Figures 13-7A and B). A Custom CAP procedure was performed, which improved the centration of the treatment zone on both axial and elevation maps (Figures 13-7C and D). A final refractive treatment improved his unaided acuity to 20/20 and decreased his symptoms of blur.

Case II

A 49-year-old man presented for consultation 4 years following LASIK with a complaint of diplopia in the left eye. Manifest refraction of -2.75 +1.75 x 135 corrected this eye to 20/30, and a rigid gas permeable (RGP) lens subjective improved the complaint of double vision. VISX CustomVue wavefront mapping revealed 43% high-order aberrations, with coma contributing most to this measurement. Axial and elevation topographies revealed an inferonasally-decentered ablation zone (Figure 13-8A and B). A Custom CAP enhancement was performed (Figure 13-8C) and postoperatively, the patient reported some improvement in the diplopia, but not total resolution.

The peripheral ablation created an increase in myopia. His refraction of -4.50 +1.50 x 120 now yielded a BCVA of 20/30 with shadows. Topographies appeared similar to preoperative measurements, though slightly improved. A repeat Custom-CAP treatment was performed

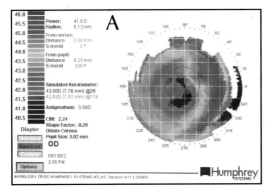
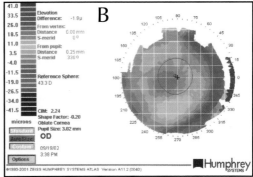
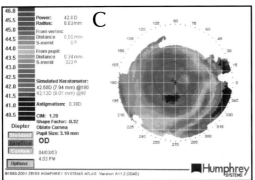
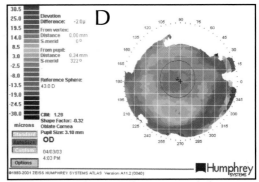

Figure 13-7. (A) The axial map reveals irregular astigmatism due to inferotemporal decentration of the ablation zone. (B) The elevation map of the same eye. A Custom CAP procedure improved the centration of the treatment, seen here on the axial map (C) and on the elevation map.

within several months (Figure 13-8D) and yielded topographies seen in Figures 13-8E and F. Despite improvement in topography, the second peripheral treatment caused even greater myopia, and the anisometropia was problematic. The patient was unable to wear glasses comfortably. The patient's refractive error was treated with PRK 2 years later following healthy renervation of the cornea. Aggressive dry eye treatment with Restasis ophthalmic emulsion (Allergan, Irvine, Calif) further smoothed the surface. His uncorrected visual acuity (UCVA) improved to 20/40, with a -1.00 D refractive error that corrects to 20/20.

Case III

A 45-year-old woman presented for an evaluation 3 years following her initial myopic LASIK procedures. Despite bilateral enhancements to correct residual refractive error, she complained of diplopia and night driving difficulty, greater in the left eye. Her topographic maps revealed a superiorly decentered treatment in the left eye (Figure 13-9A). Her UCVA was 20/30 OS and remained unchanged with refraction. An RGP resolved her complaint of monocular diplopia. The VISX CustomVue wavefront aberrometer indicated significant high-order aberrations (46.5%), with coma contributing the highest value, and the point spread function revealing the classic comet-like appearance (Figure 13-9B). A customized wavefront enhancement was performed, and her complaints of diplopia and night glare resolved as her topography improved (Figure 13-9C).

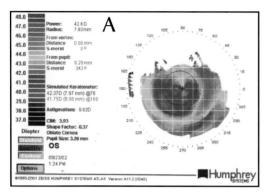
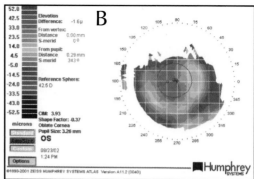

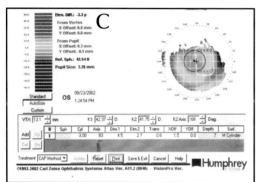
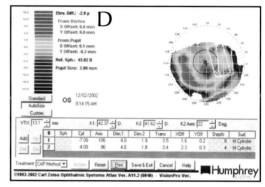

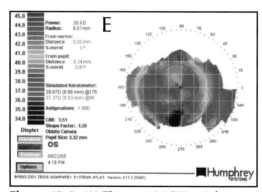
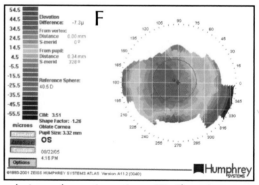

Figure 13-8. (A) The post-LASIK axial map reveals irregular astigmatism. (B) Elevation map of the same eye reveals an inferonasally-decentered ablation zone. (C) The ablation plan using the Custom-CAP device to correct the decentration. (D) The second treatment using the Custom-CAP device. Note the stronger treatment. (E) The axial map S/P 2 Custom-CAP procedures. (F) The elevation map S/P 2 Custom-CAP procedures.

Case V

A 49-year-old male presented for a second opinion evaluation 7 weeks S/P LASIK complaining of distance blur, ghosting, monocular diplopia, and foreign body sensation in his right eye. UCVA in this eye was 20/60. A manifest refraction of −2.00 +1.00 x 102 only improved his UCVA to 20/40. His axial and elevation maps are seen in Figures 13-10A and B, respectively. Although his maps suggested decentration, his complaint of foreign body sensation was suggestive of post-LASIK dry eyes, so we inserted a silicone plug into his right

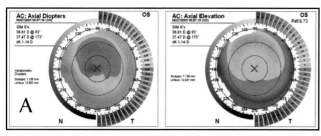

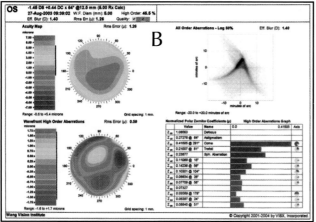

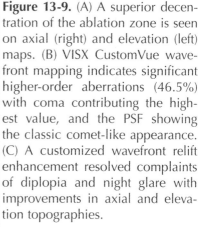

Figure 13-9. (A) A superior decentration of the ablation zone is seen on axial (right) and elevation (left) maps. (B) VISX CustomVue wavefront mapping indicates significant higher-order aberrations (46.5%) with coma contributing the highest value, and the PSF showing the classic comet-like appearance. (C) A customized wavefront relift enhancement resolved complaints of diplopia and night glare with improvements in axial and elevation topographies.

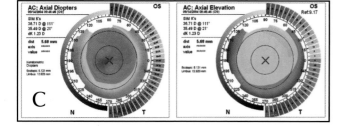

inferior lacrimal duct. We saw him at 4 months postop, when he refracted to 20/20 with a manifest of –1.50 +0.75 x 095. He reported significant improvement in shadows. His topographies also showed improvement in the appearance of decentration and can be seen in Figures 13-10C and D. A conventional enhancement with aggressive dry eye treatment yielded an UCVA of 20/20 in this eye. (see Figures 13-10C and D).

Case VI

A 29-year-old female underwent Intralase LASIK and developed DLK on Day 4. She was immediately treated with a flap lift and cleaning procedure. Slit-lamp view can be seen in Figure 13-11A. The DLK episode caused swelling of the central flaps, and when the edema resolved, striae appeared. In addition, significant inflammation resulted in collagen tissue digestion centrally causing hyperopia. We followed her topical steroid use, corneal status, and IOP frequently for weeks. Striae due to tissue expansion resulting from the DLK caused irregular astigmatism and this appeared topographically as a superonasal decentration (Figure 13-11B). PRK was recommended to smooth the striae and to treat the residual refractive error but the patient was lost to follow-up.

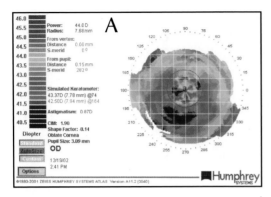
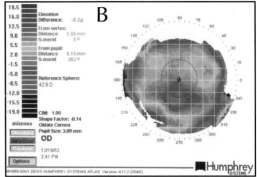
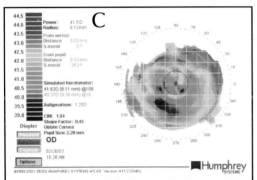
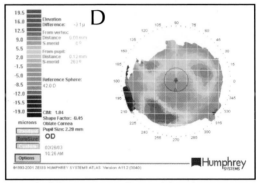

Figure 13-10. (A) Axial map of a slightly decentered ablation complicated by dry eye. (B) Elevation map shows decentration. (C) Following aggressive treatment, the irregularities were much improved. (D) Following aggressive treatment, the decentration was not significant enough to cause visually significant symptoms.

SUMMARY

When a patient with a history of refractive surgery presents with loss of BCVA and complains of glare, night vision difficulty, and diplopia, decentered ablation needs to be ruled out. An understanding of elevation topography and aberrometry is crucial for the diagnosis. Modern surgical options are presently evolving and gaining success in addressing this complication to improve visual quality in postkeratorefractive eyes.

KEY POINTS

1. Significantly decentered excimer ablations result in loss of BCVA due to irregular astigmatism and cause symptoms such as glare, night vision difficulty, ghosting, and diplopia.

2. Possible causes of decentration include poor fixation due to poor patient instruction, anxiety, oversedation, blurry vision due to high refractive error, or the exposed stromal bed causing difficulty seeing the laser's target.

3. To evaluate decentration on corneal topography, both axial curvature and elevation maps are useful. The axial algorithm provides the refractive result of ablation (ie, the optical zone). The elevation algorithm delineates the ablation zone size and location.

4. Wavefront aberrometers typically display aberrations using several methods, including PSF and Snellen letter appearance from the patient's perspective.

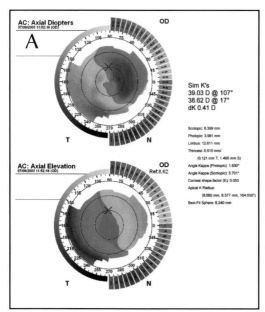

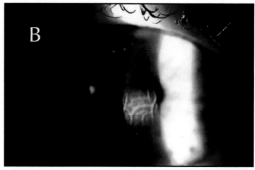

Figure 13-11. DLK can result in togographical decentration. (A) Striae due to tissue expansion appear togographically on axial and elevation maps as a superonasal decentration. (B) Note the dense central infiltrate and striae.

REFERENCES

1. Gimbel, Howard V. *Refractive Surgery: A Manual of Principles and Practice*. Thorofare, NJ: SLACK Incorporated, 2000:75-78,114

2. Mulhern M, Foley-Nolan A, O'Keefe M, Condon P. Topographic analysis of ablation centration after excimer laser photorefractive keratectomy and laser in situ keratomileusis for high myopia. *J Cataract Refract Surg.* 1997;23:488-494.

3. Salmon TO, Horner DG. Comparison of elevation, curvature, and power descriptors for corneal topographic mapping. *Optom Vis Sci.* 1995;72(11):800-808.

4. Vinciguerra P, Camesasca FI. Decentration after refractive surgery. *J Refract Surg.* 2001;17(2 Suppl): S190-191.

5. Mrochen M, Kaemmerer M, Mierdel P, Seiler T. Increased higher-order optical aberrations after laser refractive surgery: a problem of subclinical decentration. *J Cataract Refract Surg.* 2001;27(3):362-369.

6. Mulhern M, Foley-Nolan A, O'Keefe M, Condon P. Topographic analysis of ablation centration after excimer laser photorefractive keratectomy and laser in situ keratomileusis for high myopia. *J Cataract Refract Surg.* 1997;23:488-494.

Chapter 14

Post-LASIK Iatrogenic Ectasia

Amar Agarwal, MS, FRCS, FRCOphth;
Soosan Jacob, MS, FRCS, FERC, Dip NB; and Vladimir Pfeifer, MD

Introduction

The development of corneal ectasia (Figure 14-1) is a well-recognized complication following ablative refractive surgery that is induced inadvertently by the refractive surgeon. It is an insidious process and may be seen months after an originally uncomplicated refractive procedure.

The 2 well-known factors causing iatrogenic keratectasia after LASIK are the removal of excessive amounts of tissue from the posterior stromal layers and LASIK done in a previously undiagnosed forme fruste keratoconus. The progression into frank ectasia is hastened by ablating the central corneal tissue in forme fruste keratoconus and, hence, this is a definite contraindication to LASIK.

Pathogenesis

The anterior cornea is composed of alternating collagen fibrils, has a more complicated interwoven structure than the deeper stroma, and it acts as the major stress-bearing layer. The flap used for LASIK (Figure 14-2) is made in this layer and thus results in a weakening of that strongest layer of the cornea that contributes considerably to the biomechanical stability of the cornea. This, therefore, weakens the cornea, which is not able to withstand the normal intraocular pressure (IOP) of the eye. This leads to the cornea bulging outwards at the weakest area (see Figure 14-1). This outward bulging continues and leads to induction of progressively worsening myopia and irregular astigmatism. The process is irreversible once it begins.

Factors Predisposing to Iatrogenic Keratectasia

Residual Bed Thickness

The residual bed thickness (RBT) of the cornea is the crucial factor contributing to the biomechanical stability of the cornea after LASIK. The flap, as such, does not contribute much after its repositioning to the stromal bed. This is easily seen by the fact that the flap can be

Figure 14-1. Illustration depicting corneal ectasia.

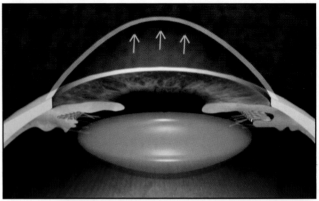

Figure 14-2. Illustration depicting LASIK.

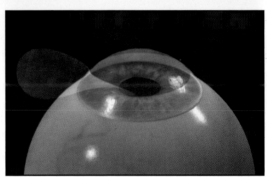

easily lifted up even up to 1 year after treatment. The decreased RBT as well as the lamellar cut in the cornea both contribute to the decreased biomechanical stability of the cornea.

A reduction in the RBT results in a long-term increase in the surface parallel stress on the cornea. The IOP can cause further forward bowing and thinning of a structurally compromised cornea. Inadvertent excessive eye rubbing, prone sleeping position, and the normal wear and tear of the cornea may also play roles. The RBT should not be less than 250 μm to avoid subsequent iatrogenic keratectasias.[1-3] Reoperations should be undertaken very carefully in corneae with RBT less than 300 μm.

Dandelion Keratectasia

Increasing myopia after every operation is known as "dandelion keratectasia." Seiler[4] has proposed retaining a minimum percentage of corneal thickness as the residual stromal bed rather than an absolute number (250 μm), taking into account biomechanical considerations and possible errors in pachymetry measurements.

Ablation Diameter

The ablation diameter also plays a very important role in LASIK. Postoperative optical distortions are more common with diameters less than 5.5 mm. Use of larger ablation diameters implies a lesser RBT postoperatively. Consider the following formula: ablation depth [μm] = 1/3 (diameter [mm])^2 x (intended correction D).[3,5] It becomes clear that a larger ablation diameter results in removal of more tissue, leading to a thinner RBT. It also leads to a larger area of thin cornea and, hence, the ectasia also occurs in a correspondingly larger zone with larger ablation diameters. Thus, to preserve a sufficient bed thickness, the range of myopic correction is limited and the upper limit of possible myopic correction may be around 12.00 D.[6]

Laser Ablation Depth

The actual laser ablation depth of the corneal stroma can also vary. Factors such as drying of the stromal bed may result in an ablation depth more than that intended.[6] Reinstein et al predict that the standard deviation of uncertainty in predicting the RBT preoperatively is around 30 μm.[7]

Miscellaneous

Patients with high myopia (-8.00 D or higher), high astigmatism, thin corneas (less than 500 μm), and primary posterior corneal elevation are at greater risk for post-LASIK ectasia. Forme fruste keratoconus and a family history of keratoconus should always be sought. Age, attempted correction, the optical zone diameter, and the flap thickness are other parameters that have to be considered.[8,9] The flap thickness may not be uniform throughout its length. In studies by Seitz et al[6], it has been shown that the Moria Model One microkeratome (Doylestown, Pa) and the Supratome cut deeper towards the hinge, whereas the Automated Corneal Shaper and the Hansatome create flaps that are thinner towards the hinge. Thus, accordingly, the area of corneal ectasia may not be in the center, but paracentral, especially if it is also associated with decentered ablation. Flap thickness has also been found to vary considerably under similar conditions (even up to 40 μm) and this may also result in a lesser RBT than intended.[10-16] It has been recommended to preoperatively calculate residual stromal bed based on 2 SD of flap thickness.[17]

Postoperative wound healing and the biochemical changes that occur during corneal thinning may also contribute to ectasia. Although iatrogenic ectasia usually occurs after deep central ablations, it has also been reported after shallow ablations.[18] In some reported cases,[19] no preoperative risk factor could be identified. Structural rigidity of the individual cornea and IOP may play major roles in these cases. The tensile strength of the normal cornea varies by as much as ±25%.[20] It has been seen that keratoconic corneas have much lower mechanical strength than normal corneas.[21] It is also known that the cornea gradually becomes thinner with age. This may cause some post-LASIK patients with borderline RBT to develop keratectasia as they get older.

CLINICAL PRESENTATION

The patient presents weeks, months, or even years later with progressively increasing myopia, irregular astigmatism, fluctuating refraction, difficulties in scotopic vision, glare, halos, ghosting of images, and, finally, loss of best-corrected visual acuity (BCVA).

TOPOGRAPHY

Topography is valuable for preoperative ophthalmic examination of LASIK candidates (see Chapter 3). Three-dimensional (3-D) imaging allows surgeons to look at corneal thickness, as well as the corneal anterior and posterior surface, and predicts the shape of the cornea after LASIK surgery. Topographic analysis using 3-D slit scan system allows us to predict which candidates would do well with LASIK and also confers the ability to screen for subtle configurations that may be contraindications to LASIK. The Orbscan (Bausch & Lomb, Rochester, NY) corneal topography system uses a scanning optical slit scan that makes it fundamentally different from the corneal topography that analyzes the reflected images from the anterior corneal surface (see Chapter 1). The slits are projected on the anterior segment of the eye: the anterior cornea, the posterior cornea, the anterior iris, and anterior lens. The data collected

Figure 14-3. Shows a patient with iatrogenic keratectasia after LASIK. Note the upper right hand corner shows the posterior float has thinning and this is also seen in the bottom right picture in which pachymetry reading is 329.

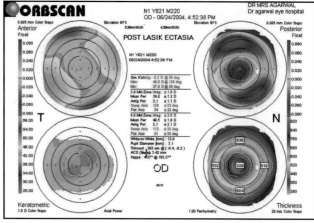

Figure 14-4. Shows the same patient with iatrogenic keratectasia after LASIK in a 3-D pattern. Notice the ectasia seen clearly in the bottom right picture.

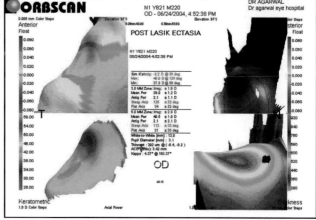

from these 4 surfaces are used to create a topographic map. This technique provides more information about the anterior segment of the eye, such as anterior and posterior corneal curvature, elevation maps of the anterior and posterior corneal surface, and corneal thickness.

DIAGNOSIS OF IATROGENIC KERATECTASIA

Detection of a mild keratectasia requires knowledge about the posterior curvature of the cornea. Posterior corneal surface topographic changes after LASIK are known (Figures 14-3 and 14-4). Increased negative keratometric diopters and oblate asphericity of the PCC, which correlate significantly with the intended correction, are common after LASIK, leading to mild keratectasia.[6,19] This change in posterior power and the risk of keratectasia were more significant with a RBT of 250 μm or less.[22] The difference in the refractive indices results in a 0.20-D difference at the back surface of the cornea becoming equivalent to a 2.00-D change in the front surface of the cornea.[6] Increase in posterior power and asphericity also correlates with the difference between the intended and achieved correction 3 months after LASIK.

It is known that corneal ectasias and keratoconus have posterior corneal elevation as the earliest manifestation.[23] The precise course of progression of posterior corneal elevation to frank keratoconus is not known. Hence, it is necessary to study the posterior corneal surface preoperatively in all LASIK candidates.

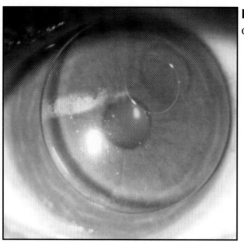

Figure 14-5. RGP lenses can be used in the early cases to treat iatrogenic ectasia.

Post-LASIK ectasia is seen on topography as a central or paracentral area of steepening that progressively worsens on follow-up evaluations. It is associated with a decreased pachymetry in the area of steepening. The earliest changes are detected on the posterior corneal surface as a posterior corneal bulging. An eccentric posterior bulge below the center of the laser-ablated area is most ominous.[24] Increasing amounts of irregular astigmatism are seen.

TREATMENT OF POST-LASIK KERATECTASIA

Rigid Gas Permeable Lenses

Rigid gas permeable (RGP) lenses can be worn to slow or halt the process of ectasia (Figure 14-5). They are a safe and reversible option for ectatic corneas and may delay the need for any surgical intervention.[25] Nonventilated, modern gas permeable scleral lenses have also been used for severe keratectasia. These may fit well due to their exclusive scleral contact zone even in cases where corneal fitted contact lenses have been unsuccessful.[26] Multicurve and reverse geometry lenses have also been used successfully in these patients.[27]

Topical Ocular Antihypertensives

These act by relieving the biomechanical strain on the cornea. Hiatt et al have attempted IOP lowering in patients with long-standing ectasia without success but have obtained good results in a patient with early ectasia.[17] They have hypothesized that the cornea may be malleable during early and active ectasia and therefore amenable to flattening from IOP reduction.[16] They have proposed that corneal shape is dependent on the balance between IOP, atmospheric pressure, and corneal rigidity. When corneal rigidity is surgically compromised as in LASIK, a delicate balance may exist that can be more easily influenced by IOP and extraocular pressure differences.

Intrastromal Corneal Ring Segments

Intrastromal corneal ring segments (Intacs [Additional Technology, Sunnyvale, Calif]) are clear microthin polymethyl methacrylate (PMMA) intracorneal inserts, hexagonal in cross-section, with an arc length of 150 degrees. They have 2 positioning holes and are implanted at an angulation of 31 degrees to follow the corneal curvature. The ring segments are placed

Figure 14-6. Postop picture of Intacs. Note the clear micro-thin PMMA intracorneal inserts.

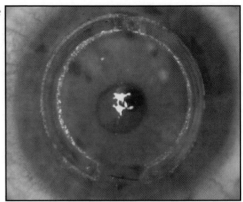

at two-thirds corneal depth (Figure 14-6). Intacs act by distending the peripheral cornea and hence flattening the central cornea, thicker segments producing a greater effect. For central ectasia, 2 segments can be inserted and in cases of inferior keratectasia, the irregular astigmatism can be corrected with a single Intacs segment placed at the site where corneal flattening was needed inferiorly or inferotemporally.[28,29] The placement of a single Intacs segment prevents overcorrection of the myopia.

The exact role of Intacs in slowing or halting the progression of ectasia is still not known. Longer follow-up studies are required. Swanson et al[30] have a 2-year follow-up of 393 patients (363 keratoconus and 30 postsurgical ectasia) using the steepest refractive axis incision technique. In this series, all mild cases and 55% of moderate-to-severe cases achieved UCVA of 20/40 or better with all cases gaining lines of vision. Maximum benefit was seen in patients with stage III keratoconus. In a series of 40 eyes of 25 keratoconus patients with placement of 2 intracorneal ring segments, Martiz[31] demonstrated improvement in both UCVA (2 to 9 lines) and BCVA, with a decrease in irregular astigmatism and improved contact lens tolerance. A unique characteristic of the Intacs refractive surgical procedure is its potential reversibility.

Ferrara Rings

Ferrara Rings, unlike Intacs, are triangular in cross section[32] and produce a prismatic effect that directs reflected light away from the visual pathway. The prismatic design prevents halos and edge glare and allows a smaller optical zone. These rings are also smaller than Intacs and positioned more centrally; therefore, they can correct the same amount of refractive error with thinner rings. Ferrara intrastromal corneal rings have reduced corneal steepening and normalize the central cornea in eyes with keratoconus.[32] It, therefore, seems very likely that they will be effective in the treatment of post-LASIK ectasia as well. Further studies are required for the same.

Collagen Crosslinking With Riboflavin (C3-R treatment)

This acts by remodeling of the cornea. The technique creates new bonds between adjacent collagen molecules, thus increasing the stiffness of the cornea 1.5 times, making it less malleable. It is, in essence, an exaggeration of the normal cross-linking that occurs with age and as a pathological process in diabetics. This utilizes combined riboflavin/UVA-induced collagen cross-linking. The procedure involves removal of the epithelium (7- to 9-mm area), application of 20% riboflavin in dextrane solution on the cornea, followed by irradiation of the cornea with UVA (365 to 370 nm, 3 mW/cm^2) at a distance of 1 cm for 30 min (Figure 14-7). These

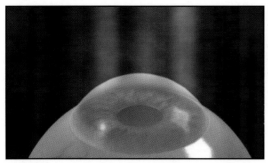

Figure 14-7. Collagen cross-linking with riboflavin (C3-R treatment). An application of 20% riboflavin in dextrane solution on the cornea is done, followed by irradiation of the cornea with UVA (365 to 370 nm, 3 mW/cm²) at a distance of 1 cm for 30 minutes.

settings have been found to be safe for the endothelium as well with a pachymetry of at least 400 µm. The study[33] noted cessation continuing keratectasia in all patients with an improvement in BCVA and maximal keratometry values in about 50% of the cases.

Chao et al[34] combined placement of single-segment Intacs technique with C3-R treatment. They report an increase in both mean UCVA and BCVA in their series. They also report a decrease in L-U ratio (difference between the sum of 5 upper keratometry values and 5 lower keratometry values referenced to the steepest lower keratometric measurement), indicating localized flattening of the inferior cornea. The vast majority of the curvature change was seen in the lower cornea, suggesting that the single-ring approach avoids unnecessary flattening of the already flat superior cornea.

Deep Anterior Lamellar Keratoplasty

Here, a full-thickness corneal stroma and epithelial button is placed into a host bed consisting of Descemet's membrane and endothelium (Figures 14-8A to E). The recovery time is faster and visual recovery quicker when compared with penetrating keratoplasty (corneal transplant). The risk of endothelial rejection is absent. It is based on adding tissue to strengthen the cornea. However, it is not known if by simply adding tissue, an already structurally compromised cornea can be strengthened. This technique requires further study.

Penetrating Keratoplasty

This is the ultimate resort for a patient with post-LASIK ectasia, with the disadvantage being interruption of the structural and immunological integrity of the eye. It is an invasive procedure (Figure 14-9) with a long rehabilitation period that carries the risk of rejection of the donor cornea. The results are especially grave considering that the ectasia developed in a previously normal patient who underwent an elective, usually cosmetic procedure.

CORNEA-SPARING LASIK

Cornea-sparing LASIK is another technique aimed at decreasing the incidence of ectasia. Here, part or all of the treatment is applied on the undersurface of the flap. This is especially useful in patients with thin corneas, high power, or in enhancement procedures where the thickness of the flap is not known. It is important not to breach the Bowman's membrane in these cases because this may lead to haze. The center of the pupil is marked first and then the flap is cut and reflected backwards onto a dome-shaped, flap-holding instrument. The eye tracker is taken off and the treatment is applied. It is ideal to apply only the spherical treatment on the undersurface. Centration of astigmatic treatments and wavefront-guided treatments are difficult or not possible as yet due to registration and orientation issues.

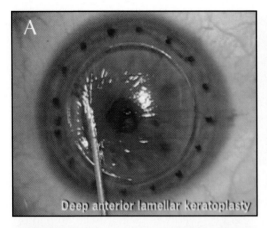

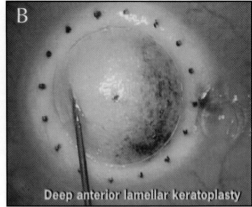

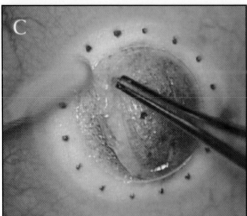

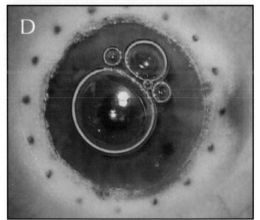

Figure 14-8. Deep anterior lamellar kera-toplasty (DALK). (A) Injection of air bub-ble starting so that one can dissect to the Descemet's membrane. (B) Air bubble inject-ed. (C) Dissection started. (D) Anterior cornea removed. Only Descemet's membrane and endothelium left behind. (E) Donor cornea placed on the recipient bed and sutured.

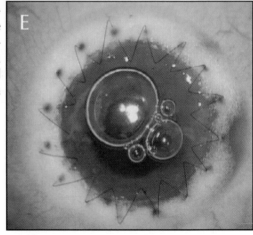

PREVENTION OF POST-LASIK KERATECTASIA

In all cases, basic investigations, such as anterior and posterior corneal evaluation and pachymetry of the entire cornea, should be done preoperatively. An Orbscan would help greatly in diagnosing thin cornea, forme fruste keratoconus, as well as other contraindica-tions to LASIK. LASIK should be avoided in corneas with a curvature greater than 48.50 D.[24]

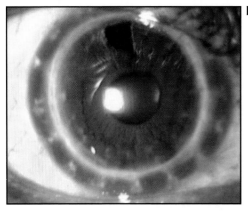

Figure 14-9. Penetrating keratoplasty.

Enhancement procedures should especially be avoided in eyes with steep topographic areas and low pachymetry.

Microkeratome head, intended correction, and ablation zone diameter should all be selected according to the patient's pachymetry, aiming for a minimum postoperative RBT of 250 μm, which should be mandatory for all cases. If the postoperative RBT threatens to be less than this value, one should consider another form of refractive surgery, including LASEK, phakic IOL, or refractive lens exchange. A postoperative RBT limit of 300 μm may be more suitable to allow for margins of error in pachymetry readings, achieved flap thickness, and laser performance. Intraoperative pachymetry to measure flap thickness and posterior stromal thickness before and after ablation is especially important to avoid ectasia because it allows for variations in flap thickness and ablation depth. New methods, such as continuous noncontact corneal pachymetry with a high-speed reflectometer[35-37] have been proposed. Intraoperative real-time optical coherence pachymetry[38] could be a very important safety mechanism. Real-time pachymetry should become a routine step in all LASIK procedures.

KEY POINTS

1. The 2 well-known factors causing onto iatrogenic keratectasia after LASIK are removal of excessive amounts of tissue from the posterior stromal layers and LASIK done in a previously undiagnosed forme fruste keratoconus.

2. The residual bed thickness (RBT) of the cornea is the crucial factor contributing to the biomechanical stability of the cornea after LASIK. The flap as such does not contribute much after its repositioning to the stromal bed.

3. Increasing myopia after every operation is known as dandelion keratectasia.

4. Topography is valuable for preoperative ophthalmic examination of LASIK candidates. Three-dimensional imaging allows surgeons to look at corneal thickness, as well as the corneal anterior and posterior surface and it can also predict the shape of the cornea after LASIK surgery.

5. Collagen crosslinking with riboflavin (C3-R treatment) acts by remodeling the cornea. This technique creates new bonds between adjacent collagen molecules, thus increasing the stiffness of the cornea one and a half times, making it less malleable.

REFERENCES

1. Seiler T, Koufala K, Richter G. Iatrogenic keratectasia after laser in situ keratomileusis. *J Refract Surg.* 1998;14(3):312-317.

2. Seiler T, Quurke AW. Iatrogenic keratectasia after laser in situ keratomileusis in a case of forme fruste keratoconus. *J Refract Surg.* 1998;24(7):1007-1009.

3. Probst LE, Machat JJ. Mathematics of laser in situ keratomileusis for high myopia. *J Cataract Refract Surg.* 1998;24.

4. Seiler T. Iatrogenic keratectasia: academic anxiety or serious risk? *J Cataract Refract Surg.* 1999;25:1307-1308.

5. McDonnell PJ. Excimer laser corneal surgery: new strategies and old enemies {review}. *Invest Ophthalmol Vis Sci.* 1995;36:4-8.

6. Seitz B, Torres F, Langenbucher A, et al. Posterior corneal curvature changes after myopic laser in situ keratomileusis. *Ophthalmology.* 2001;108(4):666-672.

7. Reinstein DZ, Srivannaboon S, Sutton HFS, et al. Risk of ectasia in LASIK: revised safety criteria. *Invest Ophthalmol Vis Sci.* 1999;40(suppl):S403.

8. Pallikaris IG, Kymionis GD, Astyrakakis NI. Corneal ectasia induced by laser in situ keratomileusis. *J Cataract Refract Surg.* 2001;27(11):1796-1802.

9. Argento C, Cosentino M J, Tytium A et al. Corneal ectasia after laser in situ keratomileusis. *J Cataract Refract Surg.* 2001;27(9):1440-1448.

10. Binder PS, Moore M, Lambert RW, et al. Comparison of two microkeratome systems. *J Refract Surg.* 1997;13:142-53.

11. Hofmann RF, Bechara SJ. An independent evaluation of second generation suction microkeratomes. *Refract Corneal Surg.* 1992;8:348-354.

12. Schuler A, Jessen K, Hoffmann F. Accuracy of the microkeratome keratectomies in pig eyes. *Invest Ophthalmol Vis Sci.* 1990;31:2022-2030.

13. Behrens A, Seitz B, Langenbucher A, et al. Evaluation of corneal flap dimensions and cut quality using a manually guided microkeratome [published erratum appears in *J Refract Surg.* 1999;15:400]. *J Refract Surg.* 1999;15:118-123.

14. Behrens A, Seitz B, Langenbucher A, et al. Evaluation of corneal flap dimensions and cut quality using the Automated Corneal Shaper microkeratome. *J Refract Surg.* 2000;16:83-89.

15. Behrens A, Langenbucher A, Kus MM, et al. Experimental evaluation of two current generation automated microkeratomes: the Hansatome and the Supratome. *Am J Ophthalmol.* 2000;129:59-67.

16. Jacobs BJ, Deutsch TA, Rubenstein JB. Reproducibility of corneal flap thickness in LASIK. *Ophthalmic Surg Lasers.* 1999;30:350-353.

17. Hiatt JA, Wachler BS, Grant C. Reversal of laser in situ keratomileusis-induced ectasia with intraocular pressure reduction. *J Cataract Refract Surg.* 2005;31(8):1652-1655.

18. Amoils SP, Deist MB, Gous P, Amoils PM. Iatrogenic keratectasia after laser in situ keratomileusis for less than −4.0 to −7.0 diopters of myopia. *J Cataract Refract Surg.* 2000;26:967-977.

19. Geggel HS, Talley AR. Delayed onset keratectasia following laser in situ keratomileusis. *J Cataract Refract Surg.* 1999;25:582–586.

20. Hoeltzel DA, Altman P, Buzard K, Choe K. Strip extensiometry for comparison of the mechanical response of bovine, rabbit, and human corneas. *J Biomech Eng.* 1992;114:202-215.

21. Andreassen TT, Simonsen H, Oxlund H. Biomechanical properties of keratoconus and normal corneas. *Exp Eye Res.* 1980;31:435-441.

22. Wang Z, Chen J, Yang B. Posterior corneal surface topographic changes after laser in situ keratomileusis are related to residual corneal bed thickness. *Ophthalmology.* 1999;106(2):406-409.

23. McDermott GK. Topography's benefits for LASIK. *Review of Ophthalmology.* YEAR; Vol: PAGES.

24. Amoils SP, Deist MB, Cilliers PLP, Keziah G. Factors causing keratectasia after LASIK. Presented at the Refr@ctive.on-line and Topogr@phy on-line symposium in Milan; September 14, 2001; Milan, Italy.

25. O'donnell C, Welham L, Doyle S. Contact lens management of keratectasia after laser in situ keratomileusis for myopia. *Eye Contact Lens.* 2004;30(3):144-146.

26. Hanisch KT, Neppert B, Geerling G. Gas permeable scleral lenses as a conservative treatment option for extreme corneal ectasias and severe dry eye. *Ophthalmologe.* 2005;102(4):387-392.

27. Choi HJ, Kim MK, Lee JL. Optimization of contact lens fitting in keratectasia patients after laser in situ keratomileusis. *J Cataract Surg.* 2004;30(5):1057-1066.

28. Pokroy R, Levinger S, Hirsh A. Single Intacs segment for post-laser in situ keratomileusis keratectasia. *J Cataract Refract Surg.* 2004;30:8:1685-1695.

29. Kymionis GD, Siganos CS, Kounis G, et al. Management of post-LASIK corneal ectasia with Intacs inserts. *Arch Ophthalmol.* 2003;121:322-326.

30. Swanson MM. Intacs for keratoconus using the steepest-axis incision technique: 2-year results. Program and abstracts from the American Society of Cataract and Refractive Surgery 2005 Symposium on Cataract, IOL, and Refractive Surgery; April 15-20, 2005; Washington, DC.

31. Martiz JR. Treatment of keratoconus using Intralase and intracorneal rings. Program and abstracts from the American Society of Cataract and Refractive Surgery 2005 Symposium on Cataract, IOL, and Refractive Surgery; April 15-20, 2005; Washington, DC.

32. Siganos D, Ferrara P, Chatzinikolas K, Bessis N, Papastergiou G. Ferrara intrastromal corneal rings for the correction of keratoconus. *J Cataract Refract Surg.* 2002;28(11):1947-1951.

33. Wollensak G, Spoerl E, Seiler T. Riboflavin/ultraviolet-A-induced collagen crosslinking for the treatment of keratoconus. *Am J Ophthalmol.* 2003;135(5):620-627.

34. Chao L. Single-segment Intacs procedure for LASIK-induced ectasia and keratoconus and the lower-upper ratio. Program and abstracts from the American Society of Cataract and Refractive Surgery 2005 Symposium on Cataract, IOL, and Refractive Surgery; April 15-20, 2005; Washington, DC.

35. Bohnke M, Chavanne P, Gionotti R, Salathe RP. Continuous non-contact corneal pachymetry with high speed reflectometer. *J Refract Surg.* 1998;14:140-146.

36. Waelti R, Boehnke N, Gianotti R. Rapid and precise in vivo-measurement of human corneal thickness with optical low-coherence reflectometry in normal human eyes. *J Biomed Opt.* 1998;3:253-258.

37. Genth U, Mrochen M, Salahedine MM, et al. Flap thickness during LASIK and its implication for the safety of LASIK. *Ophthalmology.* In press.

38. Wirbelauer C, Pham DT. Continuous monitoring of corneal thickness changes during LASIK with online optical coherence pachymetry. *J Cataract Refract Surg.* 2004;30(12):2559-2568.

Please see Battle of the Bulge video on enclosed CD-ROM.

Chapter 15

Sands of Sahara or Diffuse Lamellar Keratitis: The Refractive Emergency

Alexander Hatsis, MD, FACS

Disease Entity

The Sands of Sahara Syndrome (aka Sands) is a self-perpetuating sterile inflammation of the cornea following any intervention in which a lamellar incision has created an interface through stromal tissue. Sands is most commonly seen in the immediate postop LASIK period and is localized to the interface without directly invading the adjacent stroma. Sands affects all races equally without predilection to age or gender and has a worldwide distribution. It may vary in intensity, presenting as a white granular interface accumulation of inflammatory cells aligned in a wave pattern resembling the wind blown sands of the desert. This clinical appearance first led Robert Maddox, MD, to name it Sands of Sahara Syndrome. Since then, other authors (Ronald Smith and Robert Maloney) have also referred to the syndrome as diffuse lamellar keratitis, (DLK) and sterile interface inflammatory syndrome, (SIIS) among others. Although different names have been used to describe this stromal response to corneal lamellar surgery, Sands or DLK is quickly becoming respected as a newly described aggressive, potentially sight-threatening complication.

Clinical Features

Corneal

The corneal manifestations of Sands or DLK are characterized by an indolent sterile infiltrate. As early as 12 hours post-LASIK, inflammatory cells can be seen accumulating throughout the stromal interface. With a nasal-hinged flap, the infiltrating cells are often first seen accumulating in the superior flap interface as well as peripheral to the lamellar cut just within the limbus. With superior-hinged flaps, cells usually occupy the inferior flap interface first. As the infiltrate develops, accumulating cells become apparent throughout the interface and after only a few hours, the entire interface may be diffusely involved. As the inflammation continues, the infiltrating cells align in a characteristic "sand" pattern. This linear arrangement of inflammatory cells, seen at slit-lamp examination, is what characterizes "sands" or DLK from other keratopathies. As the infiltrate continues to accumulate, the cellular density increases, forming interface clumps, nests, or aggregates of inflammatory cells. Additionally, as the sterile infiltrate becomes more severe, other corneal signs are proportionately noted. These signs are clinical clues to the aggressive nature of the inflammation. For example, delayed re-epithelization of the keratectomy gutter, limbal edema with injection, irregular topography patterns, and superficial punctate keratitis may be seen with secondary flap edema. Topographically, edematous flap swelling causes irregular elevation patterns while thinning due to stromal melt results in geographic abnormal irregular flattening. A moderately severe infiltrate will directly affect the stroma-distorting the immediate post-LASIK normal topography. This results in a variety of atypical irregular elevation patterns that may improve with resolution.

Ocular

If the initial corneal insult is severe, the inflammatory response may not be limited to the cornea. Accompanying ocular signs such as anterior chamber cell and flare, conjunctival injection, and lid edema may be seen. The patient may complain of a foreign body sensation, reduced or cloudy vision, photophobia, or epiphoria. DLK is characterized as an indolent infiltrate because even in its severest form, with secondary iritis, patients may only complain of a mild deep ciliary discomfort without being tender to touch. Characteristically, DLK appears dramatically invasive without being painful.

Pathogenesis

DLK or Sands is the stromal response to any nonspecific insult in the presence of a corneal lamellar incision. The incision does not have to be recent, just present to allow the invading cells to accumulate within the potential interface space. Active corneal infection has not been implicated in its pathogenesis since multiple interface cultures performed at many international sites have always been negative. Polymorphonuclear neutrophils (PMNs), the hallmark of acute inflammation, accumulate in the interface as a first intent, nonspecific inflammatory reaction without directly invading the adjacent corneal tissue (Figures 15-1 and 15-2). These inflammatory cells along with injured keratocytes degranulate, releasing collagenase as well as other protease enzymes.[1] This inflammatory activity destroys the stroma by a type of cellular digestion known among ophthalmologists as stromal "melt." The enzymatic destruction of stromal tissue itself becomes as abusive to the cornea as the original insult that caused the inflammatory reaction initially. For this reason, DLK is considered a self-perpetuating inflammation. As enzymatic inflammatory stromal destruction continues to insult the cornea, more PMNs are attracted, resulting in a greater concentration of liberated enzyme. The enzymatic melting now becomes the insult that attracts more PMNs and the process self-perpetuates. It is for this reason that a moderate case of DLK can develop into a severe case overnight.

Diagnosis

Although DLK has been seen following a corneal injury as long as 1 year after LASIK surgery, the diagnosis of DLK is usually made during the immediate post-LASIK period. The characteristic white granular, wave-pattern infiltrate is most often seen at slit-lamp exam on the first postoperative day while the patient may be experiencing excellent vision. The infiltrate is limited to the interface without invading the adjacent flap stroma, while the eye is indolent and not tender to the touch. Clinically, the presentation varies according to the intensity. We have classified Sands into 4 grades based on severity. The purpose of the classification is to predict the threat to vision via enzymatic stromal digestion and corneal integrity based on the clinical signs while establishing treatment guidelines. The less severe, visually

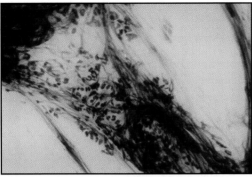

Figure 15-1. Hematoxylin and Eosin stain of harvested interface infiltrate.

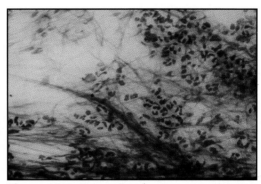

Figure 15-2. Pap stain of same.

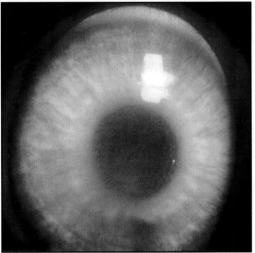

Figure 15-3. Appearance of grade II Sands.

nonthreatening cases can be treated medically while the more severe aggressive cases need immediate surgical intervention to prevent irregular astigmatism and permanent visual loss from stromal melt.

HATSIS CLASSIFICATION OF SANDS OF SAHARA SYNDROME

Grade I

The cellular infiltrate partially invades the interface. Most commonly, the superior third of the interface is involved with a nasal hinge flap and inferior with a superior hinge. In grade I, topography is normal and no other corneal signs are present. The threat of corneal melt is low.

Grade II

The cellular infiltrate is seen uniformly throughout the entire interface (Figure 15-3). Topography must be normal to be grade II and there are no associated corneal signs present. The threat of a grade II corneal melt is moderate. Grade II may progress to grade III within 24 hours with a definite threat of corneal melt.

Grade III

An overall densely opaque cellular infiltrate is seen throughout the interface with focal areas of accumulated cells appearing as nests of the inflammatory aggregate. The corneal flap is usually edematous and there is a high concentration of liberated enzyme with incomplete re-epithelization of the keratectomy gutter margin complicating matters by allowing epithelial in-growth at the flap edge. Punctate keratopathy may be present, and the patient usually complains of poor or cloudy vision. Due to flap edema and these epithelial surface irregularities, the topography is abnormal and atypical. With grade III, the threat of corneal melt is high.

Grade IV

This is represented by the extracorneal manifestation of DLK. I believe it is important to include this severe category since it implies an intense intraoperative corneal insult and management is changed. Extracorneal signs include anterior chamber flare and cell, limbal and conjunctival injection, lid edema, and epiphoria. The patient may also complain of poor vision, photophobia, and ciliary discomfort. The topography is abnormal and the threat of corneal melt is high. Stromal scarring with permanent irregular astigmatism and eventual loss of best-corrected vision is characteristic.

ETIOLOGY

Sands or DLK results from any abuse or injury to a cornea that has had a lamellar incision. Any one of several nonspecific corneal insults can cause DLK, either immediately following the lamellar incision or at any time thereafter. The acute inflammatory interface response is the same if the corneal injury is toxic, thermal, or traumatic. The nonspecific nature of the injury is recognized since DLK has been seen following various corneal insults. For example, DLK has been seen 1 day after LASIK using many different microkeratomes and lasers, both broad beam and scanning type platforms. DLK has been seen after enhancement surgery where no microkeratome was used as well as after lifting a flap to remove an epithelial in-growth[2] where neither a laser nor microkeratome was used. DLK has been reported 1 year after a LASIK procedure of a patient who sustained an embedded metallic foreign body into Bowman's layer of the cornea and in another individual who, 8 months after LASIK, sustained a traumatic partial flap avulsion. When each patient was examined, the flap was adherent to the stromal bed and the infiltrate was localized to the interface beneath the traumatized area. Debris in the interface does not singularly elicit the DLK inflammatory infiltrate; however, interface contamination with various solutions and toxins is suspected. A LASIK-induced epithelial detachment or abrasion, however, is traumatic enough to insult the cornea, producing a DLK response that can progress to grade III and eventual melt.

There has been no proof that DLK results from a genetic predisposition to overreact to LASIK surgery since the epidemiology of cases is such that they have appeared in clusters of 10 to 20 patients in a single setting. Additionally, an exaggerated immune response is unlikely since cases have been reported where DLK was seen after the initial LASIK surgery and not after laser enhancement months later on the same eye. A DLK response following LASIK surgery is not an indication that the same response will occur at enhancement surgery and an uneventful initial LASIK procedure will not guarantee an uncomplicated enhancement.

Toxic Insult

Robert Maddox, MD has done extensive research on the effects of organic esters and hydrocarbons on the cornea. These compounds are found in lubricants and machine oils. They have been identified on keratome blades as well as seen coming from various microkeratome motors. Dr. Maddox hypothesizes that as the flap tissue passes through the microkeratome head some of these toxic motor oils or silicone oils contaminate the cornea, directly provoking the insult. A secondary effect of the oils has been considered in conjunction with the energy emitted by the excimer laser. For example, little was known about sterile inflammations while thousands of automated lamellar keratoplasties (ALKs) were being performed with the same instrumentation as is used in LASIK.[3] It has been suggested that debris deposited in the interface in the form of machine oils, sterile bacterial endotoxin, cleaning solutions, or ocular lubricants can in some manor be activated by the excimer energy inciting the inflammation. If we assume that similar debris has been deposited over the years while lamellar surgery has been performed without an inflammatory response, then perhaps the excimer laser excites the interface deposit influencing the inflammation. Although this is all hypothetical, it is for this reason that some authors have hypothesized that the deposited interface debris acts as a catalyst to the inflammation.

John Doane, MD has implicated toxins in the form of endotoxin as a cause of DLK. If reusable instruments such as cannulas are cleaned and left out overnight to dry, bacteria can grow in them. Sterilization will kill the bacteria with liberation of their endotoxin. It has been hypothesized that when the sterilized cannula is used, the endotoxin is deposited in the interface provoking the insult, causing DLK. The sterile water in autoclaves can also develop a high concentration of endotoxin if not changed regularly. This sterile water laced with endotoxin can find its way into the interface, causing DLK. Although this is not the singular cause of DLK, it should be considered, and appropriate steps taken to minimize the accumulation of endotoxin in cannulas, on instruments, and in autoclaves. We suggest that instruments not be allowed to air dry overnight and that they be sterilized in sealed peal packs after the surgical day. Any moisture in the packs after sterilization indicates a violation and those instruments should be completely reprocessed. After surgery, the sterilizer water reservoir should be completely drained and immediately dried with blown air to prevent the growth of bacteria in the residual fluid. Regular maintenance of the sterilizer reservoir is mandatory if steam sterilization is used otherwise dry heat sterilization could be considered. Dry heat sterilization has, to date, not been implicated in cases of DLK since there is no moisture present to permit bacterial growth.

Traumatic Insult

DLK has been identified in several cases following corneal trauma, most commonly LASIK-induced epithelial abrasions and dehiscense. DLK must be ruled out 1 day after LASIK surgery complicated by iatrogenic corneal abrasion. The traumatized and displaced epithelium is irritating and evidently provokes more of an inflammatory reaction than the planned lamellar incision. The level of insult can potentially be severe enough to elicit a complete interface infiltrate with melt. Postoperatively, DLK has been identified 8 months after surgery in a patient who sustained an embedded metallic corneal foreign body. The small foreign body was embedded in the flap through the epithelium to the level of Bowman's layer and otherwise appeared uncomplicated. It did, however, incite an interface inflammatory response that was localized to just underneath the traumatized cornea. In another case following flap lift for epithelial in-growth, where neither laser nor microkeratome was used, DLK was seen the day after the intervention. In these cases, we must consider the trauma of the foreign body or flap lift as being potentially significant with the inciting insult being the liberation of proteolytic digestive enzymes from the keratocytes as well as, in the case of the cap lift the aberrant epithelial cyst cells.[4] The self-perpetuating nature of the DLK inflammatory response can ultimately cause an infiltrate, which potentially can progress to melt if medical therapy is not begun.

Thermal Insult

The energy released at the corneal surface by ablation may directly elevate the temperature of the stromal tissue to traumatic levels. We have demonstrated the temperature effects of the broad beam Excimer laser using an infrared thermometer. We have established that the normal corneal temperature in a 23.3°C (74°F) room is lower than the body temperature at about 33.8°C (93°F). When acted upon by the excimer laser using a 6.5-mm spot and 400 pulses at 10 Hz, the corneal temperature can rise to 41.6°C (107°F). It has also been shown that during myopic PRK ablation the corneal temperature may increase to 53.3°C (127.9°F),[5] creating more haze and prolonged reduced corneal sensitivity. The "haze" pattern of stromal thermal injury following PRK is similar in appearance to the interface infiltrate pattern, implying that the inflammatory cells orient along collagen bundle lines. The subepithelial infiltrate seen in these cases was similar to the white granular infiltrate seen with DLK but was on the surface just beneath the epithelium. It has been hypothesized that broad beam lasers running at 10 Hz could be increasing the stromal temperature especially near the end of the case when the cornea is slightly drier and the spot size is in the 5.5- to 6.5-mm range. The sudden rise in temperature could be enough to directly cause a corneal burn inciting an interface inflammatory reaction. The energy released at the corneal surface may also indirectly cause an interface inflammation by acting on deposited debris, converting this otherwise inert material into a toxin. It is for this reason that even though tens of thousands of ALKs were preformed, only 2 questionable cases of interface inflammation were reported. Other authors have also postulated that perhaps the lens and mirror coatings on the laser optics could wear with use, allowing additional quanta of energy to strike the corneal surface during ablation. Evidence to support the hypothesis that the laser energy either directly induces a stromal insult or indirectly converts an interface deposit into a toxin is seen in a nonerrodable mask case. Here we see a case of a +2.50 hyperope treated with 3 graduated nonerrodable masks in 1997. The central 3.5-mm area was masked from the laser energy throughout the entire case and has no infiltrate. The area between the 3.5- and 4.0-mm masks received a total laser energy dose of 33% and the infiltrate is mild. The ringed area between the 4.0- and the 4.5-mm masks received 66% of the total laser energy and has a moderate infiltrate. Finally, the peripheral interface received 100% of the total excimer dose and exhibits a full grade II DLK. From this example we can conclude that the degree of interface inflammation is directly proportional to the exposure of laser energy

Sterile Glove Contaminant

Diana Hatsis, BS Rn discovered that the silicone oils lubricant used in sterile surgical gloves can be transferred onto instruments and then into the interface, provoking an inflammatory DLK reaction. It has been recommended that only powderless Biogel (Regent Medical, Norcross, Ga) surgical gloves be used because they are not covered in toxic oils or talc. Shown is the imprint of a silicone-coated glove fingerprint on an adhesive drape (Figure 15-4).

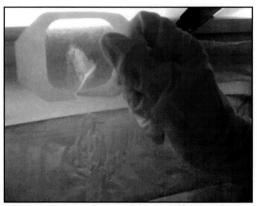

Figure 15-4. Adhesive drape silicone finger-print. (Courtesy Diana Hatsis, RN.)

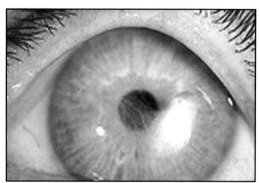

Figure 15-5. DLK-reduced flap adherence.

DIFFERENTIAL DIAGNOSIS

The diagnosis of DLK or Sands is most often made the day following LASIK surgery when the patient presents with the previously described corneal infiltrate. DLK is differentiated from epithelial ingrowth, which is dendritiform and sheet-like in appearance with slow advancement. DLK is differentiated from a bacterial keratitis since an infection is seen more commonly on the second or third postop day. DLK also has well-defined borders, is limited to the interface, and is characterized as a linear, white, granular interface infiltrate in a pattern resembling the shifting desert sands. In contrast, an infectious keratitis is usually a nebulous focal infiltrate associated with stromal extension past the limits of the interface. DLK is painless and not tender to the touch while even a small infectious infiltrate is likely to be very painful. Poor flap adherence is associated with the interface infiltrate and flap macrostriae have often been seen with DLK (Figure 15-5).

DELAYED ONSET SANDS OF SAHARA SYNDROME

The delayed onset variant is seen from the second day to within 1 week of a lamellar surgical procedure. It is believed that either an unrecognized subclinical infiltrate was present on the first postoperative day and not seen, or the infiltrate appearance was retarded by routine use of postoperative steroid medications. The indolent gradual self-perpetuating nature of the inflammation is such that the infiltrate slowly develops without the patient being aware until cloudy vision results from a dense accumulation of infiltrating cells. Although the timing of delayed onset DLK may complicate the differentiation with infected keratitis, it has the same characteristic DLK appearance is indolent, and is just as threatening.

LATE ONSET SANDS OF SAHARA SYNDROME

This is seen months after corneal lamellar surgery and has thus far only been associated with corneal injury or infection. A history of direct trauma, metallic foreign body, viral keratitis (Figure 15-6), blepharoconjunctivitis, or dry eye with keratitis precedes the characteristic sterile interface infiltrate. The inflammation begins in traumatized corneas under the area of epithelial injury that can then extend throughout the interface. This variation can behave the same as acute onset DLK. Management of the inciting injury is complicated by the necessary

Figure 15-6. Viral keratitis-induced DLK.

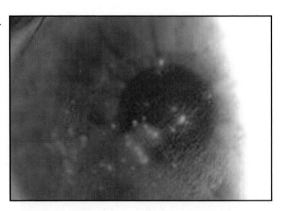

frequent application of topical steroid medication to reduce the sterile interface infiltrate. This can become a management problem if the inciting insult is a viral herpetic keratitis made worse by frequent steroid use.

CENTRAL TOXIC KERATOPATHY

One of the worst complications of LASIK is stromal melt with necrosis. This can result in a hyperopic shift with irregular astigmatism and corneal scaring with loss of best corrected visual acuity (BCVA). Due to the additional unplanned loss of tissue from stromal digestion (melt) the refractive result is usually overcorrected (hyperopic) with irregular astigmatism and loss of BCVA. Also, the resulting necrosis scars the interface and there is a loss of corneal clarity. Due to differential epithelial remodeling, there is often some resolution with an improvement in both the uncorrected visual acuity (UCVA) and BCVA over time. The cornea may clear with time, but overall central toxic keratopathy (CTK) frequently results in visual loss.

INTACS INTRALASE DIFFUSE LAMELLAR KERATITIS

The classic DLK infiltrate has been seen in the Intacs (Addition Technology, Sunnyvale, Calif) channel's following Intralase channel creation on the first postop day. The characteristic appearance of white cells surrounding the Intacs segments is accompanied by a painless expected improvement in vision. These cases have not been reported with any frequency and the infiltrate should be confined to the limited Intacs channel. Although there have been no reports of visual loss to date, we can only assume that stromal melt with irregular astigmatism is possible. We had treated this case with hourly topical steroids, but channel irrigation should be considered if there is no response to the medical therapy.

MANAGEMENT

Prevention

Prevention is the best management of DLK. Since the underlying etiology of DLK is injury to the corneal stroma, the preventative steps listed below are recommended to reduce or eliminate corneal abuse during LASIK surgery. Essentially, these 4 steps reduce the risk of exposure to toxic, thermal, and traumatic insult during LASIK surgery.

1. Clean the microkeratome motor to remove any accumulated lubricant oils. With some motor units, there is a spring-loaded eccentric rotating pin that should be depressed with a Merocel (Medtronic, Jacksonville, Fla) sponge to check for lubricant seepage. The rotating motor end should be gently cleaned then irrigated with fresh water each morning. The microkeratome head, with its accessories, is then sterilized while the motor unit is completely wiped with alcohol. After the day's surgeries, the motor unit should be cleaned and stored with the rotating tip facing up to prevent machine oils from running out.[6]

2. Consider endotoxin as a source of contamination. Do not leave cleaned reusable instruments out to air dry overnight. After surgery, clean, wrap, and sterilize cannulas for storage or preferably use disposable cannulas. Have the autoclave serviced and internally cleaned. Regularly change the water in the autoclave unit to remove potential accumulated endotoxin. Have the reservoir drained on a regular basis and then dried with pressurized canned air. An antiseptic rinse can be used on the chamber as part of the routine maintenance.

3. To reduce the risk of thermal damage from broad beam lasers, use cold balance salt solution (BSS) during the LASIK procedure.[5] Store the BSS overnight in a refrigerator maintained at its coldest setting. A Merocel pledget can be placed on the cornea and irrigated with the cold BSS for 1 minute before the ablation. This should reduce the corneal temperature to below 26.6°C (80°F) at which point laser ablation can proceed. With a broad beam platform running at 10 Hz, treat the stroma slowly to allow the cornea to cool by occasionally pausing the treatment application. As you near the end of the case, the aperture has opened wide and a greater amount of energy is being released with each pulse. Pause more often and as the ablation ends, irrigate the base stroma with the cold BSS (do not irrigate the flap stroma), then reposition the flap as usual. Small aperture flying spot platforms do not produce the same temperature rise per pulse because the diameter of the beam is small, but using cold BSS can be beneficial.

4. Take steps to minimize epithelial cell dehiscense and abrasion. During the preoperative exam, anesthetize the cornea and test the epithelium adherence by rubbing it with a moist cotton swab. Carefully examine the patient for any evidence of map-dot-fingerprint dystrophy. Check for blepharitis and treat with lid hygiene if needed. Preoperatively treat dry eye patients with omega 3, 6, and 9 fatty acid vitamins, (best choice is salmon fish oils). Artificial tears and punctal plug occlusion have been helpful and surgeons report the beneficial effects of preoperative Restasis (cyclosporine 0.05% [Allergan, Irvine, Calif]) bid for 1 month. We should also consider that contact lens intolerant patients may have a subclinical epithelialopathy. Intraoperatively maximize epithelial cell layer adhesion by cooling the cornea with BSS (see above). A cold epithelium appears to be more resistant to abrasion. Reduce anesthetic-induced epithelial toxicity by instilling 0.5% proparacaine hydrochloride just before the speculum is inserted. Absolutely avoid using 0.5% tetracaine because it reduces epithelial adherence and induces epithelial abrasion and dehiscense. Lubricate the epithelium to minimize microkeratome damage by wetting the cornea with cold BSS, artificial tears, and proparacaine just before the lamellar cut is made. After the ablation, gently float the flap into position without surface manipulation. If abrasion or dehiscense occurs, replace the loose epithelial segments. Apply a bandage contact lens after repositioning the flap to minimize direct surface manipulation. If the abrasion is large, consider treating with oral steroids such as 6 to 8 mg Decadron (Merck, Whitehouse Station, NJ) or 60 to 80 mg prednisone and have the patient wait with closed eyes for 1 hour. While waiting, artificial tears or 5% NaCl drops can be applied to the eye then examined at the slit-lamp to assure proper

tissue alignment. Prior to discharge, apply 1% prednisolone acetate drops and then resume the medication hourly at home beginning 3 hours after discharge. Prophylaxis against epithelial-induced DLK should be considered when insult from a significant corneal abrasion occurs. The previously mentioned maneuvers may indirectly prevent DLK by reducing epithelial-induced corneal insult and suppressing the inflammatory response.

Treatment

DLK was classified to predict the likelihood of stromal melt and to provide guidelines for treatment. The self-perpetuating nature of the syndrome requires daily observation, including visual acuity, corneal topography, and a slit-lamp examination. Since DLK is, by definition, a sterile infiltrate, antibiotics are not needed except if used as routine post-LASIK medication. Steroids prevent stromal digestion (melt) by stabilizing the polymorphonuclear cells (PMNs), preventing their release of collagenase and other proteolytic enzymes. Steroids will only secondarily retard or prevent the accumulation of PMNs into the interface. These drugs predominately block cellular enzymatic degranulation by suppressing the liberation of lytic enzymes from lysozymes. By stopping the enzyme-induced stromal injury that accompanies a melt, steroids will reduce the stimulus for additional PMN accumulation into the interface. The self-perpetuation of DLK is then blocked, allowing for resolution of the inflammation.[7]

For treatment guidelines, we recommend using the most potent and penetrating topical steroid available. For this reason, we have used either topical 1% prednisolone acetate or 1% prednisolone phosphate and oral Decadron (Merck, Whitehouse Station, NJ). As a rule of thumb, the frequency of topical steroid drops should be continued until the infiltrate loses its uniformity and begins to break up. The medication can then be slowly tapered, reduced, and discontinued as the infiltrate resolves.

GRADE I

Pred Forte (Allergan) every 2 to 3 hours with daily observation.

GRADE II

If there is access to an operating room, we recommend an immediate prep of the patient for surgery to lift the flap, irrigating the interface with 15 mL of BSS. If there are no operating facilities immediately available, a more conservative management can be carried out as long as the patient is monitored frequently. Pred Forte every 30 minutes continued throughout the night can be used. Daily observation with topography will detect any advancement to grade III. The infiltrate should stabilize in 48 hours and begin to improve in 72 hours. If any dense accumulation of PMNs is seen as progressing to grade III, interface irrigation should be performed without hesitation.

GRADE III

Without delay, surgically intervene. Lift the flap and irrigate the interface with cold BSS; 3 hours later begin hourly topical steroids around the clock. The therapeutic goal is to dilute the concentrated enzyme by washing out the interface and then prevent the self-perpetuation by blocking further enzymatic degranulation. Aggressive wiping to remove PMNs is not necessary and using metallic instruments to wipe the stroma is contraindicated. It must be mentioned that the infiltrate commonly returns the day after wash out, but by immediately starting hourly topical steroid after washing, the reaccumulating PMNs will enter a steroid-rich environment that prevents their enzymatic degranulation. The hourly steroid should be continued until the interface clears in 4 to 6 days.

Grade IV

Wash out the interface as described above. Treat medically with 6.0 to 8.0 mg Decadron before the washout and then 3 hours later begin topical 1% prednisolone acetate or phosphate every hour continuing throughout the night. Manage all associated symptoms with the appropriate treatment (eg, add cycloplegia for an iritis, etc). One day after wash out give a second dose of oral Decadron 8.0 mg and observe for the expected return of the infiltrate. Continue hourly Pred Forte and observe the reaccumulated infiltrate as it begins to resolve over 3 to 4 days. Taper and discontinue the Pred Forte over the next 7 to 10 days.

Central Toxic Keratopathy

One of the worst complications of LASIK is stromal melt with necrosis and opacification. This is usually seen following a grade III or IV DLK without washout. Steroid treatment should be continued and tapered and the patient should be treated with lubrication as the corneal scar resolves. The goal of DLK treatment is to prevent CTK. However, if it is present and associated with an active infiltrate, washing is recommended to prevent further melt. Care must be taken when washing out the interface because in these cases the stromal tissue has thinned and is friable. If the DLK is chronic when the CTK is first seen and there is no active infiltrate, wash out may not be necessary. These cases should be treated with lubricants and a mild topical steroid until the corneal opacification resolves. The IOP should be monitored.

Intacs Intralase

With this procedure, use Pred Forte every 2 to 3 hours with daily observation. Consider channel irrigation if there is no response to the steroids. Always treat DLK aggressively without delay and assure the patient that complete resolution is possible with patient compliance. If there is any doubt as to the classification and subsequent therapy, choose the more aggressive approach. A small infiltrate will increase if treatment is inadequate or delayed. Although washing the interface may at first seem too aggressive, the dramatic improvement of this intervention justifies its application.

PSEUDOSANDS

As ophthalmologists carefully look at the postop LASIK interface, many have noticed an entity that is easily confused with Sands or DLK. The normally clear interface appears to have a generalized granular haze in an asymptomatic patient. This entity can be seen at any time post-LASIK with excellent vision and no associated abnormalities. Surgeons have confused the interface haze with Sands and have treated patients with topical steroids for weeks only to find that the cornea remains unchanged. This haze is seen more frequently when a mechanical microkeratome is used and may only be the "frosted" ends of collagen fibrils torn by the passage of the microkeratome following excimer application. This post-LASIK stable interface haze has been named pseudosands because it has a similar appearance to and is easily confused with Sands but is not Sands or DLK. No treatment is necessary for pseudosands other than observation.

CONCLUSION

DLK or Sands of Sahara is a new syndrome that has become a common post-LASIK management problem. DLK, whose etiology is multifactorial, is a generalized corneal response to injury when a lamellar incision is present. It is not laser specific nor is it seen with any one microkeratome in particular. If not treated correctly, it will completely involve the stromal interface, causing stromal melt with a hyperopic shift, irregular astigmatism, and permanent loss of best-corrected vision. As LASIK becomes more popular, our need to recognize and manage the associated complications becomes heightened. The best treatment for DLK is prevention. The next is awareness of the problem with swift, decisive, and aggressive management. Credit must be given to Dr. Robert Maddox who first described the entity and has done so much to increase our awareness.

KEY POINTS

1. The Sands of Sahara Syndrome (aka Sands) or DLK is a self-perpetuating sterile inflammation of the cornea following any intervention where a lamellar incision has created an interface through stromal tissue.

2. The corneal manifestations of Sands or DLK are characterized by an indolent sterile infiltrate. As early as 12 hours post-LASIK, inflammatory cells can be seen accumulating throughout the stromal interface.

3. Accompanying ocular signs such as anterior chamber cell and flare, conjunctival injection, and lid edema may be seen.

4. DLK is differentiated from epithelial ingrowth, which is dendritiform and sheet like in appearance with slow advancement.

5. DLK has well-defined borders, is limited to the interface and is characterized as a linear white granular interface infiltrate in a pattern resembling the shifting desert sands. In contrast, an infectious keratitis is usually a nebulous focal infiltrate associated with stromal extension past the limits of the interface. DLK is painless and not tender to touch while even a small infectious infiltrate is likely to be very painful.

6. A post-LASIK stable interface haze has been named "pseudosands" because it has a similar appearance to and is easily confused with Sands but is not Sands or DLK. No treatment is necessary for pseudosands other than observation.

7. If DLK is not treated correctly it will completely involve the stromal interface causing stromal melt with a hyperopic shift, irregular astigmatism, and permanent loss of best corrected vision.

REFERENCES

1. Apple DJ, Rabb MF. *Ocular Pathology, Clinical Applications and Self-Assessment.* 4th ed. St Louis, Mo: Mosby Yearbook;1991:64.

2. Smith RJ, Maloney RK. Diffuse lamellar keratitis, new syndrome in lamellar refractive surgery. *Ophthalmology.* 1998;105:1721-1726.

3. Lyle WA, Jin GJC. Initial results of automated lamellar keratoplasty for correction of myopia: one year follow-up. *J Cataract Refract Surg.* 1996;22:31-43.

4. Helena MC, Meisler D, Wilson SE. Epithelial growth within the lamellar interface after laser in situ keratomileusis (LASIK). *Cornea.* 1997;16:300-305.

5. Tsubota K, Toda I, Itoh S. Reduction of subepithelial haze after photorefractive keratectomy by cooling the cornea. *Am J Ophthalmology.* 1997;115:820-821.

6. Maddox R, Hatsis AP. Interface inflammation following LASIK. In: Anderson-Penno EE, Gimbel HV, eds. *LASIK Complications Prevention and Management.* Thorofare, NJ: SLACK Incorporated; 1999:30-36.

7. Smith ME, Lewis RA. *Fundamentals and Principles of Ophthalmology, Section 1.* San Francisco, Calif: American Academy of Ophthalmology. 1987-88:293-295.

Chapter 16

Post-LASIK Infections

Soosan Jacob, MS, FRCS, DNB, MNAMS; Amar Agarwal, MS, FRCS, FRCOphth; and Nibaran Gangopadhyay, MS

Introduction

Laser in situ keratomileusis (LASIK) has become a very common refractive procedure and is generally considered very safe. The incidence of sight-threatening complications after LASIK still remains low. In this backdrop, post-LASIK infections are disastrous complications for the patient who is very often just undergoing a cosmetic procedure and usually has very high expectations (Figure 16-1). Other refractive surgeries such as radial keratotomy (RK), hexagonal keratotomy, and Ruiz procedure have been associated with infections in the past.[1-5] There have also been reports of endophthalmitis after incisional refractive surgery.[2,6–8]

Risk Factors

Infection occurring after photorefractive keratectomy (PRK) may be secondary to the defect in the epithelium (Figure 16-2) as well as the use of therapeutic contact lenses.[9-14] Unlike PRK, the integrity of Bowman's membrane and the corneal epithelium is maintained intact after LASIK, hence the risk for microbial keratitis after LASIK is considered lower than other procedures. Despite this, the occurrence of keratitis after LASIK is a reality, and numerous case reports testify this. Chang et al[15] have reported the incidence of infection after LASIK to vary widely between 0% to 1.5%.

During surgery, the corneal stroma may come into contact with infectious agents coming from the patient's own body or from contaminants present on the instruments. The surgeon and the operating room may also act as a source of infection. Breaks in the epithelial barrier and excessive surgical manipulation are other risk factors. Other factors in the postoperative period such as delayed postoperative re-epithelialization of the cornea, the use of topical steroids, therapeutic contact lenses, as well as the decreased corneal sensitivity and the dry eye situation may all contribute to post-LASIK infections.

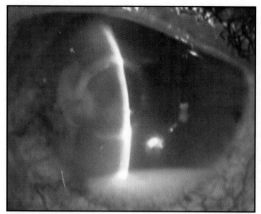

Figure 16-1. Corneal ulcer with hypopyon after LASIK.

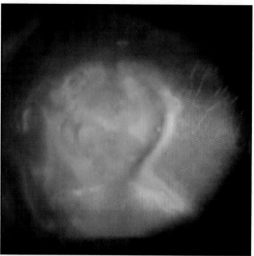

Figure 16-2. Corneal defect staining with fluorescein.

EPIDEMIOLOGY

According to a 2003 American Society of Cataract and Refractive Surgery (ASCRS) survey,[16] 116 infections were reported by 56 LASIK surgeons who had performed an estimated 338,550 procedures. Of these, 76 cases presented in the first week after surgery, 7 during the second week, 17 between the second and fourth weeks, and 16 after 1 month. Forty-seven cases were not diagnosed on initial presentation. Three clusters of mycobacteria with three or more cases in the same clinical setting within 1 month were also reported.

In a similar 2004 survey by the ASCRS,[17] 4.0% of respondents had diagnosed infectious keratitis in their LASIK practice and 2.0% in their PRK practice. There was an increase in the percentage of respondents (from 0.5% to 1.1%) who reported a LASEK patient diagnosed with infectious keratitis during the same period. The most common infectious etiologic agents reported worldwide (55.6%) were gram-positive bacteria, followed by atypical mycobacteria (19.4%) and gram-negative bacteria (13.9%). No respondent had seen a fungal infection. This was in contrast to the results in the 2003 survey, in which fungi were the third most common infectious agent (10.9%).

CLINICAL SIGNS AND SYMPTOMS

Infectious keratitis generally presents later than diffuse lamellar keratitis with which it is often confused. It traditionally presents at least 1 week after surgery and often months later. Fungal keratitis usually has a late onset (2 weeks after surgery), though *S. epidermidis*[18] and *Mycobacterium*[19-21] may also present late.

A focal area of infiltrate associated with diffuse or localized inflammation, which may extend throughout the corneal thickness, is generally seen. It may extend into the untreated area of the cornea and outside the flap. The flap may begin to melt. There may be associated ciliary congestion, secondary iritis, hypopyon, and secondary glaucoma. There is a loss in best corrected visual acuity (BCVA) as well as uncorrected visual acuity (UCVA). The patient may have symptoms such as pain, irritation, lacrimation, photophobia, etc. Atypical organisms such as fungi and mycobacteria are often responsible and therefore there may be no response to the usual antimicrobial therapy. Simultaneous or sequential bilateral involvement of both eyes and infection after flap lift enhancement have also been described.[22-25]

Infectious post-LASIK keratitis must be differentiated from sterile corneal infiltrates, which have been described after PRK[26-28] and LASIK.[29] Sterile infiltrates also present with symptoms similar to infectious keratitis. Subepithelial white infiltrates that may be associated with immune rings are seen in the first few postoperative days. Smears and cultures are negative, and it responds to topical steroids. It may result in stromal scarring and loss of BCVA. Numerous etiologies have been proposed for this, including staphylococcal-immune mediation,[22] secondary to the use of topical nonsteroidal anti-inflammatory drugs (NSAIDs) without concomitant use of topical steroids and contact-lens-induced hypoxia.[28]

HISTOPATHOLOGY

The corneas of the patients who had to undergo penetrating keratoplasty often show partial or complete dehiscense of the flap, signs of acute inflammation affecting all the corneal layers, and evidence of the pathogenic organism such as bacteria or fungi.

MICROBIOLOGY OF POST-LASIK INFECTIONS

Unusual organisms are often responsible for post-LASIK keratitis. The first post-LASIK infection reported was due to Nocardia asteroids.[30] Later, bacterial keratitis due to *Staphylococcus*,[25,31,32] *Streptococcus*,[33,34] *Mycobacterium*,[19-21,24,35] and anaerobes[36;] fungal keratitis due to *Aspergillus*,[37-39] *Curvularia*,[40] *Scedosporium*,[41] and *Acremonium*[42] and also multifocal, polymicrobial keratitis[38,43] have been reported. *Staphylococcus aureus*[25,31,32] and *Mycobacterium*[19-21,24,35] are most commonly observed. Many cultures do become negative[18,44-48] possibly due to antibiotic pretreatment, inadequate culture methods, true culture negativity and misdiagnosis.

The *ASCRS White Paper*[49] on post-LASIK infectious keratitis divides the entity into early onset (occurring within the first 2 weeks of surgery) and late onset (occurring 2 weeks to 3 months after surgery). The organisms seen in early-onset infectious keratitis are common bacterial pathogens such as staphylococcal and streptococcal species. Gram-negative organisms are rare. The organisms seen in late-onset infectious keratitis are usually opportunistic such as fungi, nocardia, and atypical mycobacteria.

Corneal samples should be inoculated in several media, including thioglycolate broth, blood agar, chocolate agar, MacConkey, Löwenstein-Jensen (LJ), and Sabouraud's dextrose agar to facilitate the growth of bacteria, mycobacteria, and fungi. Middlebrook 7H-9 agar may also be used for atypical mycobacteria in addition to LJ media. Appropriate smears should also be taken at the time. Scrapings should also be stained with Gram, Gomori's methenamine silver, and Ziehl-Neelsen to rule out unusual pathogens such as *Nocardia*, atypical mycobacteria, and fungi. Acid-fast staining should include the auramine-rhodamine fluorochrome method and the Kinyoun acid-fast stain.

COMPLICATIONS

The infection can spread to involve all the layers of the cornea and can cause flap and stromal melting and scarring, AC reaction, hypopyon, secondary glaucoma, anterior and posterior synechiae, irregular astigmatism, and loss of BCVA and UCVA.

PREVENTION OF POST-LASIK KERATITIS

It is important to take every possible measure to prevent this sight-threatening complication. Preoperative evaluation of the adnexa and the lacrimal apparatus and treatment of any pre-existing condition should become routine for all patients just as it is for cataract surgery. Some surgeons do advocate performing surgery in only one eye at a time or using completely different sets for the two eyes in case of simultaneous bilateral procedures[50] even though the ASCRS Cornea Clinical Committee does not make this recommendation. It is highly advisable to maintain rigid asepsis throughout the surgical procedure including the use of sterile drapes, etc. Good sterilization techniques are a must and can prevent the use of contaminated instruments. Povidone–iodine solution should be used to paint the lids preoperatively. All fluids applied to the eye before, during, and after LASIK should be sterile as atypical mycobacteria epidemics have originated from the use of nonsterile water used to clean instruments or to the ice used during LASIK.[51-53]

TREATMENT OF POST-LASIK KERATITIS

Early diagnosis and institution of appropriate therapy are of prime importance in the treatment of post-LASIK infections. Any focal infiltrate should be considered infectious until proven otherwise. Flap elevation and culturing should be performed as early as possible in all cases in which post-LASIK infectious keratitis is suspected. Smears help in deciding on immediate treatment that is then changed according to the culture and sensitivity reports. Polymerase chain reaction testing is also helpful in diagnosis. A corneal biopsy may be required in some cases. Empiric therapy is not helpful because opportunistic and atypical organisms with unusual antimicrobial sensitivities are common and these are not responsive to conventional therapy.

The *ASCRS White Paper*[49] recommends elevation of the flap, culture, and irrigation of the stromal bed with antibiotic solution (fortified vancomycin 50 mg/mL for rapid-onset keratitis and fortified amikacin 35 mg/ml for delayed-onset keratitis) for all post-LASIK infectious keratitis.

For rapid-onset keratitis, it recommends a fourth-generation topical fluoroquinolone such as gatifloxacin 0.3% or moxifloxacin 0.5% given in a loading dose every 5 minutes for 3 doses and then every 30 minutes, alternating with an antimicrobial that is rapidly bacteriocidal and has increased activity against gram-positive organisms, such as fortified cefazolin 50 mg/ml every 30 minutes. In patients working in a hospital environment with added risk for methicillin-resistant *Staphylococcus aureus* (MRSA), it recommends the substitution of fortified vancomycin 50 mg/ml for cefazolin every 30 minutes to provide more effective therapy against MRSA. Oral doxycycline 100 mg twice a day to inhibit collagenase production and discontinuation of corticosteroids is also advised. Treatment should be modified according to culture and sensitivity reports.

For delayed-onset keratitis, which is commonly due to atypical mycobacteria, nocardia, and fungi, the *ASCRS White Paper*[49] recommends therapy with amikacin 35 mg/ml every 30 minutes, alternating with a fourth-generation fluoroquinolone (gatifloxacin 0.3% or moxifloxacin 0.5%) every 30 minutes along with oral doxycycline 100 mg twice a day, and discontinuation of corticosteroids.

This treatment is ineffective for fungal infections and often presents late with more extensive keratitis. Appropriate antifungal agents should be started and modified according to sensitivity reports. Fungal infections are often difficult to treat because of the lack of potent antifungal agents, low penetration through intact corneal epithelium, ocular toxicity, and

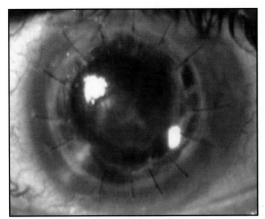

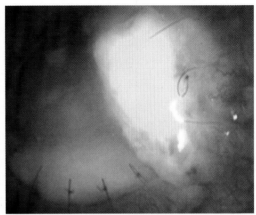

Figure 16-3. Status postpenetrating kerato-plasty.

Figure 16-4. Reinfection with hypopyon after penetrating keratoplasty.

decreased solubility. The flap may often need to be amputated for better penetration of the antifungal agents. In unresponsive cases with extensive involvement of the cornea, a penetrating keratoplasty may often become necessary (Figures 16-3 and 16-4).

Nontuberculous mycobacteria are also indolent and difficult-to-treat pathogens. Giaconi et al[24] recommend a combination of intensive fortified topical amikacin and topical and oral clarithromycin with LASIK flap amputation. Other potentially useful agents include topical tobramycin, the fluoroquinolones ciprofloxacin and ofloxacin,[54,55] and the macrolide azithromycin.[56]

RECENT ADVANCES

The polymerase chain reaction testing can be used to diagnose the causative organism, especially in cases with limited availability of samples.[36] Confocal microscopy can also be of diagnostic use. Muallem et al use confocal microscopy to describe diagnosing yeast infection as highly reflective, round organisms, 3.0 to 4.5 µm in diameter.[23]

KEY POINTS

1. Breaks in the epithelial barrier and excessive surgical manipulation, delayed postoperative re-epithelialization of the cornea, the use of topical steroids and therapeutic contact lenses as well as the decreased corneal sensitivity and the dry eye situation may all contribute to post-LASIK infections.

2. Infectious keratitis traditionally presents at least 1 week after surgery and often months later.

3. A focal area of infiltrate associated with diffuse or localized inflammation, which may extend throughout the corneal thickness is generally seen. It may extend into the untreated area of the cornea and outside the flap. The flap may begin to melt.

4. Atypical organisms such as fungi and mycobacteria are often responsible and therefore, there may be no response to the usual antimicrobial therapy.

5. The organisms seen in early-onset (within the first 2 weeks of surgery) infectious keratitis are common bacterial pathogens such as staphylococcal and streptococcal species. Gram-negative organisms are rare. The organisms seen in late-onset (occurring 2 weeks to 3 months after surgery) infectious keratitis are usually opportunistic such as fungi, *Nocardia*, and atypical *Mycobacteria*.

6. Corneal samples should be inoculated in several media and appropriate smears should be taken. Polymerase chain reaction testing and corneal biopsy may also be required in some cases.

7. Early diagnosis and institution of appropriate therapy are of prime importance in the treatment of post-LASIK infections. Any focal infiltrate should be considered infectious until proven otherwise.

8. The treatment protocol has been described in the *ASCRS White Paper*[49] on post-LASIK infectious keratitis.

REFERENCES

1. Rashid ER, Waring GO III. Complications of radial and transverse keratotomy [review]. *Surv Ophthalmol.* 1989;34:73-106.

2. Jain S, Azar DT. Eye infections after refractive keratotomy [review]. *J Refract Surg.* 1996;12:148-155.

3. Szerenyi K, McDonnell JM, Smith RE, et al. Keratitis as a complication of bilateral simultaneous radial keratotomy [case report]. *Am J Ophthalmol.* 1994;117:462-467.

4. Beldavs RA, al-Ghamdi S, Wilson LA, Waring GO III. Bilateral microbial keratitis after radial keratotomy [case report]. *Arch Ophthalmol.* 1993;111:440.

5. Duffey RJ. Bilateral Serratia marcescens keratitis after simultaneous bilateral radial keratotomy. *Am J Ophthalmol.* 1995;119:233-236.

6. Manka RL, Gast TJ. Endophthalmitis following Ruiz procedure [case report]. *Arch Ophthalmol.* 1990;108:21.

7. McLeod SD, Flowers CW, Lopez PF, et al. Endophthalmitis and orbital cellulitis after radial keratotomy [case report]. *Ophthalmology.* 1995;102:1902-1907.

8. Heideman DG, Dunn SP, Haimann M. Endophthalmitis after radial keratotomy enhancement [case report]. *J Cataract Refract Surg.* 1997;23:951-953.

9. Amayem A, Ali AT, Waring GO III, Ibrahim O. Bacterial keratitis after photorefractive keratectomy. *J Refract Surg.* 1996;12:642-644.

10. Wee WR, Kim JY, Choi YS, Lee JH. Bacterial keratitis after photorefractive keratectomy in a young, healthy man [case report]. *J Cataract Refract Surg.* 1997;23:954-956.

11. Fulton JC, Cohen EJ, Rapuano CJ. Bacterial ulcer 3 days after excimer laser phototherapeutic keratectomy. *Arch Ophthalmol.* 1996;114:626-627.

12. Sampath R, Ridgway AEA, Litherbarrow B. Bacterial keratitis following excimer laser photorefractive keratectomy: a case report [letter]. *Eye.* 1994;8(Pt 4):481-482.

13. Aron-Rosa DS, Colin J, Aron B, et al. Clinical results of excimer laser photorefractive keratectomy: a multicenter study of 265 eyes. *J Cataract Refract Surg.* 1995;21:644-652.

14. Malling S. Keratitis with loss of useful vision after photorefractive keratectomy. *J Cataract Refract Surg.* 1999;25:137-139.

15. Chang MA, Jain S, Azar DT. Infections following laser in situ keratomileusis: an integration of the published literature. *Surv Ophthalmol.* 2004;49:269-280.

16. Solomon R, Donnenfeld ED, Azar DT et al. Infectious keratitis after laser in situ keratomileusis: results of an ASCRS survey. *J Cataract Refract Surg.* 2003;29:2001-2006.

17. Sandoval HP, Castro LF, Vroman DT et al. Refractive Surgery Survey 2004. *J Cataract Refract Surg.* 2005;31:221-233.

18. Karp KO, Hersh PS, Epstein RJ. Delayed keratitis after laser in situ keratomileusis. *J Cataract Refract Surg.* 2000;26:925-928.

19. Solomon A, Karp CL, Miller D, et al. Mycobacterium interface keratitis after laser in situ keratomileusis. *Ophthalmology.* 2001;108:2201-2208.

20. Garg P, Bansal AK, Sharma S, Vemuganti GK. Bilateral infectious keratitis after laser in situ keratomileusis; a case report and review of the literature. *Ophthalmology.* 2001;108:121-125.

21. Chung MS, Goldstein MH, Driebe Jr WT, Schwartz BH. Mycobacterium chelonae keratitis after laser in situ keratomileusis successfully treated with medical therapy and flap removal. *Am J Ophthalmol.* 2000;129:382-384.

22. Rao SK, Fogla R, Rajagopal R, et al. Bilateral corneal infiltrates after excimer laser photorefractive keratectomy. *J Cataract Refract Surg.* 2000;26:456-459.

23. Muallem MS, Alfonso EC, Romano AC, et al. Bilateral *Candida parapsilosis* interface keratitis after laser in situ keratomileusis. *J Cataract Refract Surg.* 2003;29:2022-2025.

24. Giaconi JA, Pham R, Ta CN. Bilateral *Mycobacterium abscessus* keratitis after laser in situ keratomileusis. *J Cataract Refract Surg.* 2002;28:887-890.

25. Suresh PS, Rootman DS. Bilateral infectious keratitis after a laser in situ keratomileusis enhancement procedure. *J Cataract Refract Surg.* 2002;28:720-721.

26. Sher NA, Frantz JM, Talley A, et al. Topical diclofenac in the treatment of ocular pain after excimer photorefractive keratectomy. *Refract Corneal Surg.* 1993;9:425-436

27. Sher NA, Krueger RR, Teal P, et al. Role of topical corticosteroids and nonsteroidal antiinflammatory drugs in the etiology of stromal infiltrates after excimer photorefractive keratectomy (letter). *J Refract Corneal Surg.* 1994;10:587-588.

28. Teal P, Breslin C, Arshinoff S, Edmison D. Corneal subepithelial infiltrates following excimer laser photorefractive keratectomy. *J Cataract Refract Surg.* 1995;21:516-518.

29. Haw WW, Manche EE. Sterile peripheral keratitis following laser in situ keratomileusis. *J Refract Surg.* 1999;15:61-63.

30. Pérez-Santonja JJ, Sakla HF, Abad JL, et al. Nocardial keratitis after laser in situ keratomileusis. *J Refract Surg.* 1997;13:314-317.

31. Rudd JC, Moshirfar M. Methicillin-resistant *Staphylococcus aureus* keratitis after laser in situ keratomileusis. *J Cataract Refract Surg.* 2001;27:471-473.

32. Rubinfeld RS, Negvesky GJ. Methicillin-resistant *Staphylococcus aureus* ulcerative keratitis after laser in situ keratomileusis. *J Cataract Refract Surg.* 2001;27:1523-1525.

33. Dada T, Sharma N, Dada VK, Vajpayee RB. Pneumococcal keratitis after laser in situ keratomileusis. *J Cataract Refract Surg.* 2000;26:460-461.

34. Ramírez M, Hernández-Quintela E, Beltrán F, Naranjo-Tackman R. Pneumococcal keratitis at the flap interface after laser in situ keratomileusis. *J Cataract Refract Surg.* 2002;28:550-552.

35. Chandra NS, Torres MF, Winthrop KL, et al. Cluster of *Mycobacterium chelonae* keratitis cases following laser in-situ keratomileusis. *Am J Ophthalmol.* 2001;132:819-830.

36. Ferrer C, Abad JL, Alio J. Unusual anaerobic bacteria in keratitis after laser in situ keratomileusis: diagnosis using molecular biology methods. *J Cataract Refract Surg.* 2004;30:1790-1794.

37. Sridhar MS, Garg P, Bansal AK, Gopinathan U. *Aspergillus flavus* keratitis after laser in situ keratomileusis. *Am J Ophthalmol.* 2000;129:802-804.

38. Ritterband D, Kelly J, McNamara T, et al. Delayed-onset multifocal polymicrobial keratitis after laser in situ keratomileusis. *J Cataract Refract Surg.* 2002;28:898-899.

39. Kuo IC, Margolis TP, Cevallos V, Hwang DG. *Aspergillus fumigatus* keratitis after laser in situ keratomileusis. *Cornea.* 2001;20:342-344.

40. Chung MS, Goldstein MH, Driebe Jr WT, Schwartz B. Fungal keratitis after laser in situ keratomileusis: A case report. *Cornea.* 2000;19:236-237.

41. Sridhar MS, Garg P, Bansal AK, Sharma S. Fungal keratitis after laser in situ keratomileusis. *J Cataract Refract Surg.* 2000;26:613-615.

42. Alfonso JF, Santos J, Astudillo A, et al. Acremonium fungal infection in 4 patients after laser in situ keratomileusis. *J Cataract Refract Surg.* 2004;30:269-274.

43. Gupta V, Dada T, Vajpayee RB, et al. Polymicrobial keratitis after laser in situ keratomileusis. *J Refract Surg.* 2001;17:147-148.

44. Quiros PA, Chuck RS, Smith RE, et al. Infectious ulcerative keratitis after laser in situ keratomileusis. *Arch Ophthalmol.* 1999;117:1423-1427.

45. Aras C, Özdamar A, Bahçecioglu H, Sener B. Corneal interface abscess after excimer laser in situ keratomileusis. *J Refract Surg.* 1998;14:156-157.

46. Stulting RD, Carr JD, Thompson KP, et al. Complications of laser in situ keratomileusis for the correction of myopia. *Ophthalmology.* 1999;106:13-20.

47. Lam DSC, Leung ATS, Wu JT, et al. Culture-negative ulcerative keratitis after laser in situ keratomileusis. *J Cataract Refract Surg.* 1999;25:1004-1008.

48. Lin RT, Maloney RK. Flap complications associated with lamellar refractive surgery. *Am J Ophthalmol.* 1999;127:129-136.

49. Donnenfeld ED, Kim T, Holland E,J et al. ASCRS White Paper: Management of infectious keratitis following laser in situ keratomileusis. *J Cataract Refract Surg.* 2005;31:2008-2011.

50. Kohnen T. Infections after corneal refractive surgery: can we do better? (editorial). *J Cataract Refract Surg.* 2002;28:569–570.

51. Fulcher SFA, Fader RC, Rosa RH, Holmes GP. Delayed-onset mycobacterial keratitis after LASIK. *Cornea.* 2002;21:546–554.

52. Freitas D, Alvarenga L, Sampaio J, et al. An outbreak of *Mycobacterium chelonae* infection after LASIK. *Ophthalmology.* 2003;110:276–285.

53. Winthrop KL, Steinberg EB, Holmes G, et al. Epidemic and sporadic cases of nontuberculous mycobacterial keratitis associated with laser in situ keratomileusis. *Am J Ophthalmol.* 2003;135:223–224.

54. Hu F-R, Luh K-T. Topical ciprofloxacin for treating nontuberculous mycobacterial keratitis. *Ophthalmology.* 1998;105:269-272

55. Hu F-R, Wang I-J. Comparison of topical antibiotics for treating *Mycobacterium chelonae* keratitis in a rabbit model. *Curr Eye Res.* 1998;17:478-482

56. Tabbara KF, Al-Kharashi SA, Al-Mansouri SM, et al. Ocular levels of azithromycin. *Arch Ophthalmol.* 1998;116:1625-1628.

Chapter 17

EPITHELIAL INGROWTH

Amar Agarwal, MS, FRCS, FRCOphth and
Soosan Jacob, MS, FRCS, DNB, MNAMS

INTRODUCTION

Epithelial ingrowth after LASIK is a known complication occurring in up to 0.2[1] to 0.4% of cases.[2] The incidence may be higher, up to 15% of cases[3-9] where adherence to meticulous surgical technique is not followed. It may remain as an innocuous, nonprogressive condition or may progress to become a potentially sight-threatening condition. In a study of 1245 LASIK cases, there was a 14.7% rate of epithelial ingrowth and a 1.7% rate of clinically significant epithelial ingrowth.[10] In a study by Wang and Maloney, the incidence of significant epithelial ingrowth after primary treatment was 0.92%, and 1.7% after enhancement. Clinically significant ingrowth recurred in 10 of 43 eyes after the initial surgical removal.[11]

HISTOPATHOLOGY

Epithelial cell ingrowth (Figure 17-1) may be secondary to one of two mechanisms in a post-LASIK patient. The cells may be introduced into the interface either during the microkeratome pass or during other steps such as irrigation of the bed or repositioning of the flap. The other possible mechanism for epithelial ingrowth is due to loss of contact inhibition of the epithelial cell layer. Epithelial cells on the surface of the cornea have contact inhibition. Therefore, as long as a cell is surrounded on all sides with other epithelial cells, it does not have any stimulus to migrate. On the other hand, once this contact is gone, the epithelial layer starts to migrate to fill in this defect due to loss of contact inhibition. In LASIK, the discontinuity in the epithelium at the margin of the flap acts as a stimulus for epithelial ingrowth. This is overcome in the large majority of patients by the firm adhesion of the flap to the stromal bed. In cases with poor adhesion, the epithelial cells actively proliferate and begin to move centrally into the interface to cover the perceived defect.[12]

Figure 17-1. Epithelial ingrowth after LASIK.

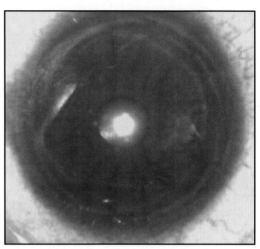

RISK FACTORS

The very nature of LASIK as a lamellar surgery predisposes it to the development of epithelial ingrowth. In uncomplicated LASIK, it may occur either during surgery because of implantation of epithelial cells during the surgical steps or it may occur postoperatively as an ingrowth occurring from the edges of the flap. It may occur in cases with complications such as torn buttonholes or irregular flaps (Table 17-1).

CLASSIFICATION

Machat[13,14] has classified epithelial ingrowth based on its severity and treatment strategy.

Grade 1

This presents as an early, nonprogressive faintly visible ingrowth within 2 mm of the flap edge with a demarcation line and no changes in the overlying flap. This requires observation only.

Grade 2

The ingrowth is a greyish white, slowly progressive nest within 2 mm of the flap edge, which is thickened or may be rolled up or grey with no clear demarcation line. This requires treatment within 2 to 3 weeks if there is evidence of further progression.

Grade 3

This exceeds 2 mm from the flap edge, showing thick, opaque, and whitish nests of epithelial cells. It extends toward the visual axis and shows erosion or melting of the flap with exposure of the stromal bed. This grade requires urgent treatment and intensive follow-up.

> ### Table 17-1
> ## *Risk Factors for Epithelial Ingrowth After LASIK*
>
> *Patient Factors*
>
> - Older patient
> - History of recurrent corneal erosions
> - Basement membrane epithelial dystrophy
> - Diabetes
> - Blepharospasm
> - Forcible eye rubbing
> - Similar complication in the other eye
>
> *Surgical Factors*
>
> - Excessive usage of topical anesthetics
> - Excessive manipulation and/or drying of the corneal epithelium
> - Excessive irrigation with hydration of the flap
> - Flap edema due to any cause
> - Poor quality blade
> - Epithelial defect during surgery
> - Hyperopic LASIK
> - Transition zones extending beyond the flap edge
> - Displaced, improperly aligned flap
> - Flap striae
> - Unstable flap
> - Thin, torn, irregular flaps with ragged edges
> - Free caps
> - Buttonholes, partial flaps
> - Enhancement procedure
> - Flap lift for the treatment of any other complication
> - LASIK over previous radial keratotomy, penetrating keratoplasty

CLINICAL FEATURES

Symptoms

Epithelial ingrowth may be mild, which is usually asymptomatic and seen on routine evaluation. In moderate cases, the patient may have foreign body sensation, photophobia, congestion, pain, irritation, ghosting, glare, halos, and loss of best-corrected visual acuity (BCVA). The dry eye symptoms may be worse in these patients as compared to others due to the irregular ocular surface leading to a decreased tear break-up time. In very severe cases, the patient may present with loss of vision, intense pain, and other symptoms due to stromal melting. It can cause haze and discomfort, especially if the lifted edge is sensed when blinking.

Signs

The epithelial ingrowth may be seen as white or gray nests of cells or as finger-like extensions extending inwards from the flap edges. Epithelial ingrowth may also be seen as a thin sheet within the interface or sometimes as a combination. Indirect slit-lamp illumination is sometimes required to see the sheet-like proliferation. It can also be seen on retroillumination. Epithelial ingrowth is usually located at the periphery but may occasionally begin from the center of the flap, especially in cases secondary to buttonhole or central epithelial defects. In nasally-hinged flaps, it is seen most commonly at the temporal margin, whereas in superiorly hinged flaps, it is seen commonly at the inferior margin and at the border of the hinge.[12] Fluorescein solution when instilled into the flap stains the involved area. It may also delineate the area of ingrowth. An increase in staining at the area of impending flap melt may also be seen.[12] One can also detect the potential for ingrowth by instilling fluorescein. This demonstrates areas of the cut in the cornea that have yet to be epithelialized.

Epithelial ingrowth can cause a decrease in vision by growing into the visual axis or secondary to irregular astigmatism via interface elevations.[15] Progressive epithelial ingrowth may induce astigmatism by causing flattening of the meridian, where the ingrowth is located, and steepening of the meridian 90 degrees away.[12] Very severe cases may present with flap or stromal necrosis.

FORMS

Epithelial ingrowth can exist in 2 forms, benign and aggressive.[12]

Benign Form

It is seen within 2 mm of the flap edge and may occur as a diffuse or localized form. It may be slowly progressive or nonprogressive and may sometimes disappear after a few months, leaving a residual haze in the interface.

Aggressive Form

It appears in the shape of cell nests—pearl-like small islands, sheaths, colonies, strands, or cysts—without any demarcating white line. As the condition progresses, these nests become whitish and tend to merge together.

FOLLOW-UP

All patients with epithelial ingrowth must be monitored regularly for the development of any complications. All patients who have undergone LASIK should have a postoperative visit scheduled at around the third month to look for the onset of any epithelial ingrowth.

COMPLICATIONS

Epithelial ingrowth may induce regular and irregular astigmatism with resulting decreased vision. It may also result in melting of the flap or the stromal bed. Epithelial fistulas may form near the flap margin. Clinically significant ingrowth may interfere with diffusion of nutrients between aqueous and flap tissue. Collagenase and protease enzymes that are released by necrotic epithelial cells may result in stromal and flap melting. The presence of stromal inflammation may be an early sign of necrosis.

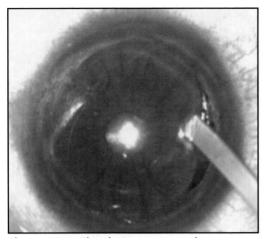

Figure 17-2. Flap being separated to remove the epithelial ingrowth.

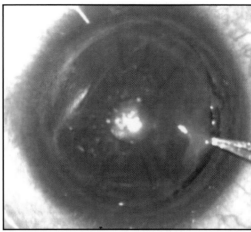

Figure 17-3. Forceps used to grasp the epithelial ingrowth.

Figure 17-4. Epithelial ingrowth removed.

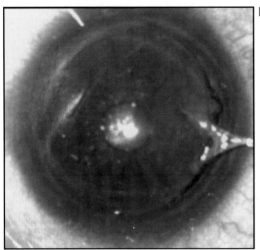

TREATMENT

The limited, benign form of epithelial ingrowth, less or equal than 2 mm in diameter, does not require treatment. Treatment is required only when epithelial ingrowth interferes with, or threatens to interfere with, visual acuity by encroaching onto the visual axis, causing other complications such as irregular astigmatism, or threatening to cause stromal necrosis or flap melt. Treatment is also indicated in case of symptomatic ingrowth. Numerous techniques have been described for the management of epithelial ingrowth. Techniques for removal include scraping of epithelial ingrowth and excimer laser phototherapeutic keratectomy (PTK).[15] The flap is reflected and the ingrowth is peeled off like a sheet using fine forceps (Figures 17-2 to 17-4) or by scraping both the stromal bed and the undersurface of the flap (Figures 17-5 and 17-7). The bed is then well irrigated before replacing the flap. Excimer laser PTK may also be used to remove the epithelial cells.[16] Adjuncts such as cryotherapy, cocaine, Nd:YAG laser, mitomycin-C, and sutures may lead to a decreased incidence of recurrence. Some authors[15,17] have reported success with ethanol and laser therapy for recurrences. The major difficulty in

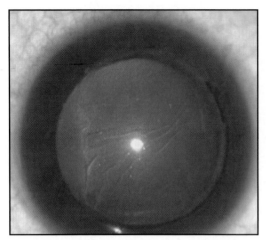

Figure 17-5. Patient with an epithelial ingrowth after a nasal hinge flap.

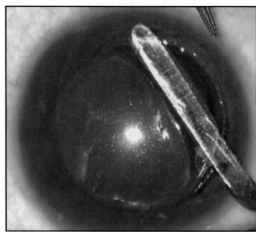

Figure 17-6. Flap is being lifted with a spatula. One should be careful when one does this so that a flap tear does not occur.

Figure 17-7. Epithelial ingrowth from the undersurface of the flap is removed.

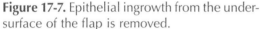

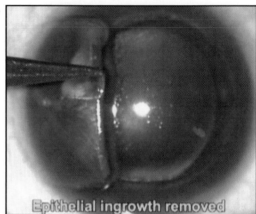

the management of epithelial ingrowth is the high incidence of recurrences even after treatment. Recurrence of epithelial ingrowth after treatment has been reported to be as high as 44%.[11] In the same study, 23% of patients treated for epithelial ingrowth had to undergo a second procedure because the recurrence was deemed clinically significant.

Recurrence of ingrowth can be caused by improper adhesion of the flap to the bed, which leaves behind a potential space for the cells to grow. It has been suggested to place interrupted sutures[18,19] at the site of ingrowth after epithelial removal with just enough tension to oppose the flap to the bed without inducing striae. The sutures can be removed after 1 month.

PREVENTION

Extra care in patients with known risk factors, minimal and careful use of local anesthetics, avoiding excessive flap manipulations, careful relifts, using new blades, and careful attention to meticulous technique all play a very important role in decreasing the incidence of epithelial ingrowth. It is important to avoid large transition zones on small beds and shield the hinge area as necessary.

RECENT ADVANCES

Cryotherapy of the cornea[20] at the area of the epithelial ingrowth has been described as a noninvasive, nonaggressive, and efficacious method to destroy epithelial ingrowth.

KEY POINTS

1. Epithelial ingrowth after LASIK is a known complication occurring in up to 0.2% to 0.4% of cases. The incidence may be higher up to 15% in cases where adherence to meticulous surgical technique is not followed.

2. The cells may be introduced into the interface either during the microkeratome pass or other steps such as irrigation of the bed or repositioning of the flap.

3. In LASIK, the discontinuity in the epithelium at the margin of the flap acts as a stimulus for epithelial ingrowth.

4. Collagenase and protease enzymes that are released by necrotic epithelial cells may result in stromal and flap melting.

5. Treatment is required only when epithelial ingrowth interferes with or threatens to interfere with visual acuity by encroaching onto the visual axis or by causing other complications such as irregular astigmatism or threatening to cause stromal necrosis or flap melt.

REFERENCES

1. Kornmehl EW. *Management of Striae and Epithelial Ingrowth Following LASIK*. Presented to: New England Ophthalmological Society; October 1999.

2. Walker MB, Wilson SE. Incidence and prevention of epithelial growth within the interface after laser in situ keratomileusis. *Cornea*. 2000;19:170-173.

3. Lindstrom RL, Hardten DR, Houtman DM, et al. Six-month results of hyperopic and astigmatic LASIK in eyes with primary and secondary hyperopia. *Trans Am Ophthalmol Soc*. 1999;97:241-255.

4. Stulting RD, Carr JD, Thompson KP, Waring GO III, Wiley WM, Walker JG. Complications of laser in situ keratomileusis for the correction of myopia. *Ophthalmology*. 1999;106:13-20.

5. Yildirim R, Devranoglu K, Ozdamar A, et al. Flap complications in our learning curve of laser in situ keratomileusis using the Hansatome microkeratome. *Eur J Ophthalmol*. 2001;11:328-332.

6. Helena MC, Meisler D, Wilson SE. Epithelial growth within the lamellar interface after laser in situ keratomileusis (LASIK). *Cornea*. 1997;16:300-305.

7. Wang MY, Maloney RK. Epithelial ingrowth after laser in situ keratomileusis. *Am J Ophthalmol*. 2000;129:746-751.

8. Spigelman AV. Complications of LASIK. *J Refract Surg*. 2001;17:475.

9. Melki SA, Azar DT. LASIK complications: etiology, management, and prevention. *Surv Ophthalmol*. 2001;46:95-116.

10. Carr JD, Nardon R Jr, Stulting RD, et al. Risk factors for epithelial ingrowth after LASIK. *Invest Ophthalmol Vis Sci*. 1997;28(4):S232.

11. Wang MY Maloney RK. Epithelial ingrowth after laser in situ keratomileusis. *Am J Ophthalmol*. 2000;129:746-751.

12. Chawla JS. Complications of LASIK part 2—Epithelial ingrowth. Available online at: http://www.optometry.co.uk/files/25a4db11c71b7215d414770adb90a9b6_chawla20031003.pdf. Accessed August 24, 2006.

13. Buratto L, Brint S. *LASIK: Surgical Techniques and Complications*. 2nd ed. Thorofare, NJ: SLACK Incorporated; 2000.

14. Probst LE, Machat JJ. Epithelial ingrowth following LASIK. In: Machat JJ, Slade SG, Probst LE, eds. *The Art of LASIK*. 2nd ed. Thorofare, NJ: SLACK Incorporated; 1999:427-433.

15. Lahners WJ, Hardten DR, et al. Alcohol and mechanical scraping for epithelial ingrowth following laser in situ keratomileusis. *J Refract Surg*. 2005;21(2).

16. Fagerholm P, Molander N, et al. Epithelial ingrowth after LASIK treatment with scraping and phototherapeutic keratectomy. *Acta Ophthalmol Scand*. 2004;82(6):707-713.

17. Haw WW, Manche EE. Treatment of progressive or recurrent epithelial ingrowth with ethanol following laser in situ keratomileusis. *J Refract Surg*. 2001;17:63-67.

18. Kohnen T. Refractive surgical problem. Consultation Section. *J Cat Refract Surg*. 2003;29(5).

19. Rojas MC, Lumba JD. Treatment of epithelial ingrowth after laser in situ keratomileusis with mechanical debridement and flap suturing. *Arch Ophthalmol*. 2004;122(7):997-1001.

20. Murube J, Murube E, et al. New treatment by cryotherapy of the sublamellar epithelial ingrowth after lasik. *Arch Soc Canar Oftal*. 2000;11.

Chapter 18

DEALING WITH IRREGULAR ASTIGMATISM: STATE OF THE ART

Jorge L. Alió, MD, PhD and José I. Belda, MD, PhD

DEFINITION

Irregular astigmatism (IA) is one of the most frequent complications of corneal injuries, corneal surgery (especially refractive surgery), and corneal grafting. It also complicates certain corneal diseases such as keratoconus. Its incidence was relatively unnoticed and underestimated until computerized videokeratography showed that the prevalence of some patterns were as high as 40%.[1,2]

IA has been variously defined. The astigmatism is defined as irregular if the principal meridians are not 90 degrees apart, usually because of an irregularity of the corneal curvature, and it cannot be completely corrected with a spherocylindrical lens. Duke-Elder defines IA as a refractive condition in which the refraction in different meridians conforms to no geometric plan and the refracted rays have no planes of symmetry.[3] Clinically, IA is only correctable by a contact lens.[1] However, contact lens fitting is not the unique choice to treat these patients, but rather an alternative to new surgical approaches—the aim of which is to correct the irregular cornea.

EXAMINATION

The most common clinical symptoms of induced IA are decrease in best corrected vision and visual distortion, together with night and/or day glare. Other subjective symptoms reported by the patient are haloes, dazzling, monocular diplopia, or polyopia.

When managing IA patients, a meticulous preoperative evaluation is mandatory, including previous medical reports and a complete ocular examination: uncorrected visual acuity (UCVA) and best-corrected visual acuity (BCVA), pinhole visual acuity and cycloplegic refraction, retinoscopy, keratometry, and contact ultrasonic pachymetry. Successful correction of the IA by hard contact lens fitting may also help to assure the presence of corneal IA.

Clinically, IA will present with a typical *retinoscopy* pattern, the most common being spinning and scissoring of the red reflex. On attempting *keratometry*, the mires will appear distorted. *Corneal topography* shows certain patterns and numerical indices for IA that will be useful for the diagram and follow-up. With this technology, it is possible to define different patterns for IA, which have been essential to develop different surgical techniques to treat it. The elevation topography of the Orbscan system is probably less useful than the placido disk tangential maps when studying, understanding, and classifying corneal IA.

The most recent and sophisticated technique is the application of *wavefront examination* (aberrometers),[4] especially corneal wavefront analysis. This method measures the refractive status of the whole internal ocular light path. By comparing the wavefront of a pattern of several small beams of coherent light projected through to the retina with the emerging reflected light wavefront, it is possible to measure the refractive path taken by each beam and to infer the specific spatial correction required on each path. Corneal wavefront analysis is performed by a mathematical transformation of the corneal topography data and it is much more meaningful than global wavefront for the purposes of corneal IA study and correction.

Another method for determining higher-order aberrations of the eye is *ray-tracing*.[5] A laser beam is delivered parallel to the optical axis onto the retina sequentially through different pupil locations. The retinal images of each spot are viewed by a charge-coupled device (CCD) camera and put together to a spot diagram in pupillotopic arrangement. Wavefront errors are computed by analyzing the spot diagram. Although this simulated ray tracing does not provide information about the true aberrations of the eye, it is a useful tool for assessing corneal surface irregularities before and after refractive surgery.

In addition to the topographic parameters, the study of IA could be expanded by means of the introduction of *Fourier analysis*.[6] Fourier analysis is a mathematical procedure that breaks any function into a sum of sine wave components with different frequencies, amplitudes, and phases (Figure 18-1). Fourier analysis allows more precise and detailed corneal irregularities, and makes it possible to quantify the level of corneal irregularity in normal and irregular corneas, stabilizing the standard irregularity parameters for any cornea.

In order to classify the severity of the IA, it is suitable to use a grading system (Table 18-1).

ETIOLOGY

Primary Idiopathic

There is a general prevalence of low levels of IA of unknown cause within the population.[1] Wavefront analysis with aberrometers reveal in these cases some degree of high-order aberrations, especially coma and coma-like aberrations.

Secondary

POSTSURGICAL

With the increase of refractive surgery procedures, this is probably the main cause of IA. Irregular corneal astigmatism can complicate any of the following refractive surgical procedures: photorefractive keratectomy (PRK), laser epithelial keratomileusis (LASEK), epithelial laser assisted in situ keratomileusis (Epi-LASIK), laser in situ keratomileusis (LASIK), radial keratotomy (RK), arcuate keratotomy (AK), intracorneal segments (Intacs [Addition Technology, Sunnydale, Calif]), laser thermokeratoplasty (LTK), conductive keratoplasty (CK), lamellar or penetrating keratoplasty, and cataract incisions. Scleral retinal detachment surgery may also induce to some extent IA.[1]

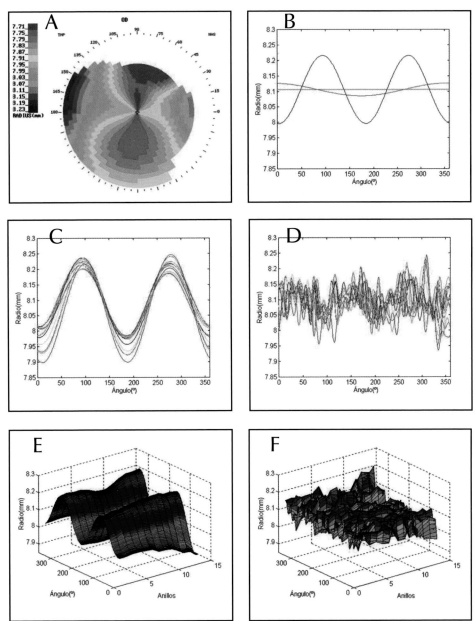

Figure 18-1. Fourier analysis of videokeratography data. (A) Corneal topography. (B) First three frequencies of one ring. (C) Regular component, sum of the first three frequencies. (D) Irregular component, sum of higher frequencies. (E) Regular 3-D corneal surface. (F) Irregular 3-D corneal surface. Figures B, C and D are plotted radius (mm) vs angle (degrees). Note that each ring of the topography is color-coded in Figures C and D. 3-D surfaces are plotted in radius (X-axis, mm), angle (Z-axis, degrees), and rings (Y-axis).

Table 18-1
Grading of IA

Grade 1	Mild symptoms at night or daylight conditions
	Loss of 1 to 2 lines of BCVA
	Useful vision for reading, driving, and walking
	No disability for normal life, but uncomforted
	No monocular diplopia
	Ray-tracing abnormal. Distortion = 2 to 8 mm
	Aberrometry: RMS = 2 to 3 μm
Grade 2	Moderate disability
	Loss of 3 to 4 lines of BCVA
	Reading and driving partially affected, especially in dim light conditions
	Some patients prefer not to use the eye
	Moderate monocular diplopia
	Ray-tracing affected. Distortion = 8 to 14 mm
	Aberrometry: RMS = 3 to 6 μm
Grade 3	Severe disability. Eye not useful for visual performance
	Loss of >5 lines of BCVA
	Patients prefer not to use the eye
	Reading and driving affected, all light conditions
	Severe monocular diplopia or polyopia
	Ray-tracing disaster. Distortion >14 mm
	Aberrometry: RMS >6 μm
Grade 4	Eye not useful, legally blind
	BCVA =20/200 or less
	Aberrometry, ray-tracing, and topography not possible to caption due to the severity of irregularities

DYSTROPHIC

Keratoconus describes a condition in which the cornea assumes a conical shape as a result of noninflammatory corneal thinning. The thinning in keratoconus induces IA, myopia, and protrusion, resulting in mild to marked impairment in the quality of vision. It is a progressive disorder ultimately affecting both eyes, though only one eye may be affected initially.[7]

Pellucid marginal degeneration and keratoglobus may also be associated with posterior corneal surface irregularity, causing IA. In the lens, lenticonus may cause IA; and in the retina, posterior staphyloma.[1]

TRAUMATIC

Corneal irregularity is caused commonly by corneal wounds (incision or excision) or burns (chemical, thermal, or electrical).[1]

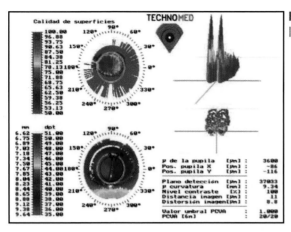

Figure 18-2. IA with pattern (macroirregular): decentered ablation.

POSTINFECTIVE

Postherpetic keratitits is the most common form of postkeratitic healing and scarring that may lead to an irregular surface.[1] Another source of postinfective IA is infectious keratitis in contact lens wearers.[9]

CLINICAL CLASSIFICATION

According to its anatomical location, the IA after LASIK is classified as:
- *Superficial*: Caused by irregularities in the corneal surface, due to problems with the microkeratome creating the flap or bad flap position (folds).
- *Stromal*: Induced by corneal bed irregularities caused during LASIK surgery (microkeratome or excimer ablation problems such as decentration).
- *Mixed*: Due to irregularities in both flap and stroma.

CORNEAL TOPOGRAPHY CLASSIFICATION

Based on the topography, the following classification was proposed for IA[9]:

Irregular Astigmatism With Defined Pattern (or Macroirregular)

The corneal topography shows a steep or flat area of at least 2 mm of diameter, at any location of the corneal topography, which is the main cause of the IA (Figure 18-2).

Irregular Astigmatism With Undefined Pattern (or Microirregular)

The corneal topography shows a surface with multiple irregularities, big and small, and steep and flat areas. Macroirregular astigmatism may be associated with some degree of microirregularity in some cases (Figure 18-3).

Figure 18-3. IA without pattern (microirregular): irregularly irregular.

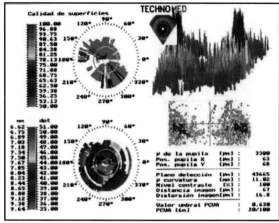

Treatment

Contact Lens Correction of Irregular Astigmatism

There are very few reports on contact lens fitting in patients suffering from induced IA.[10,11] Although contact lens fitting provides a good visual acuity in patients with induced IA, this is not the preferred option for a patient that had refractive surgery to get rid of their glasses and contact lenses. However, in some cases, contact lenses can be a temporary alternative—and sometimes the unique solution—to correct IA. Four types of contact lenses can be used in these patients: hard (polymethylmethacrylate, PMMA), gas-permeable (silicone fluorometacrylate and silicone acrylate), hybrid (synergicon, SoftPerm {CibaVision, Duluth, Ga]), and hydrophilic. The preoperative keratometry (when available), the fluorescein pattern, and the topographic pattern of the IA should be used to select the trial contact lens.

In cases of lamellar refractive surgery (LASIK), the diameter of the lens depends on the diameter of the flap, and the lens should lean on a zone not affected by refractive surgery (ie, corneal periphery). In cases of incisional surgery (eg, RK), toric hydrophilic lenses and SoftPerm were preferred because these lenses have larger diameters, so they rest on the scleral rim and avoid the corneal periphery, which is usually affected by the healing effect of the incision, and leads to poor stability of the lens. Contact lens fitting could be a good alternative in cases that had undesirable results after corneal refractive surgery due to induced IA.[11]

Excimer Laser Surgery

There have been several methods used to correct IA. At this moment, we divide these procedures with excimer laser into the following surgical groups:
- Zonal Ablations
- Masking solutions
- Topography-linked excimer laser ablation (TOPOLINK)
- Wavefront-oriented excimer laser

Zonal Ablations

In 1994, Gibralter and Trokel applied excimer laser in PTK mode to treat surgically-induced IA in 2 patients. They used the corneal topographic maps to plan focal treatment

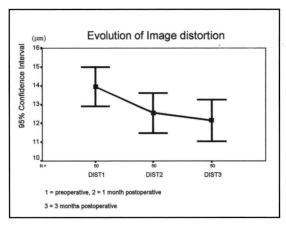

Figure 18-4. Evolution of peak distortion preop, 3 months, and 6 months after ELASHY.

areas with good results, achieving a more regular surface.[12] This was the first attempt performing a customized laser excimer ablation. Later, Alió and coworkers described a technique to correct cases of postsurgical IA using a broad-beam excimer laser in PTK mode, the so-called selective excimer laser zonal ablations (SELZA).[9] The observed results in this study showed that all cases of IA without a defined pattern (microirregular) had very poor outcome, but only those in which a clearly defined pattern of macroirregularity was present had a better visual outcome.

MASKING SOLUTIONS

The use of a viscous masking agent during the ablations of an irregular cornea aims to protect the valleys between the irregular corneal peaks, leaving these peaks of pathology exposed to laser treatment. Of the different masking agents that have been evaluated, methylcellulose is the most commonly used and is available in different concentrations. However, it turns white during ablation due to its low boiling point and was not ideal for treatment.[15] Other attempts to improve IA with a masking substance were made by Pallikaris and colleagues, applying their photoablatable lenticular modulator (PALM) technique to smooth the corneal surface. However, this technique was abandoned due to its lack of reproductibility.[16] Alió and coworkers described a new technique using sodium hyaluronate 0.25% as the masking solution, so called excimer laser assisted by sodium hyaluronate (ELASHY). The physical characteristics of sodium hyaluronate confer important rheological properties to the product and the photoablation rate is similar to that of corneal tissue, forming a stable and uniform coating on the surface of the eye, filling depressions on the cornea and effectively masking tissues to be protected against ablation by the laser pulses in PTK mode. They performed a prospective clinically controlled study performed on 50 eyes of 50 patients with induced IA.[17-22] The safety index was equal to 1.1 and the efficacy index was 0.74. The ray-tracing parameters improved, and most of the patients (89.3%) subjectively noted improvement of the visual acuity and disappearance of the visual aberrations that previously impaired their quality of vision. This coincided with the improvement in the peak distortion (Figure 18-4) and the ray-tracing (Figure 18-5). The clinical indications for this procedure include IA caused by irregularity in flap or irregularity on stromal base induced by LASIK.[23]

A different approach to treat cases in which IA is associated with a superficial corneal opacity—such as post-PRK haze—is a combination of a superficial lamellar keratectomy and ELASHY. In those cases, a 8.5-mm free cap is obtained with the automated lamellar keratectomy (ALK) microkeratome and then sent out for pathological analysis. From a complete set of footplates with different depths, the footplate based on the depth of the opacity calculated

Figure 18-5. Pre- (A) and postoperative (B) topography and ray-tracing analysis of a patient with IA that was treated with ELASHY. Note the improvement of the irregular pattern as well as the ray-tracing parameters.

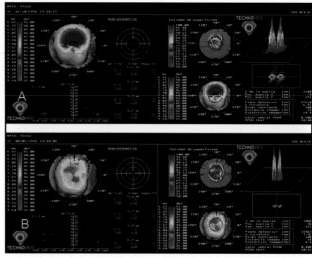

by confocal microscopy is selected. The ELASHY technique helps to improve the corneal surface irregularity on the stromal surface. A bandage contact lens is used after the treatment until complete re-epithelization. Topical steroids must be used for a long period after the treatment to modulate scarring and haze formation.

TOPOGRAPHY-LINKED EXCIMER LASER ABLATION (TOPOLINK)

About 40% of human corneas show some irregularities that cannot be taken into account in a standard basis treatment with excimer laser.[24] For these patients, and for those suffering from IA after trauma or refractive surgery, a custom-tailored, topography-based ablation, which has been adapted to the corneal irregularity, would be the best approach to improve not only their refractive problem but also to improve their quality of vision. This treatment was the first step in customized ablation depending mainly on the corneal topography as well as the refraction for calculating the treatment. It aimed to obtain the BCVA attained by wearing hard contact lenses. Its requirements were an excimer laser with spot scanning technology, in which a small laser spot delivers a multitude of single shots fired in diverse positions to fashion the desired ablation profile. The laser spot is programmable and, thus, any profile could be obtained. A videokeratography system that provides an elevation map at high resolution is needed, and specific software is used to create a customized ablation program for the spot scanner laser.

The earlier studies with this technology proved that those patients with an IA with pattern improved the visual acuity, the refractive error, and the quality of vision[25,26] (Figure 18-6). In a similar study, Knorz and Jendritza[27] evaluated the predictability and safety of topographically guided LASIK. They studied 27 patients (29 eyes) with postsurgical corneal irregularities using the same TOPOLINK procedure. They reported improvement of the corneal regularity in 66% of eyes in the postkeratoplasty group, whereas 34% remained irregular. In the post-trauma group, 83% improved and 17% remained irregular. In the decentered/small optical zone group, 91% improved and 9% remained irregular. In the central islands group, 50% improved and 50% remained irregular.

A different attempt to correct IA using a similar technology was made by Alessio et al.[28] This study evaluated the efficacy, predictability, stability, and safety of a software program (Corneal Interactive Programmed Topographic Ablation [CIPTA], LIGI, Taranto, Italy) that, by transferring programmed ablation from the corneal topography to a flying-spot excimer laser,

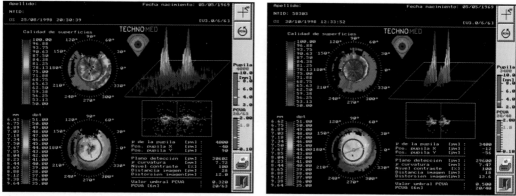

Figure 18-6. Pre- (A) and postoperative (B) topography and ray-tracing analysis of a patient with macroirregular astigmatism that was treated with TOPOLINK. Note the disappearance of the central irregularity after the treatment.

provides customized laser ablation. Forty-two eyes of 34 subjects had CIPTA. Twenty-eight eyes were treated for hyperopic astigmatism and 14 for myopic astigmatism. All the subjects had IA. These data were processed to obtain a customized altimetric ablation profile, which was transferred to a flying-spot laser. At the last postoperative examination, 26 eyes (92.8%) in the hyperopic group and 12 eyes (85.7%) in the myopic group had UCVA superior to 20/40. Twelve hyperopic eyes (42.8%) and 5 myopic eyes (35.7%) had a UCVA of 20/20.

All these studies conclude that the combination of topographic data with computer-controlled flying-spot excimer laser ablation is a suitable solution for correcting IA due to different causes. But those patients that present microirregular astigmatism (small irregularities) such as central islands or undefined patterns of IA are not suitable for these treatments, as the results were sufficiently poor to advise against the use of our technique in these patients.

WAVEFRONT-ORIENTED EXCIMER LASER

Wavefront-assisted excimer laser surgery is an emerging technology based on the concept of correcting high-order aberrations. Such aberrations are largely increased in abnormal irregular corneas. Aberrometers available today are capable of measuring to a limited degree such optical anomalies and their performance at this regard is thus also limited. Other pitfalls for standard aberrometers is that measurements include whole eye aberrations and cannot distinguish corneal aberrations separately so the wavefront-oriented surgery is today limited to very mild forms of IA. Large amounts of macro- or microirregularities are not measurable by today's devices, which will be better treated by corneal wavefront-assisted excimer laser surgery.

Corneal wavefront screening of IA offers much more reliable information on a larger number of points studied on the cornea, allowing more precise information to build the customized program required for the correction of cases of IA with defined macroirregular pattern and also to some extent the microirregular component.[29] Corneal aberrations contribute to approximately 80% of the total ocular aberrations in normal eyes and to an even greater value in corneas with IA.

This technique to treat corneal IA has been evaluated in a prospective, nonrandomized pilot study by Alió and coworkers. They evaluated 18 patients (18 eyes) diagnosed with macroirregular or mixed (macro and micro) IA caused by the previous corneal refractive surgery. For this process, both the alignment and the stability of the precorneal tear film are extremely important. The CSO topographer is able to convert the elevation data in terms of Zernike

Figure 18-7. Treatment ablation profile based on corneal wavefront aberrations.

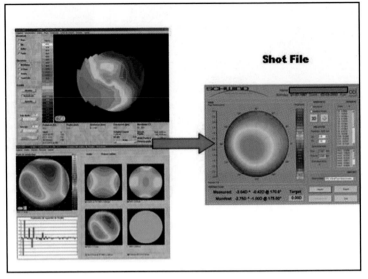

polynomials to quantify the corneal wavefront aberrometry. The root-mean-square (RMS) was used as a measure of the optical quality before and after customized corneal wavefront analysis. After capturing and analyzing corneal aberrations up to the 7th Zernike order, these data are processed by the ORK-W software (Schwind), which transforms corneal aberration data into an adequate ablation profile (Figure 18-7). The software enables the surgeon to take an active part in the decision-making process, selecting the best solution for each patient. The software also allows the exclusion of specific aberrations according to specific surgical criteria and the choice of wide optical and transition zones. Finally, customized ablation was performed with the Schwind ESIRIS Excimer-Laser. UCVA improved in 81% of the patients with a safety index of 1.16. The mean gain of lines of postoperative BCVA was 1.09 ± 0.7 lines. After ORK-W, there was a statically significant decrease in total higher-order aberration and in total higher-order corneal wavefront aberration. Total higher-order aberration was reduced by a factor of 1.45 at 3 months after surgery ($p<0.005$). Corneal wavefront-guided laser may be an excellent tool for correction of IA induce by previous corneal refractive surgery.

Nonlaser Corneal Surgery

AUTOMATED ANTERIOR LAMELLAR KERATOPLASTY

This technique was originally designed to treat superficial stromal disorders, but it has also been used for the treatment of difficult cases of IA, with very poor results.[30] The surgeon performs PTK or a microkeratome or femtosecond laser lamellar resection to 250 to 400 µm stromal depth, followed by transplantation of a donor lamella of the same dimension onto the recipient bed. It is a good option for patients with thin corneas, and with the preservation of the Descemet's membrane, the complications of rejection should be extremely minimized if not eliminated. Results are very good if lenticules are over 300 µm. Visual recovery is fast, occurring between 2 and 4 months. Sutures are removed during the third month and astigmatism can be retreated with LASIK (Figure 18-8). Although complications are rare, some epithelial invasion has been observed with thin tissues that have been inadequately sutured.

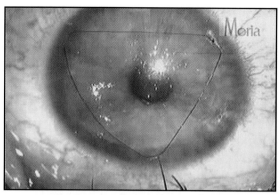

Figure 18-8. Automated anterior lamellar keratoplasty (ALTK) result at the end of the surgery. Thin flap with one triangular stitch.

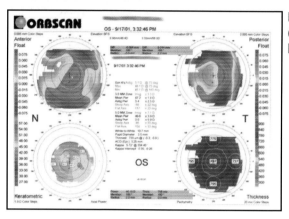

Figure 18-9. Orbscan corneal topography 6 months after deep anterior lamellar keratoplasty (DALK).

Deep Anterior Lamellar Keratoplasty

Deep Anterior Lamellar Keratoplasty (DALK) is an alternative surgical technique in which optically abnormal corneal tissue is substituted by a donor normal cornea, leaving the corneal endothelium and Descemet's membrane of the recipient cornea untouched. This allows a large decrease in the risk of immunological rejections. The technique has been made popular by Melles and Terry, but it has been practiced by a few ophthalmologists due to technical surgical difficulties and the limitations in visual recovery that is associated with DALK.[31]

Apparently, the presence of residual corneal stroma over the Descemet's membrane and the irregular surface left by the handmade surgery creates a wound-healing surface and optical irregularities that are responsible for the limited visual functional outcome in some cases of DALK (Figure 18-9). Although the clinical results of DALK vary with the indication, the final visual acuity averaged 20/25.[30] However, about one-third of these patients still needed hard contact lens fitting to achieve this result. DALK is, therefore, reserved for those patients who suffer from postrefractive surgery IA that cannot be managed with other forms of treatment or from astigmatism combined with scarring, near or within the optical axis.

Penetrating Keratoplasty

Penetrating keratoplasty (PK) is the first option in the management of IA associated with full-thickness corneal opacities. However, it may also be indicated in a clear cornea (after trauma or previous surgery) as a last resort, when all other treatments have failed. The difficulty lies in deciding when a PK is required (ie, when we should stop trying the remaining, more-conservative approaches that may spare both the patient and the surgeon the frustrating time and energy invested in ineffective attempts with milder techniques).

Although a lamellar keratoplasty has a much lower risk of rejection, this is counterbalanced by a greater technical complexity and the above-discussed difficulties in effectively eliminating all irregularity. A PK provides, at least, a corneal "brand new start." As long as topography-guided laser ablation is not widely available and time tested, PK will remain an option for some IA, even in the absence of significant leucoma.

KEY POINTS

1. Irregular astigmatism (IA) is defined as irregular if the principal meridians are not 90 degrees apart, usually because of an irregularity of the corneal curvature, and it cannot be completely corrected with a spherocylindrical lens.
2. The most common clinical symptoms of induced IA are decreases in best-corrected vision and visual distortion, together with night and/or day glare.
3. Clinically, IA will present with a typical retinoscopy pattern, the most common being spinning and scissoring of the red reflex.
4. The most recent and sophisticated technique in examination is the application of wavefront examination (aberrometers),[4] especially corneal wavefront analysis.
5. In addition to the topographic parameters, the study of IA could be expanded by means of the introduction of Fourier analysis.

REFERENCES

1. Goggin M, Alpins N, Schmid LM. Management of IA. *Curr Opin Ophthalmol.* 2000;11:260-266.
2. Alió JL, Artola A, Claramonte PJ, et al. Complications of photorefractive keratectomy for myopia: two year follow-up of 3000 cases. *J Cataract Refract Surg.* 1998;24:619-626.
3. Duke-Elder S, Abrams D, eds. Pathological refractive errors. In: *System of Ophthalmology. Vol V. Ophthalmic Optics and Refraction.* St Louis, Mo: Mosby; 1970:363.
4. Harris WF. Wavefronts and their propagation in astigmatic optical systems. *Optom Vis Sci.* 1996;73:606–612.
5. Moreno-Barriuso E, Merayo-Lloves JM, Marcos S, Navarro R. Ocular aberrations after refractive surgery measured with a laser ray tracing technique. *Invest Ophthalmol Vis Sci.* 2000;41:S303.
6. Goodman JW. *Introduction to Fourier Optics.* San Francisco, Calif: McGraw-Hill; 1968:75.
7. Rabinowitz YS. Definition, etiology and diagnosis of keratoconus. In: Alio JL, Belda JI, eds. *Treating IA and Keratoconus.* Panama: Highlights of Ophthalmology; 2004:241-260.
8. Alió JL, Pérez-Santonja JJ, Tervo T, et al. Postoperative inflammation, microbial complications, and wound healing following laser in situ keratomileusis. *J Refract Surg.* 2000;16:523-538.
9. Alió JL, Artola A, Rodríguez-Mier FA. Selective Zonal Ablations with excimer laser for correction of IA induced by refractive surgery. *Ophthalmology.* 2000;107:662-673.
10. Chou B, Wachier BS. Soft contact lenses for IA after laser in situ keratomileusis. *J Refract Surg.* 2001;17:692-695.
11. Alio JL, Belda JI, Artola A, García-Lledó M, Osman A. Contact lens fitting in the correction of IA after corneal refractive surgery. *J Cataract Refract Surg.* 2002;28:1750-1757.
12. Gibralter R, Trokel SL. Correction of IA with the excimer laser. *Ophthalmology.* 1994;101:1310-1315.
13. Munnerlyn C, Koons S, Marshall J. Photorefractive keratectomy: a technique for laser refractive surgery. *J Cataract Refract Surg.* 1988;14:46-52.
14. Buzard K, Fundingsland B. Treatment of IA with a broad beam excimer laser. *J Refract Surg.* 1997;13:624-636.

15. Thompson V, Durrie DS, Cavanaugh TB. Philosophy and technique for excimer laser phototherapeutic keratectomy. *J Refract Corneal Surg.* 1993;9:81-85.

16. Pallikaris IG, Katsanevaki VJ, Ginis HS. The PALM technique for the treatment of corneal IA. In: Alió JL, Belda JI, eds. *Treating IA and Keratoconus.* Panama: Highlights of Ophthalmology; 2004:97-101.

17. Alio JL, Belda JI, Shalaby AMM. Excimer laser assisted by sodium hyaluronate for correction of IA (ELASHY). *Ophthalmology.* 2001;108:1246-1260.

18. Kornmehl EW, Steiner RF, Puliafito CA. A comparative study of masking fluids for excimer laser photo-therapeutic keratectomy. *Arch Ophthalmol.* 1991;109:860-863.

19. Kornmehl EW, Steinert RF, Puliafito CA, Reidy W. Morphology of an irregular corneal surface following 193 nm ArF excimer laser large area ablation with 0.3% hydroxypropyl methylcellulose 2910 and 0.1% dextran 70.1% carboxy-methylcellulose sodium or 0.9% saline. *Invest Ophthalmol Vis Sci.* 1990;31: 245.

20. Trokel SL, Srinivasan R, Braren B. Excimer laser surgery of the cornea. *Am J Ophthalmol.* 1983;96:705-710.

21. Orndahl M, Fagerholm P, Fitzsimmons T, Tengroth B. Treatment of corneal dystrophies with excimer laser. *Acta Ophthalmol.* 1994;72:235-240.

22. Seiler T, Bendee T, Wollensak J. Ablation rate of human corneal epithelium and Bowman's layer with the excimer laser (193nm). *J Refract Corneal Surg.* 1990;6:99-102.

23. Artola A, Alió JL, Bellot JL, Ruiz JM. Protective properties of viscoelastic substances (sodium hyaluronate and 2% hydroxymethyl cellulose) against experimental free radical damage to the corneal endothelium. *Cornea.* 1993;12:109-114.

24. Klyce SD, Smolek MK. Corneal topography of excimer laser photorefractive keratectomy. *J Cataract Refract Surg.* 1993;19:122-130.

25. Alió JL, Belda JI, Osman AA, Shalaby AMM. Topography-guided laser in situ keratomileusis (TOPOLINK) to correct IA after previous refractive surgery. *J Refract Surg.* 2003;19:516-527.

26. Wiesinger-Jendritza B, Knorz M, Hugger P, Liermann A. Laser in situ keratomileusis assisted by corneal topography. *J Cataract Surg.* 1998;24:166-174.

27. Knorz MC, Jendritza B. Topographically-guided laser in situ keratomileusis to treat corneal irregularities. *Ophthalmology.* 2000;107:1138-1143.

28. Alessio G, Boscia F, La Tegola MG, Sborgia C. Topography-driven photorefractive keratectomy: results of corneal interactive programmed topographic ablation software. *Ophthalmology.* 2000;107:1578-1587.

29. Cáliz A, Montes-Micó R, Belda JI, Alió JL. Corneal aberrometry as a guide for the correction of IA. In: Alio JL, Belda JI, ed. *Treating IA and Keratoconus.* Panama: Highlights of Ophthalmology; 2004:121-133.

30. Alió JL, Uhah J, Barraquer C, et al. New techniques in lamellar keratoplasty. *Curr Opin Ophthalmol.* 2002;13:224-229.

31. Melles GRJ, Lander F, Rietveld FJR, et al. A new surgical technique for deep stromal, anterior lamellar keratoplasty. *Br J Ophthalmol.* 1999;83:327-333.

Chapter 19

GLARE AND HALOS AFTER REFRACTIVE SURGERY

Guillermo Simón-Castellví, MD; Sarabel Simón-Castellví, MD; José María Simón-Castellví, MD; Cristina Simón-Castellví, MD; and José María Simón-Tor, MD

PHYSICS

The current concept of light states that it is an electromagnetic radiation to which the organs of sight react. Visible light comes primarily from the sun. The propagation direction of a ray of light changes when this ray passes from one medium (eg, air) to a different medium (eg, cornea or aqueous humour), or vice versa. Entering the eye, each ray suffers different phenomena: dispersion, reflection, and diffraction. Dispersion is an optical phenomenon whereby the optical properties of a medium (eg, the cornea) vary according to the wavelength of light passing through the medium. Reflection is a phenomenon that causes a portion of the light striking the surface of a medium (eg, the cornea) to break off and propagate in an entirely new direction. Diffraction is a phenomenon in which light waves enter the shadow area of an object. The amount of light entering the eye is adjusted by varying the pupil size. Diffraction can occur with small pupils (miosis), when the pupil border obstructs and bends the straight-line path of advancing light waves into the eye. Diffraction causes reductions in image contrast and resolution.

REFRACTIVE SURGERY

In young healthy eyes, dioptric media are functionally transparent and these phenomena have poor or not noticeable impact in image quality, despite the fact that 10% of the incident light is scattered. The above-mentioned optical phenomena, together with the 5 aberrations of Seidel (spherical aberrations, coma or chromatic aberrations, astigmatism, curvature of field, and distortion), may be responsible for a decrease in quality and comfort of vision after refractive surgery.[1] Most subjects are satisfied with their vision after LASIK.[2] Nevertheless, each day, the practitioner is confronted with a sample of patients in the consulting room, each patient exhibiting individual personality traits and having visual problems not easily understood or explained. Especially important are patients who underwent successful (or sometimes unsuccessful) refractive surgery but are not pleased with the functional results and ask for active listening and for a prompt solution.

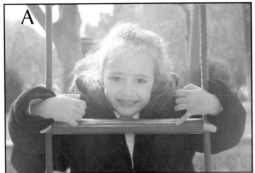 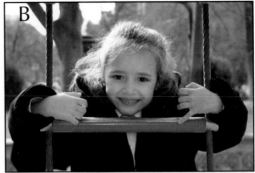

Figure 19-1. (A) This figure depicts a computer simulation of glare, a condition of discomfort in the eye (with contrast reduction and decreased central vision), produced when a bright light enters the field of view. The amount of glare is proportional to the power of the light: the brighter (and closer) the light, the stronger the glare. Notice that (B) shows the same image as seen by a healthy patient.

GLARE

Glare (Figure 19-1) is a condition of discomfort in the eye (with contrast reduction and decreased central vision), produced when a bright light enters the field of view, especially when the eye adapts to the dark (at night). The amount of glare is proportional to the power of the light: the brighter (and closer) the light, the stronger the glare. Glare from the lights of an approaching automobile can be measured with a glarometer (eg, Larson Glarometer). Glare testers can measure sensitivity to glare by means of a variable contrast series of slides. Clinical practice shows that glare is amplified as corneal or lens scattering are increased. A patient with a poorly fitted contact lens or dirty contacts who develops corneal epithelial edema reports unusual glare from automobile headlights. Glare may interfere with the patient's ability to drive at night and to enjoy outdoor activities on hazy or bright days.

There are actually 2 kinds of post-LASIK glare: daytime glare and dim-light or nighttime glare. A postrefractive surgery patient in daylight sees the first type. Instead of the usual glare from the sun reflecting off the bumper of a car, this post-LASIK glare is brighter on the eyes. It is different from the glare seen by a virgin eye. The second type of glare is a low light and night disturbance that a post-LASIK patient describes it as starbursts and halos. Most patients, including those that have not undergone refractive surgery, experience greater vision difficulty at night than during the day. This is due to the larger pupil size in the dark. As the pupil gets larger, and that is the case for most myopic patients, the optical quality of every eye worsens.

HALO

A halo is an annular flare of light (Figure 19-2) surrounding a luminous body or image, seen in varicolored patterns or as a brightness gradient, as a result of aberrations (after refractive surgery), internal reflections (after cataract surgery with some intraocular lenses [IOLs]), diffraction (with multifocal IOLs) or scattering (corneal oedema or corneal scars). Common causes of halos are listed in Table 19-1. Laser assisted in situ keratomileusis (LASIK), photorefractive keratectomy (PRK), radial keratotomies (RK), and other forms of refractive surgery can cause visual aberrations[3,4] (Figure 19-3 and 19-4).

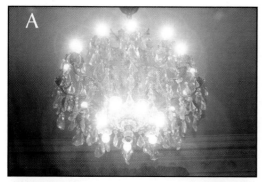

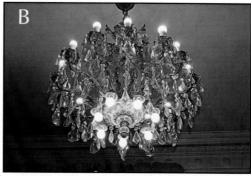

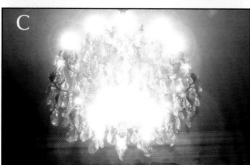

Figure 19-2. This figure (A) depicts a computer simulation of halos, annular flare of light surrounding points of light. Notice that picture B shows the same image as would be seen by a healthy patient (crisp clear image). Most times, halos and glare come together (C), since they have the same origin (optical aberrations), and can severely damage visual function under certain light conditions.

GLARE, HALOS, AND PUPIL SIZE

Despite what is stated in some recent publications, it is very clear from the published reports and from our own clinical experience that a large pupil is the predominant factor leading to glare and halos. If you compare patients with the same prescriptions, the larger the pupil size, the bigger the chance to have more night vision problems. Residual refractive error and irregularity or pattern of ablation zones also play a role, as does the age of the patient (the older the patient, the higher the risk).

It is widely accepted that small optical zone treatments in LASIK increase a patient's risk of glare, halos, and other optical anomalies, especially during low or dim light settings. Glare and halo disturbance is subjective; this can explain why some patients with large pupils and that have had laser surgery do not experience halos, glare, or night vision problems. We believe from their aberrometer measurements that they do suffer them, as they probably did before surgery, but are so happy with the fact that they do not have to wear glasses, that it is not an important issue for them. Nevertheless, we have noted that big pupils do not always necessarily experience glare at night, and on the contrary, we have also seen glare and halos with small pupils.

Accurate pupillometry (especially in low-light conditions) is an essential part of the evaluation for refractive surgery.[5] What causes starbursts and halos? If the patient's dark-adapted (scotopic) pupil size exceeds the size of the planned ablation zone (effective optical zone) created by the laser, light will pass through the ablated area of the cornea as well as through the transition zone and the untreated area of the cornea. Light will scatter across this transition zone and reach the retina, making the patient see this light scatter as a ring (or halo) of light around any light (colored and reflective objects) and/or starbursts from light sources. Refraction (amount of spherical correction), pupil size, flap size, ablation zone size, and the laser used are the main factors that determine the risk of glare and halos. Notice that the

Table 19-1

Causes of Colored Halos Around Lights

Nonpathological Causes

- Environmental (lights seen through a steamy window [driving])
- Physiological (from the radial structure of crystalline lens halo disappears in part as the slit—of the slit lamp—passes over the pupil)

Pathological Causes

- Acute or subacute angle closure (halo remains intact but diminishes in intensity as slit passes over the pupil)
- Edematous cornea (postcataract surgery, in severe uveitis, etc)
- Corneal dystrophies or degenerations (including keratoconus and amiodarone keratopathy[6]
- Severe dry eye
- Corneal epithelial defect (in intensive contact lens wear, or secondary to eye drugs like topical carbon anhydrase inhibitors)
- Headache (migraine)
- As complication of refractive surgery (any technique):
    - RK
    - LASIK
    - Irregular astigmatism
    - Epithelialization of the stromal interface
    - Mydriasis (paralitic)
    - Loss or damage of the corneal cap
    - Multifocal intraocular lens (after cataract or clear lens extraction)

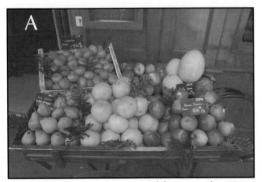 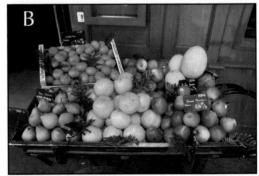

Figure 19-3. Another possible complication after refractive surgery is reduced contrast: the ability to see well in low contrast situations (eg, in a rainy day or driving at night) can fall below normal levels following laser eye surgery, reducing the patient's ability to see clearly. After several weeks or months, contrast sensitivity usually returns to normal and vision becomes clearer in low contrast conditions. However, in some cases, contrast sensitivity will not return to normal. This figure depicts a computer simulation of reduced contrast (A), with mild posterior capsule opacification and normal contrast (B), after Nd-YAG laser posterior capsulotomy. Notice that the fruit price is more readable in the normal contrast example.

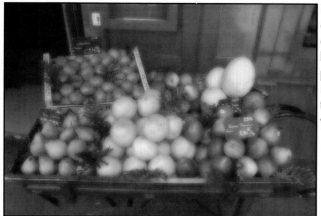

Figure 19-4. This figure depicts a computer simulation of reduced contrast and halos, as probably seen by a complicated post-LASIK myopic patient suffering from severe interstitial keratitis. Notice that neither fruit price nor fruit details are visible with clarity.

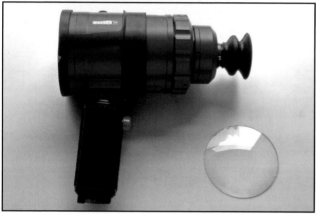

Figure 19-5. Pupil size must be carefully measured preoperatively in a dark room (under scotopic conditions) with an infrared pupillometer. This measurement is critical. If the pupil dilates larger than the planned ablation zone (not including a blend or transition zone), the patient should not have LASIK or should be specially aware of LASIK risks. This image shows a self-made pupillometer, made from a night vision device (image intensifier) and a graduated scale in millimeters. Many commercial devices available for accurate preoperative pupil size assessment (eg, PupilScan II [Keeler/Fairville Medical Optics, Newark, Del], the Colvard pupillometer [Oasis Medical, Glendora, Calif], the NeurOptics pupillometer [BD Medical Ophthalmic Systems, Waltham, Mass], the P2000SA pupillometer [Keeler Instruments, Broomall, Pa], and the Procyon Instruments Limited system [Montrose, United Kingdom]) store dynamic pupil measurements in a laptop computer.

healing process affects effective ablation zone; a planned 6-mm ablation may result in an effective optical zone of 5 mm after corneal healing.

We believe that the most important factors in night vision complaints are pupil size and preoperative refraction. In general, patients with large pupils and high corrections are at greater risk of developing glare and halos: the higher the degree of correction, the smaller the central optical zone. High degrees of myopia and/or astigmatism can create a sharper junction zone between treated and untreated cornea to potentially scatter light. If the ablation is not perfectly centered, or if the refractive treatment includes correction for medium to high astigmatism, there is more risk of glare and halos. An astigmatic ablation pattern is elliptical in shape rather than round like the pupil, and this difference in shape can cause visual disturbances under certain light conditions; hence, pupil size and prescription must be considered together (not separately) to evaluate if the patient is at low, medium, or high risk for developing glare and halos (Figure 19-5).

Figure 19-6. An intense capsule opacification following cataract surgery produces glare symptoms and/or reduced contrast sensitivity. The reduced visual acuity and glare disability require a posterior Nd-YAG laser capsulotomy, the size of which must be considered: the optimal capsulotomy equals the size of the pupil in scotopic ambience.

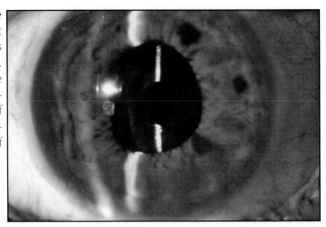

PREVENTION

By replacing the microkeratome blade with the Pulsion FS laser (IntraLase, Irvine, Calif), we virtually eliminate the most severe, sight-threatening complications associated with the use of microkeratomes (eg, free cap). It uses a rapidly firing femtosecond (Nd:YLF) laser to cause photodisruption of the corneal tissue at a predetermined depth and size. Instead of mechanically cutting the cornea, the Pulsion FS IntraLase laser acts as a bladeless keratome and creates in about 30 seconds thousands of microscopic bubbles that link together to define the precise shape and depth of the flap. We can program factors that can be varied to meet patients' needs: precise flap diameter to reduce the risk of glare and halos, flap depth to reduce the risk of folds, hinge width and location, and side-cut architecture. Bladeless LASIK is particularly beneficial for patients with thin corneas, a factor that might otherwise disqualify them for LASIK. Advantages of Pulsion FS IntraLase laser include fewer intraoperative complications, increased vision quality by creating an optimal corneal surface under the flap, lower incidence of high and low spots, and irregular hydration on the corneal surface; factors that can compromise the tissue ablation and may be responsible for glare and halos. Glare and halos are the rule just following the use of IntraLase, but soon disappear with vision recovery. Microkeratomed LASIK patients' visual recovery is almost immediate. When using the Pulsion FS IntraLase laser, complete visual recovery may take a bit longer—a few days (or weeks), the time taken for the "bubbles" to completely disappear.

Since the borders of the flap are more vertically oriented when compared to those created by traditional mechanical keratomes, they lower the risk of flap slippage and epithelial ingrowth.

TREATMENT

When a patient has glare disability, laser or surgical removal of the scattering lesion has to be considered. For example, significant corneal edema refractory to medical topical medication may need a corneal transplant, a significant cataract should be operated, and an intense capsule opacification following cataract surgery may require a laser Nd-YAG capsulotomy (Figures 19-6 through 19-8).

Identifiable postoperative complications, like diffuse lamellar keratitis or DLK (an inflammatory condition of unknown cause that can occur in about 0.2% of LASIK procedures, also called Sands of the Sahara syndrome) have to be recognized and treated promptly with intensive topical steroid drops; it usually resolves without further complication (see Chapter

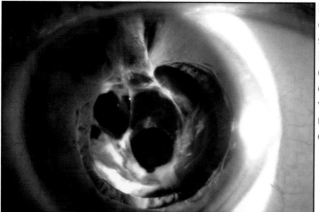

Figure 19-7. An intense capsule opacification following extracapsular clear lens extraction without IOL implant in a high myope produced glare symptoms and reduced contrast sensitivity. The reduced visual acuity and glare disability required a posterior Nd-YAG laser capsulotomy.

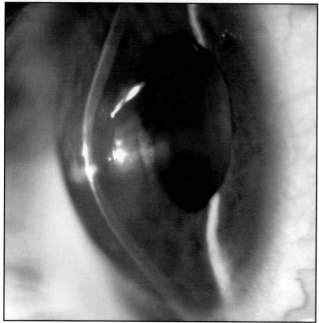

Figure 19-8. A keratoconus can produce glare symptoms and reduced contrast sensitivity with reduced visual acuity: treatment of the symptoms may require a successful corneal graft.

15). Other refractive complications (like decentered ablations or infection) need specific treatment (see Chapters 13 and 16).

The problem arises when dealing with a refractive surgery patient who underwent laser correction surgery to avoid the use of lenses or contacts and increase the quality of vision. For patients complaining of persisting glare and halos after refractive surgery, different therapeutic strategies (although none is perfect) can be tried, as single therapeutic approach or in combination.

Waiting

This is the main rule: the vast majority of LASIK or refractive patients experience some temporary glare and halos during the immediate recovery. This visual discomfort can last for weeks and is due to corneal swelling and reorganization of the corneal architecture. Patients in the healing phase need to understand that these phenomena are normal and different from

Figure 19-9. Classic signs of dry eye include eye redness, conjunctival hyperemia, decreased tear meniscus, increased debris in the tear film, superficial punctate keratopathy (with fluorescein, lissamine green, and/or rose Bengal positive staining), mucous plaques and discharge, and corneal filaments (in severe cases). Symptoms depend on the severity of the sicca and include foreign body sensation, sensation of ocular dryness and grittiness (initially at the end of the day, and 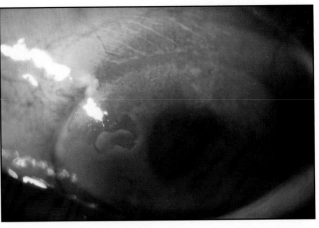 later, the whole day), hyperemia and ocular irritation (exacerbated by smoky or dry environments, indoor heating systems, prolonged reading, or use of computers), mucous discharge, and excessive tearing (secondary to reflex secretion). Picture shows tear film break as seen at the slit lamp with cobalt blue light after instillation of fluorescein dye.

the persistent variety of night vision problems to which we refer in this chapter. The surgeon's first rule is waiting for spontaneous resolution.

Corneal Dryness Treatment

Dry eye after refractive surgery was described early[8] and may strongly interfere with the patient's satisfaction and quality of vision if not properly and early addressed (Figure 19-9). After refractive surgery, an unstable tear film may be responsible for optical aberrations. In such cases, visual acuity improves after each blink or after artificial tear instillation. We strongly recommend intensive pre- and postoperative ocular lubrication at least 2 months after surgery (the time tear film takes to recover complete stability after refractive surgery). Indeed, the incidence of postoperative complications is higher in patients who have intraoperative epithelial defects.

Long-Term Topical Steroid Therapy

Some (if not all) refractive patients experience a very mild interstitial keratitis, responsible for optical aberrations, vision fluctuations, and—in the long term—for regression. We have noticed that refractive patients strongly benefit from long-term (1 month) steroid therapy (dexamethasone), at decreasing doses. Patients suffering from glare or halos may benefit from topical instillation of fluorometholone, 2 or 3 times a day, for 1 to 3 months at decreasing dosage (ie, tapering of the dosage).

Correction of Residual Refractive Defects by Means of Multicoated Glasses

Refractive error after refractive surgery is a very important cause of poor night vision. Since some refractive patients suffering from glare and halos also suffer from over- or undercorrection, we advocate—at least temporarily—the correction of the refractive error with multicoated glasses until laser retreatment can be performed. About 4% of the visible light is reflected from either the front or back surface of a glass lens, causing ghost images.

Multicoating helps to reduce the perception of glare and halos. Most times, the refractive error correction alone significantly reduces patient complaints. Inexpensive clip-on sunglasses may be added for more comfort.

Multicoated Sunglasses (Blue-Grey Tinted 10% to 40%)

In certain high-illumination situations, sunglasses allow better visual function. A tint alone only helps in reducing glare and improving visibility. The major function of dark sunglasses (grey, green, or brown) is to return the retina to a level of maximal contrast sensitivity.

Customized Wavefront-Guided Lenses

Recently, a new range of customized wavefront-guided lenses, the Ophthonix iZon Wavefront-Guided Lenses, can correct the aberrations of the eye itself. They are fully customized spectacle lenses and correct for both conventional, sphere, cylinder, and axis as well as high-order aberrations of the eye. They are individually customized lenses, offering true wavefront correction of any individual's unique eye optical irregularities.

Polarizing Sunglasses

Polarized sunglasses are designed to filter out a component of the sun's broad range of frequencies of radiation. The lights of electromagnetic fields point at many different angles. Polarizing lenses will only allow the transmission of the light waves that are at a certain angle. While normal sunglasses decrease the intensity of everything by the same amount, polarizing sunglasses can selectively reduce or eliminate reflected light from road surfaces, glass windows, lake or river surfaces, or metal surfaces.

For daily living, polarizing glasses greatly improve contrast and color saturation and increase quality of vision under bright sun, but have also the effect of greatly attenuating the brightness of the light, which results in a disadvantage when the light turns dim or in case of cloudy weather. While polarizing lenses work as antiglare glasses with bright sun, they must be forbidden for night driving!

The glare of the sun on the sea and other surfaces is highly horizontally polarized depending on the height of the sun. Polarized sunglasses make water appear darker and more transparent, which allows one to see what is underwater. Because polarization has the effect of cutting down the glare of reflected light, these glasses are ideal for people participating in watersports or driving into the sun, when the light reflects from the dashboard, onto the windshield, and into the eyes, making daylight driving almost impossible. With polarized sunglasses, the reflections are almost totally filtered away.

Some polarized glasses made for sportsmen, with UV protection and water-resistant lenses, have detachable plastic or leather side panels that reduce the amount of side light entering the eye.

Yellow Glasses for Night Driving (eg, Kodak Wratten 12)

Sodium yellow efficiently absorbs wavelengths in the purple through blue-green range and provides excellent contrast and depth perception in low intensity light.

Acting on Pupil Size: Pupil Constriction

There are several treatments for pupil-related night vision problems, although none is perfect. Driving at night with the dome light on can help constrict the pupils, although this practice is not legal in certain states. Alternatively, you can prescribe drops to shrink the pupil.

Figure 19-10. Instilling 1 drop of Alphagan in each eye at twilight to restrict pupil expansion for better night vision can effectively reduce the starbursts that otherwise create after-dark visual interferences. Long-term side effects include follicular conjunctivitis, either chronic (picture) or acute (simulating an adenoviral infection). Treatment of this complication requires cessation of topical treatment with brimonidine tartrate, and topical 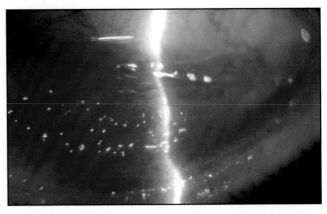 steroids combined with topical antihistamine medications with mast cells stabilizing effects (dual action antihistamines, like Ketotifen fumarate 0.025% [Zaditor Zaditen]). Acute follicular conjunctivitis is less frequent with Alphagan P (with the new preservative Purite), which has reduced pupil expansion restriction.

1. *Dilute pilocarpine* (0.5%): This can reduce glare, but patients rarely use it for a long period of time. With pilocarpine, the pupil turns so small that the patient has ineffective night vision. Other drawbacks of pilocarpine are eye redness, ciliary spasm (headache), and pinpoint pupil. In certain patients, it may cause focusing spasm and increase the risk of retinal detachment.

2. *Brimonidine tartrate* 0.2% (Alphagan, Allergan, Irvine, Calif) or brimonidine tartrate 0.15% (Alphagan P, Allergan, Irvine, Calif) can be prescribed to control pupil dilation at night and thus alleviate some of the symptoms (Figure 19-10). Brimonidine tartrate 0.15% ophthalmic solution produces a significant miotic effect[9] under 3 luminance conditions (scotopic, mesopic, photopic). The reproducible miotic effect under scotopic and mesopic conditions may help postoperative refractive patients who report night-vision difficulties related to a large pupil.[10] It works by inhibiting the sphincter dilator, with no apparent effect on the constrictor pupil muscle. This keeps the pupil from dilating fully, which is noticeable in dim light. We have found a significant decrease in the night-time pupil (scotopic conditions), with very little or no effect on daytime (photopic) pupil. With brimonidine tartrate, we avoid the drawbacks of pilocarpine: no eye redness, no ciliary spasm, and no pinpoint pupil.

   In our clinical practice, we have found that instilling 1 drop in each eye at twilight to restrict pupil expansion for better night vision can effectively reduce the starbursts that otherwise create after-dark visual interferences. We instruct our patients to use it not more than 2 or 3 times a week to avoid tachyphylaxis and the effect wearing off. This is not an FDA approved indication for brimonidine tartrate. Nevertheless, when perioperatively used, brimonidine tartrate 0.2% may adversely affect proper flap adherence after LASIK surgery[11] and may result in an increased rate of postoperative retreatment procedures. Since the publication of these data, we avoid perioperative use of brimonidine tartrate, and wait a couple of months before prescribing to face glare and halos.

3. *Dapiprazole*: This drop is expensive, makes the eyes appear red, and stings on instillation.

Eye Color-Changing Soft Contact Lenses

With an annular ring of color, these may reduce glare and halos by making the functional pupil smaller.

Rigid Gas Permeable Lenses

Rigid gas permeable lenses (RGPs) can also help in establishing a larger functional optical zone and offer the BCVA with minimal complications after radial keratotomies or other refractive procedures.

Wavefront Analysis Customized Ablation

When everything fails and the patient asks for a prompt solution, some surgeons have suggested performing an enhancement procedure using a laser to enlarge the original treatment zone. Wavefront technology (aberrometry) is applicable in certain situations in repairing eyes that have undergone previous nonoptimal or complicated surgeries (eg, decentered ablations).

Wavefront analysis customized ablation treatment helps[7] (but may not be enough) to reshape the cornea; expand the ablation zone; and reduce or eliminate glare, halos, double vision, night vision problems, and other vision loss that may result from complications of refractive surgery.

KEY POINTS

1. Glare is a condition of discomfort in the eye (with contrast reduction and decreased central vision) produced when bright light enters the field of view, especially when the eye is adapted to dark (at night).
2. The amount of glare is proportional to the power of the light: the brighter (and closer) the light, the stronger the glare.
3. A halo is an annular flare of light surrounding a luminous body or image, seen in varicolored patterns or as a brightness gradient, as a result of aberrations (after refractive surgery), internal reflections (after cataract surgery with some intraocular lenses, IOLs), diffraction (with multifocal IOLs), or scattering (corneal edema or corneal scars).
4. A large pupil is the predominant factor leading to glare and halos.
5. Small optical zone treatments in LASIK increase the patient's risk of glare, halos, and other optical anomalies especially during low or dim light settings.

REFERENCES

1. McCormick GJ, Porter J, Cox IG, MacRae S. Higher-order aberrations in eyes with irregular corneas after laser refractive surgery. *Ophthalmology.* 2005;112(10):1699-1709.
2. Bailey MD, Mitchell GL, Dhaliwal DK, Boxer Wachler BS, Zadnik K. Patient satisfaction and visual symptoms after laser in situ keratomileusis. *Ophthalmology.* 2003;110(7):1371-1378.
3. Chalita MR, Krueger RR. Correlation of aberrations with visual acuity and symptoms. *Ophthalmol Clin North Am.* 2004;17(2):135-42, v-vi.

4. Chalita MR, Xu M, Krueger RR. Correlation of aberrations with visual symptoms using wavefront analysis in eyes after laser in situ keratomileusis. *J Refract Surg*. 2003;19(6):S682-686.

5. Haw WW, Manche EE. Effect of preoperative pupil measurements on glare, halos, and visual function after photoastigmatic refractive keratectomy. *J Cataract Refract Surg*. 2001;27(6):907-916.

6. Dovie JM, Gurwood AS. Acute onset of halos and glare: Bilateral corneal epithelial edema with cystic eruptions-atypical presentation of amiodarone keratopathy. *Optometry*. 2006;77(2):76-81.

7. Hiatt JA, Grant CN, Wachler BS. Complex wavefront-guided retreatments with the Alcon CustomCornea platform after prior LASIK. *J Refract Surg*. 2006;22(1):48-53.

8. Simón-Castellví GL., Simón-Castellví S, Simón-Castellví JM, Simón-Tor JM. Tips and tricks for successful refractive surgery. In *Refractive Surgery*. New Delhi, India: Jaypee Brothers; 1998.

9. Thordsen JE, Bower KS, Warren BB, Stutzman R., Miotic effect of brimonidine tartrate 0.15% ophthalmic solution in normal eyes. *J Cataract Refract Surg*. 2004;30(8):1702-1706.

10. McDonald JE II, El-Moatassem Kotb AM, Decker BB. Effect of brimonidine tartrate ophthalmic solution 0.2% on pupil size in normal eyes under different luminance conditions. *J Cataract Refract Surg*. 2001; 27:560–564.

11. Walter KA, Gilbert DD. The adverse effect of perioperative brimonidine tartrate 0.2% on flap adherence and enhancement rates in laser in situ keratomileusis patients. *Ophthalmology*. 2001;108(8):1434–1438.

COMPLICATIONS CREATING LASIK FLAPS WITH THE INTRALASE FEMTOSECOND LASER

William W. Culbertson, MD

INTRODUCTION

The near infrared femtosecond laser is a unique instrument that can produce incisions and lamellar interface planes in the cornea by the process of photodisruption. Contiguous plasma gas bubbles are created in the cornea and expands causing microdelamination of the corneal collagen. A cone-shaped female suction ring is placed on the eye to stabilize it and a male cone-shaped applanation plate is "docked" to it. The cornea is flattened over the area of the intended treatment and the eye is held stationary by the suction ring. A scanning pattern of laser pulses is placed at a predetermined depth and diameter by moving the beam in either a raster pattern for the lamellar interface or a circular spiral pattern for the side (or edge) cut of the flap. Nothing moves across the cornea and the resection is performed out by only scanning the laser beam. The flap interface still has some thin tissue attachments to the underlying bed that are broken when the flap is lifted. In comparison to a blade microkeratome, the Intralase flap has a more predictable thickness and diameter and has a planar contour from side to side. The flap diameter is not influenced by corneal curvature, and the flap centration can be adjusted by the laser software prior to activation of the laser. As a result of its inherent precision and the fact that nothing moves across the cornea during the process of flap creation, minor complications and side effects are minimal and transient and serious complications are rare.[1]

INTRAOPERATIVE COMPLICATIONS

Suction Loss

During the creation of the flap, the Intralase suction ring may lose vacuum and the applanation plate may become separated from the cornea. If this occurs during the propagation of the lamellar interface, there is no serious consequence to the flap except that the interface is incomplete. In this case, the suction ring is reapplied, the interface cut is performed again, and the side cut is made at the end. If suction is lost during the side cut, then the diameter of the side cut is decreased by 1.0 mm, the suction ring is reapplied, and the side cut is performed just inside the outside diameter of the lamellar cut.

Figure 20-1. Gas bubbles in the anterior chamber obscuring the patient's view of the laser fixation light.

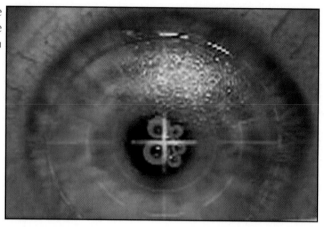

Interference by Gas Bubbles

GAS BUBBLES IN THE ANTERIOR CHAMBER

Occasionally, the gas bubbles generated from the intrastromal photodisruption can dissect from the interface through the peripheral cornea and into the anterior chamber via the trabecular meshwork.[2] With the patient supine and the anteroposterior axis of the eye oriented vertically in preparation for flap lifting and excimer laser treatment, the bubble(s) collects and coalesces in the apex of the anterior chamber, partially obscuring the pupil and the patient's view of the fixation light (Figure 20-1). If the bubble(s) is large enough, it may prevent pupil margin tracking by the laser and inhibit the patient's ability to fixate. The bubble(s) absorbs into the aqueous humor in 2 to 3 hours and treatment may be completed. Often the bubble(s) is small, the edge of the pupil is not obscured, and the patient is able to fixate around the bubble. In this event, the treatment may proceed without waiting for the bubble(s) to absorb. The gas bubble(s) is otherwise innocuous and does not cause any subsequent effect to the eye.

GAS BUBBLES IN THE CORNEA

Gas bubbles are routinely formed in the LASIK interface by femtosecond laser photodisruption (opaque bubble layer [OBL]). These interface bubbles are released when the flap is lifted and therefore they do not interfere with treatment. However, sometimes the bubbles dissect into the superficial layers of the stromal bed during propagation of the laser interface (deep OBL) (Figure 20-2). These deep bubbles are not released when the flap is lifted. Depending on the location of the deep OBL, the pupil or iris landmarks may be obscured, preventing either pupil localization for tracking and/or iris landmark-based iris registration. In addition, if the bubbles are distributed confluently in the peripheral cornea adjacent to the limbus, they may form a false limbus and as a consequence decenter the laser treatment by excimer lasers (such as VISX) that use the limbal ring to center the treatment zone (Figure 20-3). These superficial stromal bed bubbles usually resolve within 30 to 45 minutes. If the OBL interferes in pupil tracking or iris registration, then the laser treatment should be delayed until the OBL resolves.

Unliftable Flap

Occasionally, the interface is insufficiently dissected and it is difficult or impossible to separate the flap from the underlying stromal bed. Attempts to forcefully open the interface

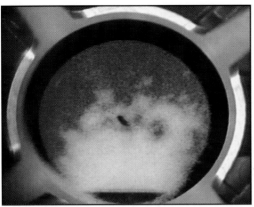

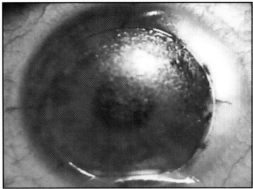

Figure 20-2. Gas bubbles deep to the interface in the anterior stromal bed (deep OBL).

Figure 20-3. Deep OBL in the peripheral cornea producing a "false limbus" or scleral rim that may be misidentified as the true limbus during iris registration and centration.

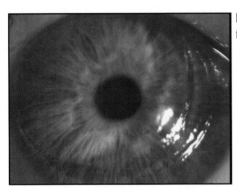

Figure 20-4. Flap torn during an attempt to forcefully dissect the flap with a spatula.

with spatulas and blades may lead to torn flaps or rough or irregular surfaces (Figure 20-4). The etiology of the inadequate dissection is uncertain but appears to occur bilaterally in individual patients. When the ophthalmologist is actually able to forcefully elevate the flap, there often is some keratocyte activation and associated interface haze. The haze is corticosteroid sensitive and resolves with treatment within 3 to 4 months. There is no effect on vision. If the flap appears difficult to lift, then it is reasonable to abort the procedure and replace the already lifted edges of the flap to allow for healing over approximately a 1-month period. The procedure may be reattempted with a blade microkeratome set to cut the flap 50 μm deeper than the original femtosecond flap interface. If the flap were to be recut with the femtosecond laser, then the plasma gas bubbles may percolate through to the level of the old unlifted interface, preventing passage of the laser light through to the newly programmed interface level.

Nondissected Islands

If gas bubbles dissect through the stroma anteriorly, the bubbles will come to lie between the applanation plate and the corneal surface. The bubbles will spread ahead of the advancing propagation of the laser raster pattern and block the focused femtosecond laser light. This blocking leaves an undissected zone wherever it occurs. The interface then is not separable in this area. Forceful attempts to delaminate the corneal collagen fibers in this area can result in a tear through to the surface, leaving an isolated "island" of undissected tissue similar to the central islands that may occur with blade microkeratome-created flaps. This phenomenon of dissection of gas bubbles through the anterior stroma can occur with thin flaps (anterior stromal component less than 50 µm), through incisions such as following radial keratotomy or penetrating keratoplasty, and through scars such as following previous microbial keratoplasty or conductive keratoplasty. A similar process may occur when there has been a previous surgical lamellar plane created in the cornea such as from previous LASIK or keratomileusis. In this event, the gas may dissect along this existing intralamellar plane anterior to the intended plane and block the laser. The new plane is not dissected under this area, resulting in what amounts to a partial flap cut. Again, the management in these cases is to not initially attempt to lift the flap; but allow it to heal for 6 weeks and then recut the flap with a blade microkeratome at a level at least 50 µm deeper or more superficial to the original femtosecond laser plane.

POSTOPERATIVE COMPLICATIONS

Transient Light Sensitivity

There are 2 minor complications that are encountered following LASIK with the Intralase laser. The first is the transient light sensitivity (TLS) syndrome or Good Acuity–Photophobia Syndrome (GAPS) in which patients with good vision develop photophobia in the absence of any apparent finding on examination.[3] Corticosteroid drops are prescribed and symptoms improve within 1 week of treatment. Invariably, symptoms resolve with or without treatment, leaving no residual abnormality or symptoms. Its etiology is unknown and speculation has varied among keratocyte activation to laser-induced iritis, scleritis, or neuritis. The majority of patients feel more comfortable wearing sunglasses during the 2 to 6 weeks that it takes to resolve. The incidence of this symptom is approximately 1%.

Keratitis

The second complication is intrastromal inflammation localized around the edge of the flap that occurs 2 to 7 days following flap creation.[4] The corneal stromal tissue becomes hazy or white along the side cut and there is associated cellular infiltration in the interface and in the superficial cornea in a narrow band along the edge of the flap. There may be some associated photophobia. Presumably, this inflammation results from microscopic cornea tissue damage caused by the laser photodisruption perhaps exaggerated by exogenous inflammatory factors in the tear film. Although this process may share some features with diffuse lamellar keratitis syndrome (DLK), it is differentiated by its later onset and the stromal inflammation outside of the edge of the flap. Treatment consists of frequent topical corticosteroid drops and adjunctive measures such as oral doxycycline. In mild to moderate cases, the process resolves without sequelae. In rare cases, the inflammation is severe and scarring may develop in the area of the side cut and haze in the interface. Since the majority of the inflammation occurs in the peripheral area of the flap outside the visual axis, there is typically minimal, if any, effect on visual acuity. The frequency of cases appears to have declined with lower side cut energies.

Diffuse Lamellar Keratitis

Typical DLK is occasionally observed in femtosecond laser-created flaps, but the clinical course is benign and self-limited (Figure 20-5). Treatment is with topical corticosteroids until resolution. Higher laser repetition rates such as 30,000 or 60,000 hertz and smaller spot energies (1.7 mj) appear to decrease the incidence of both GAPS and DLK.

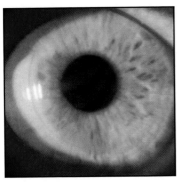

Figure 20-5. Diffuse lamellar keratitis.

CONCLUSION

The femtosecond laser is very dependable and predictable for creating lamellar interfaces and side cuts for LASIK. Striae, epithelial ingrowth, and displaced flaps are uncommon in femtosecond laser-created LASIK flaps.[5,6] Side effects and complications are rare and when they occur the outcome is usually not compromised. Careful attention to factors such as corneal scars that may be interfere with laser photodisruption can usually be anticipated and alternative treatments such as using a blade microkeratome or performing surface ablation could be considered in these cases.

KEY POINTS

1. During the creation of the flap, the Intralase suction ring may lose vacuum and the applanation plate may become separated from the cornea.
2. Occasionally, the gas bubbles generated from the intrastromal photodisruption can dissect from the interface through the peripheral cornea and into the anterior chamber via the trabecular meshwork.
3. Gas bubbles are routinely formed in the LASIK interface by femtosecond laser photodisruption (opaque bubble layer [OBL]).
4. Transient light sensitivity (TLS) syndrome or good acuity-photophobia syndrome (GAPS) is a condition in which patients with good vision develop photophobia in the absence of any apparent finding on examination. Corticosteroid drops are prescribed and symptoms improve within 1 week of treatment.
5. Typical diffuse lamellar keratitis (DLK) is occasionally observed in femtosecond laser-created flaps but the clinical course is benign and self-limited.

REFERENCES

1. Stonecipher KG, Dishler JG, Ignacio TS, Binder PS. Transient light sensitivity after femtosecond laser flap creation: clinical findings and management. *J Cataract Refract Surg.* 2006;32:91-94.
2. Lifshitz T, Levy J, Mahler O, Levinger S. Peripheral sterile corneal infiltrates after refractive surgery. *J Cataract Refract Surg.* 2005;31:1392-1395.
3. Biser SA, Bloom AH, Donnenfeld ED, Perry HD, Solomon R, Doshi S. Flap folds after femtosecond LASIK. *Eye Contact Lens.* 2003;29:252-254.

4. Durrie DS, Kezirian GM. Femtosecond laser versus mechanical keratome flaps in wavefront-guided laser in situ keratomileusis: prospective contralateral eye study. *J Cataract Refract Surg.* 2005;31:120-126.

5. Kim JY, Kim MJ, Kim TI, Choi HJ, Pak JH, Tchah H. A femtosecond laser creates a stronger flap than a mechanical microkeratome. *Invest Ophthalmol Vis Sci.* 2006;47:599-604.

6. Lifshitz T, Levy J, Klemperer I, Levinger S. Anterior chamber gas bubbles after corneal flap creation with a femtosecond laser. *J Cataract Refract Surg.* 2005;31:2227-2229.

Please see Flap Wars video on enclosed CD-ROM.

Chapter 21

LASIK OVER- AND UNDERCORRECTIONS

Luis Escaf Jaraba, MD; Alejandro Tello, MD; and Victor Rojas Hernandez, MD

INTRODUCTION

Refractive surgery procedures have progressively increased their efficacy and safety, and that, in turn, has caused patients' expectations to grow. In terms of safety and efficacy, several studies have proven that laser-assisted in situ keratomileusis (LASIK) is better than photorefractive keratectomy (PRK),[1] although surface ablation using new techniques, like Laser epithelial keratomileusis (LASEK)[2,3] and Epi-LASIK[4,5] has shown to have similar outcomes. However, LASIK is still the preferred procedure, as it has been during the past 10 years.[6,7] The risk of visual loss is significantly less and results are better in currently-applied LASIK techniques than some years ago due to advances in the surgical technique, better selection of surgery candidates, improvements in the microkeratomes, and in the laser's performance (including better eye-tracking systems and improved ablation profiles) and the advent of the clinical use of wavefront-customized ablations.[8-10]

LASIK PREDICTABILITY FACTORS

Factors Influencing Early Refractive Outcomes

LASIK outcomes depend on multiple factors, many of them still unknown or barely recognized. The change in the refractive power of the cornea is based on mathematical calculations like Munnerlyn's,[11] which modified according with empirical experience, and has been relatively successful in correcting refractive errors (lower-order aberrations) for the majority of patients treated to date. However, in this formula, the cornea is modeled as sphere and its behavior considered as if it were a piece of plastic being sculpted, which as we will see later, is not true.[12,13] Hydration of the cornea will also influence the ablation rate of the laser.[14-16]

Wavefront-guided customized ablations have shown promising results, but they are still not optimized for reasons that range from technological to biological, including the corneal biomechanical response to ablative surgery, and evidence is limited that it outperforms conventional modern conventional LASIK.[9,17-21] Moreover, it has been demonstrated that the corneal flap induces changes in corneal topography and both lower- and higher-order optical aberrations, and this factor is not taken into account in current LASIK software.[22,23]

Currently, we are using the Schwind ESIRIS (Kleinostheim. Germany) laser system (200Hz pulse frequency, 330 Hz active high-speed eyetracking and 0.8-mm scanning spot with Gaussian beam profile). It offers a treatment based on corneal wavefront data. A high-resolution topography system (Optikon Keratron [Rome, Italy] or CSO Eye-Top [Florence, Italy]) captures the data from the cornea and software (ORK CAM Custom Ablation Manager [Schwind]), realizes the transformation of the cornea into an individual, customized ablation profile. We use this option in 70% of the cases. Advantages of working with a corneal wavefront include reliable measurement results especially with irregular corneas, accommodation does not influence measuring results, and the treatment zone is not limited by the pupil. We are also using the option of the complete eye wavefront-guided customized ablations in 30% of our patients. In the future, we will compare the outcomes of these two groups of patients.

LONG-TERM STABILITY AND REGRESSION

Besides these factors in the laser-tissue interaction, the healing response of every cornea may be different and corneal biomechanics play a critical role.[18] The surgical plan is based upon an average healing response of a group of patients, but in a particular case, the patient may heal in a different way, leading to under- or overcorrection.[12,24] In order to improve LASIK predictability, it is important to realize that the cornea is not a piece of plastic.[12,13] Evidence shows that biomechanical corneal properties are an important source of individual variation that influence treatment response. The only way to improve outcomes will be to measure and predict them accurately, which is still not readily possible in vivo, although new techniques to investigate corneal biomechanical properties, not yet commercially available, have been used in clinical research studies, representing the critical first step in not only understanding biomechanical response to ablative procedures, but also predicting it on an individual basis.[25-27] In the field of stability and regression, postoperative stroma remodeling and corneal epithelial hyperplasia are factors that play a role.[28,29]

In conclusion, since the vast majority of modern refractive surgical procedures are based in large part on a population-based normative response, the possibility of individual differences and over- or undercorrections is real, so surgeons and patients must be aware of that.

Long-term stability of modern LASIK seems to be related to preoperative refractive error magnitude. A study in moderate myopic patients (mean preoperative spherical equivalent -4.85) showed that 5 years postoperatively, 60% of eyes were within ± 0.50 D of attempted correction with 83% within ±1.00 D. Eighty-nine percent of eyes had a vision of 6/12 or better at 5 years. Best spectacle-corrected visual acuity (BSCVA) was unchanged or improved in 51%. No eye lost more than 1 line of BSCVA. Overall, there was regression towards myopia with a mean change in refraction of -0.50 D over the 5 years. As expected, severely myopic patients regressed more with a mean change of -1.06 D.[30] In a series of higher myopes (mean spherical equivalent -13.65 D) followed for a mean of 76 months (range 50 to 84 months) after primary LASIK, only 46% of eyes were within ±1.00 D of the attempted correction and 88% were within ±3.00 D.[31] In hyperopia, the behavior of stability is similar, having poor long-term stability in cases higher than +4.50 or +5.00 D, although the most recent technologies show better results.[32-38]

Nomograms

Optimizing refractive surgery outcomes requires personalized nomograms that account for variations in equipment, surgical technique, the operating environment, and some features of each individual patient, so each surgeon has to refine his or her formula based upon real practical experience with a particular set of parameters.[39,40]

UNDER- OR OVERCORRECTION MANAGEMENT

In many cases, undercorrection and regression can be managed with a retreatment, but it is critical to study every case individually and avoid making decisions due to the pressure of the patient. Remember that myopic enhancements are common in eyes with post-LASIK ectasias.[41] Using ultrasound to measure central pachymetry postoperatively to determine if a patient can undergo an enhancement is inaccurate because epithelial hypertrophy may contribute to the postoperative reading. New technologies like anterior segment optical coherence tomography (OCT) are promising. Visante OCT (Carl Zeiss Meditec, Dublin, Calif) is the first noncontact device to image, measure, and document both corneal flap thickness and residual stromal thickness immediately following LASIK surgery (see Chapter 4), with the capability of quick measurements of flap and residual stromal thickness at any location.[42-44]

Hyperopic enhancements for undercorrections also need to be evaluated carefully because a too-steep cornea (higher than 50.00 D) may increase dry eye symptoms and cause epithelial problems in the apex, and their results seem to be not as good as myopic retreatments.[45,46] Moreover, the quality of vision in very steep corneas is directly related to the optical zone and the pupillary diameter.

An overcorrection of myopia may be corrected by performing a hyperopic LASIK enhancement and although its results have been considered safe and predictable, one series reported at the end of a 3-month follow-up that only 69% of eyes were within ±0.50 D and not all (96%) were within ±1.00 D of emmetropia.[47] A hyperopic overcorrection would in most cases be correctable via a myopic LASIK enhancement, but since regression may occur, it is important to wait until the stability is confirmed.

Since in many cases, the patient may not be a good candidate for a retreatment due to residual stromal bed thickness, corneal curvature or high refractive residual error, every patient undergoing LASIK should be aware about the possibility of a residual refractive error that can not be surgically corrected.

ENHANCEMENT TECHNIQUE

Not every post-LASIK refractive error is an indication for a retreatment. It depends on the symptoms of the patient and the level of satisfaction. Sometimes, if the eye with the residual ammetropia is not the dominant one and the fellow eye is close to emmetropia, the patient will feel good enough and it is not necessary to risk retreatment.

In our cases, undercorrections are usually enhanced 2 (or preferably 3) to 6 months from the original procedure. Meanwhile, the patient is managed with spectacles. Contact lenses should not be prescribed before 1 month after the LASIK and even then, patients must be instructed on careful insertion and removal to avoid affecting the flap. In overcorrections, we tend to wait a little more to be sure the patient has corneal and refractive stability.

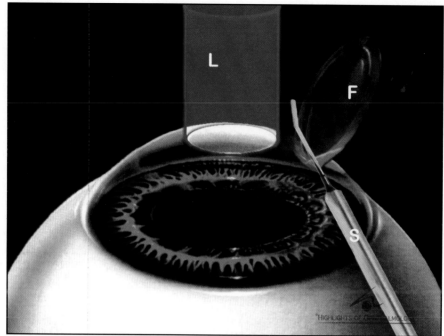

Figure 21-1. Enhancement with LASIK. After lifting the flap (F), the stromal bed is irrigated with BSS to eliminate any epithelial cells that may have moved when lifting the flap. The stromal bed is then dried with a sponge. After adequate centration and calibration of the laser, the excimer laser beam (L) is applied to obtain the desired ablation. (Courtesy of Benjamin F. Boyd, MD, FACS, Editor-in-Chief, *Atlas of Refractive Surgery* with permission from Highlights of Ophthalmology, English Edition, 2000.)

If the retreatment is done before 12 weeks post-LASIK, we prefer to lift the flap (Figure 21-1), unless the original one has had any problem (too thin, buttonhole, too small, too decentered). When lifted less than 8 weeks after the first procedure, it is easy to locate the edge under the microscope and then advancing a blunt spatula under the flap, usually beginning inferotemporally, it is easy to detach it. When lifted more than 8 weeks following the primary LASIK, we prefer to use a needle to mark the edge at the slit lamp, scratching a small amount of epithelium in that point so that it is easier to find it under the microscope.

If the enhancement is performed later than 12 weeks postoperatively, we use the microkeratome to recut a new flap. In this case, we leave the suction ring a little long to be sure the vacuum is very good, and decenter the new flap a little to avoid cutting exactly in the same position than the original. After passing the microkeratome with the same plate used originally, we use a 0.12 toothed forceps to gently lift the flap, since cutting at a depth close to the previous interface and using a spatula to lift the flap can sometimes mobilize a sheet of stromal tissue between the two cuts.

Other authors have described a technique to lift LASIK flaps up to 3 years after the initial surgery.[48] We do not recommend performing PRK over a LASIK because the risk of haze is very high.

AVOIDING DIFFICULTIES

Since our goal as refractive surgeons is to improve our patients' quality of life, exposing them to the lowest risk possible, it is crucial that we are well prepared as refractive surgeons and have an updated excimer laser system and microkeratome. Some other important points are discussed next.

Rational Advertising

Patients' expectations may be unrealistically high because of all the promotional material available. In advertising, it is important to attract public attention, but in our field of work it is essential to maintain a balance between enthusiasm and moderation in order to avoid disappointments when things do not go as expected.

Patient Counseling

Given the limitations of LASIK in its current form, it is crucial to counsel patients realistically.

One very important point is to always maintain a very good doctor-patient relationship. It is necessary to talk with the patients, to understand their fears, and to make them feel confident in our knowledge and skills.

Patient Selection

Several characteristics may make a patient not a good case for LASIK, so it is crucial to determine who is suitable for surgery and, importantly, who is not. It is becoming more evident that patients with keratoconus are not good candidates for LASIK, so every effort must be made to discover them.

Currently, it is known that high refractive errors have a higher incidence of under- or overcorrections, and late regression.[10,32-38,50-56] Most surgeons, including us, currently consider that the upper limit for myopic LASIK correction is -10.00 D.[54] For astigmatism our upper limit is a cylinder value of 6.00 D. For hyperopia we consider the upper limit to be +6.00 D.

ACCURATE REFRACTION

Many of the patients who are candidates for refractive surgery wear contact lenses, and it is very important that they stop using them before performing the preoperative exams because they can change the refraction (due to corneal warpage as a result of either mechanical deformation, chronic metabolic insult, or a combination of those 2 conditions).[57] In our protocol, we instruct the patients to discontinue wearing rigid or soft extended-wear contact lenses at least 3 weeks before the refraction and the surgery. If they have been wearing the contact lenses for more than 5 years, a second visit 1 to 3 weeks later is scheduled to confirm stability.[58,59] For soft daily wear contact lenses, we suggest discontinuation for 2 weeks before the surgery.

In young myopes, it is important to rule out an accommodative effect, using cycloplegia when there is any doubt. In young hyperopes, it is mandatory to perform cycloplegia. If the subjective refraction and the cycloplegic refraction are very different, it may be a good idea to make this patient wear the intended correction in spectacles for several weeks, so that the accommodation relaxes. The use of autorefractors may be helpful as a complementary tool when performing refraction in these patients.[60]

Accurate Programming

One possibility that has lead to many unexpected results is the improper programming of the laser, treating the wrong eye, or even treating the wrong patient.

Preoperative verification of a patient's identity, refractive error, and treatment parameters is critical and must be considered a step in the LASIK procedure.

CASE REPORT OF A NIGHTMARE

A 51-year-old woman had a preoperative refraction of OD: +4.75 –2.25 x 90 degrees and OS: + 4.50 –1.25 x 90 degrees. Pachymetry was OD: 544 µm and OS: 545 µm. The patient underwent LASIK, with a monovision approach (right eye for near vision). The next day her refraction was OD:+12.00 and OS: +10.50 –0.50 x 90 degrees. In that moment, it was evident that a misprogramming situation had occurred: the signs of the sphere in the planned treatment had been changed. A second wavefront-guided LASIK treatment was programmed, planning a total correction of her refractive error, and performed 1 week after the first procedure. Ten days following the retreatment her UCVA was OD: 20/60 and OS: 20/30. Her refraction OD:+1.75 and OS: +0.50.

We have taken all the measures described to avoid a recurrence of these cases happening again.

KEY POINTS

1. Prior myopic enhancement is a common risk factor in eyes with post-LASIK ectasias.
2. Using ultrasound to measure central pachymetry postoperatively to determine if a patient can undergo an enhancement is inaccurate because epithelial hypertrophy may contribute to the postoperative reading.
3. New technologies like anterior segment optical coherence tomography (OCT) are promising. Visante OCT is the first noncontact device to image, measure, and document both corneal flap thickness and residual stromal thickness immediately following LASIK surgery, with the capability of quick measurements of flap and residual stromal thickness at any location.
4. Many of the patients who are candidates for refractive surgery wear contact lenses, and it is very important that they stop using them before performing the preoperative exams because they can change the refraction
5. Not every post-LASIK refractive error is an indication for a retreatment.

REFERENCES

1. Hersh P, et al. Photorefractive keratectomy versus laser in situ keratomileusis for moderate to high myopia. *Ophthalmology*. 1998;105:1512-1523.
2. Camellin M. Laser epithelial keratomileusis for myopia. *J Refract Surg*. 2003;19(6):666-670.
3. Taneri S, Zieske JD, Azar DT. Evolution, techniques, clinical outcomes, and pathophysiology of LASEK: review of the literature. *Surv Ophthalmol*. 2004;49(6):576-602. Review. Erratum in: *Surv Ophthalmol*. 2005;50(5):502-504.
4. Pallikaris I. Epi-LASIK vs LASEK for the treatment of myopia. *Highlights of Ophthalmology*. 2006;Jan-Feb(1):2-3.

5. Pallikaris IG, Kalyvianaki MI, Katsanevaki VJ, Ginis HS. Epi-LASIK: preliminary clinical results of an alternative surface ablation procedure. *J Cataract Refract Surg.* 2005;31(5):879-885.

6. Sánchez-Thorin JC, Barraquer-Granados JI. Myopic laser assisted keratomileusis: an overview of published results. *Int Ophthalmol Clin.* 1996;36(4):53-63.

7. Duffey RJ, Leaming D. US trends in refractive surgery: 2002 ISRS survey. *J Refract Surg.* 2003;19(3):357-363.

8. Jacobs JM, Taravella MJ. Incidence of intraoperative flap complications in laser in situ keratomileusis. *J Cataract Refract Surg.* 2002;28(1):23-28.

9. Nuijts RM, Nabar VA, Hament WJ, Eggink FA.Wavefront-guided versus standard laser in situ keratomileusis to correct low to moderate myopia. *J Cataract Refract Surg.* 2002;28(11):1907-1913.

10. Watson SL, Bunce C, Allan BDS. Improved Safety in Contemporary LASIK. *Ophthalmology.* 2005; 112:1375-1380.

11. Munnerlyn CR, Koons SJ, Marshall J. Photorefractive keratectomy: a technique for laser refractive surgery. *J Cataract Refract Surg.* 1988;14(1):46-52.

12. Roberts C. Future challenges to aberration-free ablative procedures. *J Refract Surg.* 2000;16:S623-S629.

13. Roberts C. The cornea is not a piece of plastic. *J Refract Surg.* 2000;16(4):407-413.

14. Dougherty PJ, Wellish KL, Maloney RK. Excimer laser ablation rate and corneal hydration. *Am J Ophthalmol.* 1994;118:169–176.

15. Kim WS, Jo JM. Corneal hydration affects ablation during laser in situ keratomileusis surgery. *Cornea.* 2001;20:394–397.

16. Patel S, Aló JL, Perez-Santonja JJ. Refractive index change in bovine and human corneal stroma before and after LASIK: a study of untreated and re-treated corneas implicating stromal hydration. *Invest Ophthalmol Vis Sci.* 2004;45(10):3523-3530.

17. Roberts C. Biomechanical customization: the next generation of laser refractive surgery. *J Cataract Refract Surg.* 2005;31(1):2-5.

18. Roberts C. Biomechanics of the cornea and wavefront-guided laser refractive surgery. *J Refract Surg.* 2002;18(5):S589-592.

19. Aizawa D, Shimizu K, Komatsu M, et al. Clinical outcomes of wavefront-guided laser in situ keratomileusis: 6-month follow-up. *J Cataract Refract Surg.* 2003;29(8):1507-1513.

20. Caster AI, Hoff JL, Ruiz R. Conventional vs wavefront-guided LASIK using the LADARVision4000 excimer laser. *J Refract Surg.* 2005;21(6):S786-791.

21. Netto MV, Dupps W Jr, Wilson SE. Wavefront-guided ablation: evidence for efficacy compared to traditional ablation. *Am J Ophthalmol.* 2006;141(2):360-368.

22. Potgieter FJ, Roberts C, Cox IG, et al. Prediction of flap response. *J Cataract Refract Surg.* 2005;31:106-114.

23. Guell JL, Velasco F, Roberts C, Sisquella MT, Mahmoud A. Corneal flap thickness and topography changes induced by flap creation during laser in situ keratomileusis. *J Cataract Refract Surg.* 2005; 31(1):115-119.

24. Ambrosio, R, Wilson, SE. Complications of laser in situ keratomileusis: etiology, prevention, and treatment. *J Refract Surg.* 2001;17.

25. Jaycock PD, Lobo L, Ibrahim J, Tyrer J, Marshall J. Interferometric technique to measure biomechanical changes in the cornea induced by refractive surgery. *J Cataract Refract Surg.* 2005;31(1):175-184.

26. Luce DA. Determining in vivo biomechanical properties of the cornea with an ocular response analyzer. *J Cataract Refract Surg.* 2005;31(1):156-62.

27. Grabner G, Eilmsteiner R, Steindl C, Ruckhofer J, Mattioli R, Husinsky W. Dynamic corneal imaging. *J Cataract Refract Surg.* 2005;31(1):163-174.

28. Lohmann CP, Guell JL. Regression after LASIK for the treatment of myopia: the role of the corneal epithelium. *Semin Ophthalmol.* 1998;13(2):79-82.

29. Spadea L, Fasciani R, Necozione S, Balestrazzi E. Role of the corneal epithelium in refractive changes following laser in situ keratomileusis for high myopia. *J Refract Surg.* 2000;16(2):133-139.

30. M O'Doherty, M O'Keeffe, C Kelleher. Five year follow up of laser in situ keratomileusis for all levels of myopia. *Br J Ophthalmol.* 2006;90:20–23.

31. Sekundo W, Bonicke K, Mattausch P, Wiegand W. Six-year follow-up of laser in situ keratomileusis for moderate and extreme myopia using a first-generation excimer laser and microkeratome. *J Cataract Refract Surg.* 2003;29(6):1152-1158.

32. Kanellopoulos AJ, Conway J, Pe LH. LASIK for hyperopia with the WaveLight excimer laser. *J Refract Surg.* 2006;22(1):43-47.

33. Spadea L, Sabetti L, D'Alessandri L, Balestrazzi E. Photorefractive keratectomy and LASIK for the correction of hyperopia: 2-year follow-up. *J Refract Surg.* 2006;22(2):131-136.

34. Zaldivar R, Oscherow S, Bains HS. Five techniques for improving outcomes of hyperopic LASIK. *J Refract Surg.* 2005;21(5 Suppl):S628-632.

35. Ditzen K, Fiedler J, Pieger S..Laser in situ keratomileusis for hyperopia and hyperopic astigmatism using the Meditec MEL 70 spot scanner. *J Refract Surg.* 2002;18(4):430-434.

36. Esquenazi S. Five-year follow-up of laser in situ keratomileusis for hyperopia using the Technolas Keracor 117C excimer laser. *J Refract Surg.* 2004;20(4):356-363.

37. Jaycock PD, O'Brart DP, Rajan MS, Marshall J. 5-year follow-up of LASIK for hyperopia. *Ophthalmology.* 2005;112(2):191-199.

38. Zadok D, Maskaleris G, Montes M, et al. Hyperopic laser in situ keratomileusis with the Nidek EC-5000 excimer laser. *Ophthalmology.* 2000;107:1132–1137.

39. Mrochen M, Hafezi F, Iseli HP, Loffler J, Seiler T. [Nomograms for the improvement of refractive outcomes.] *Ophthalmologe.* 2006;103(4):331-339.

40. Ditzen K, Handzel A, Pieger S. Laser in situ keratomileusis nomogram development. *J Refract Surg.* 1999;15(2 Suppl):S197-201.

41. Randleman JB, Russell B, Ward MA, Thompson KP, Stulting RD. Risk factors and prognosis for corneal ectasia after LASIK. *Ophthalmology.* 2003;110(2):267-275.

42. Packer M. Visante OCT Applications for the Anterior Segment Surgeons. Presented at AAO; October 15, 2005; Chicago, Ill.

43. Kohnrn T. First Clinical Results with the Anterior Segment OCT: Evaluation of Patients for Refractive Surgery. Presented at AAO; October 15, 2005; Chicago, Ill.

44. Huang D. *Physical Principles of Corneal and Anterior Segment Optical Coherence Tomography Anterior Segment Imaging: New Advances in OCT Technology.* Available online at: http://www.osnsupersite. com/default.asp?ID=11746. Accessed August 28, 2006.

45. Mulhern MG, Condon PI, O'Keefe M. Myopic and hyperopic laser in situ keratomileusis retreatments: indications, techniques, limitations, and results. *J Cataract Refract Surg.* 2001;27(8):1278-1287.

46. McGhee CN, Ormonde S, Kohnen T, et al. The surgical correction of moderate hypermetropia: the management controversy. *Br J Ophthalmol.* 2002;86:815-822.

47. Jacobs JM, Sanderson MC, Spivack LD, et al. Hyperopic laser in situ keratomileusis to treat overcorrected myopic LASIK. *J Cataract Refract Surg.* 2001;27(3):389-395.

48. Hersh PS, Fry KL, Bishop DS. Incidence and associations of retreatment after LASIK. *Ophthalmology.* 2003;110(4):748-754.

49. Salah T, Waring GO, Magraby AE, et al. Excimer laser in situ keratomileusis under a corneal flap for myopia of 2 to 20 diopters. *Am J Ophthalmol.* 1996;121:143–255.

50. Stulting RD, Carr JD, Thompson KP, et al. Complications of laser in situ keratomileusis for the correction of myopia. *Ophthalmology.* 1999;106(1):13-20.

51. Dada T, Sudan R, Sinha R, et al. Results of laser in situ keratomileusis for myopia of -10 to -19 diopters with a Technolas 217 laser. *J Refract Surg.* 2003;19(1):44-47.

52. Magallanes R, Shah S, Zadok D, et al. Stability after laser in situ keratomileusis in moderately and extremely myopic eyes. *J Cataract Refract Surg.* 2001;27(7):1007-1012.

53. Han HS, Song JS, Kim HM. Long-term results of laser in situ keratomileusis for high myopia. *Korean J Ophthalmol.* 2000;14(1):1-6.

54. Sugar A, Rapuano CJ, Culberston WW, et al. Laser in situ kerartomileusis for myopia and astigmatism: safety and efficacy: a report by the American Academy of Ophthalmology. *Ophthalmology.* 2002;109:175-87.

55. Arbelaez MC, Knorz MC. LASIK for hyperopia and hyperopic astigmatism. *J Refract Surg.* 1999;15:406–414.

56. Choi RY, Wilson SE. Hyperopic laser in situ keratomileusis: primary and secondary treatments are safe and effective. *Cornea.* 2001;20(4):388-393.

57. Schornack M. Hydrogel contact lens-induced corneal warpage. *Cont Lens Anterior Eye.* 2003;26(3):153-159.

58. Tsai PS, Dowidar A, Naseri A, McLeod SD. Predicting time to refractive stability after discontinuation of rigid contact lens wear before refractive surgery. *J Cataract Refract Surg.* 2004;30(11):2290-2294.

59. Wang X, McCulley JP, Bowman RW, Cavanagh HD. Time to resolution of contact lens-induced corneal warpage prior to refractive surgery. *CLAO J.* 2002;28(4):169-171.

60. Salmon TO, West RW, Gasser W, Kenmore T. Measurement of refractive errors in young myopes using the COAS Shack-Hartmann aberrometer. *Optom Vis Sci.* 2003;80(1):6-14.

Chapter 22

TOPOGRAPHIC AND WAVEFRONT ABERROMETRY DISASTERS

Tracy Swartz, OD, MS, FAAO and Ming Wang, MD, PhD

When patients suffer reduced visual quality, or in more severe cases, reduced best corrected vision, the etiology of the visual complaint may be identified as topographic irregularities measured by corneal topography or increased higher-order aberrations (HOAs) measured by wavefront aberrometry.

CORNEAL TOPOGRAPHY

Topographically, irregular astigmatism, defined as astigmatism in which the principle meridians are not 90 degrees apart and associated with decreased best spectacle-corrected visual acuity (BSCVA), represents one of the most serious and frequent complications of corneal refractive surgery. While regular astigmatism is correctable using a cylindrical spectacle lens, irregular astigmatism occurs when the orientation of the principal meridians changes from one point to another across the pupillary zone. The astigmatism may be easily seen on topography, such as in the case of a central irregularity or decentered ablation (Figure 22-1), or be diffusely irregular, such as from dry eye (Figure 22-2).

Simulated keratometry (SimK) provides the power and axis of the steepest and flattest meridian similar to values provided by the keratometer. They are calculated from rings 7 to 9 corresponding to the position on the cornea at which keratometry measurements are obtained. This calculation assumes the posterior surface mirrors the anterior, and contributes about one-eighth the power of the cornea, which may not be true following keratorefractive surgery.

Statistical indices employed by various topographic systems, such as SimK, surface asymmetry index (SAI), shape factor (SF), and the corneal irregularity measurement may not be helpful in determining the nature of the abnormality in eyes with a history of keratorefractive surgery. Common indices are listed in Table 22-1. Since topographical systems assume a virgin prolate cornea, these programs often misdiagnose irregular astigmatism as keratoconus or generalize the curvature changes as simply "irregular." An example is shown in Figure 22-3.

Topography can often be misinterpreted when clinicians confuse curvature maps for elevation maps, and vice versa. For example, using curvature maps to identify irregular

Figure 22-1. A decentered ablation as displayed on an axial (bottom) and elevation (top) map.

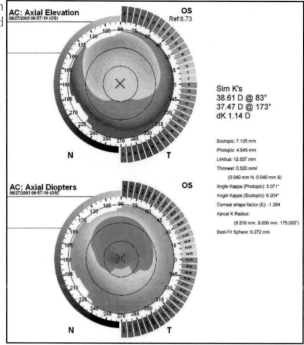

Figure 22-2. General irregularities with no pattern, such as this presentation of dry eye on the instantaneous curvature map.

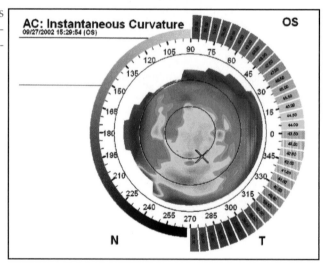

astigmatism may actually exaggerate the defect, as shown in Figure 22-4. When evaluating maps for decentration, it is best to use elevation rather than curvature maps.

As refractive surgery became more advanced, and the problems it created required improved technology for surgical correction, corneal topography became more precise. Greater computer capabilities enabled machines to handle complicated algorithms, allowing greater precision in corneal topography. Elevation mapping, an improvement over curvature mapping for surgical correction of loss of visual quality following refractive surgery,[1,2] made surgical planning using corneal topography a reality. Unfortunately, irregular surfaces may cause data capture failure, and algorithms may be less accurate for highly irregular surfaces.

Table 22-1

Common Index Used to Describe Irregular Astigmatism Using Corneal Topographical Systems

Simulated keratometry (SimK)	Provides the power and axis of the steepest and flattest meridian similar to values provided by the keratometer. They are calculated from rings 7 to 9 corresponding to the position on the cornea at which keratometry measurements are obtained.
Surface asymmetry index (SAI)	A centrally-weighted summation of differences in corneal power between corresponding points 180 degrees apart on 128 equally spaced meridians. The SAI approaches zero for a perfectly radially symmetrical surface and increases as the corneal shape becomes more asymmetrical.
Shape factor (SF)	The measurement of corneal asphericity. A negative SF usually indicates a postrefractive surgery eye with the center flatter than the periphery (oblate).
Corneal irregularity measurement (CIM)	An index that represents the irregularity of the corneal surface. High irregularity index often predicts irregular astigmatism.
Mean toric keratometry (MTK)	An index that uses elevation data to compare the toric reference to the actual cornea. The mean apical curvature value helps select the best toric fit using a spherocylinder design. This provides the most accurate toric representation of a patient's cornea.

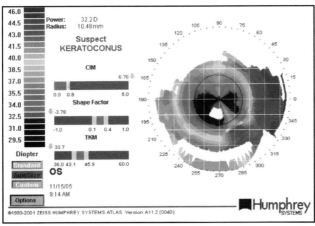

Figure 22-3. Indices may not yield useful information when the patient is S/P refractive surgery. This patient suffers from irregular astigmatism secondary to radial keratotomy (RK) surgery, not keratoconus.

Figure 22-4. Using curvature maps to identify irregular astigmatism may actually exaggerate the defect. Here the ablations look significantly larger on the curvature map then what is depicted in the elevation map.

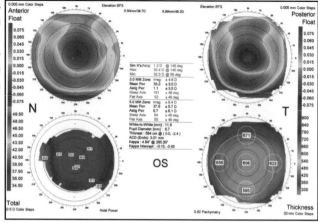

Figure 22-5. The Zernicke polynomial pyramid. (Courtesy of Naoyuki Maeda, MD.)

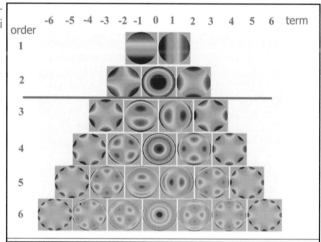

WAVEFRONT ABERROMETRY

Just as the advancement of computer technology facilitated topographic analysis, it likewise facilitated measurement of optical aberrations. This advance in technology occurred slightly later and parallel to the growth of topography. The most common models of aberrometry are Hartmann-Shack (Zywave, Milwaukee, Wis) and ray-tracing. Hartmann-Shack models utilize several hundred lenslets to measure the wavefront. Ray-tracing models utilize individual rays of light to measure the wavefront. Both models measure aberrations as a deviation from the plane wave in microns, and measurements are limited by pupil size. This is problematic in eyes with smaller pupils.

The shape of the wavefront is then mathematically described, most commonly using Zernicke polynomials—a combination of radial trigometric functions that describe the wavefront mathematically. Figure 22-5 shows this polynomial pyramid. While second-order terms of defocus and astigmatism are addressed by the manifest refraction, the irregular astigmatism resulting from higher-order aberrations primarily attributed to the cornea can be described by terms such as coma, spherical aberration, and trefoil.

Just as topographers exhibit difficulty capturing irregular corneal surfaces, aberrometers falter on irregular wavefronts (typically due to irregular astigmatism). This is especially true

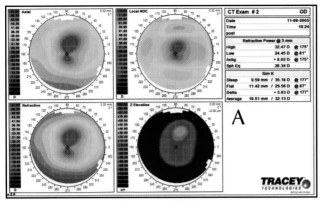

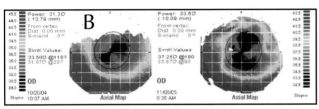

Figure 22-6. (A) The corneal wavefront of a patient S/P RK followed by LASIK with severe irregular astigmatism. (B) The topography of the same eye pre- and post-LASIK.

for diseased eyes and those with a history of keratorefractive procedures. Smolek and Klyce studied Zernicke-fitting methods for corneal elevation and reported fourth-order Zernike polynomials may not be adequate in their description of corneal aberrations in significantly aberrant eyes.[3]

CORNEAL WAVEFRONT

Because the majority of the eye's refraction occurs where the tear film meets the cornea's anterior surface, corneal distortion always significantly affects the total ocular wavefront aberration. The corneal wavefront is the component of the total ocular wavefront due to the corneal surface, calculated from corneal topographic height data. The corneal wavefront can be described using Zernike polynomials in the same manner as the total wavefront. Comparing the two Zernike representations enables isolation of corneal irregularities in reference to the total ocular wavefront.

For example, in Figure 22-6A, the corneal topography and wavefront maps are shown for a patient who underwent RK followed by LASIK. Note the irregular astigmatism. LASIK surgery increased the irregularity, shown in Figure 22-6B, which manifested as higher-order aberrations that did not improve with aggressive dry eye treatment. The following rule is generally accepted with regard to the deviation of elevation from the ideal shape: 3 μm of distortion from the ideal shape of the cornea results in about a –1.0-μm difference in the wavefront error map.

Using corneal wavefront enables better understanding of corneal irregularities because it presents corneal optics in the same "language" as wavefront systems. While elevation maps may be difficult for doctors to interpret, the pictorial representations of point spread functions (PSF) and Snellen letters are more easily understood. Results can be displayed in simulated visual acuity, PSF, modulated transfer functions (MTF), and other quantities that assess quality of vision.

IRREGULAR ASTIGMATISM S/P KERATOREFRACTIVE SURGERY

Clinical causes of irregular astigmatism as measured using aberrometry or topography following keratorefractive surgery (RK, AK, LASIK, PRK, LTK, CK) include extreme curvature changes; decentered ablation; small optical zone; posterior corneal changes; and irregular astigmatism due to flap complications such as incomplete flaps, tears, or diffuse lamellar keratitis (DLK). Nonsurgical treatment options are limited to gas permeable contact lenses (also called rigid gas permeables or RGPs), especially reverse geometry lenses or aspheric lenses. Surgical management of stable corneae include VISX Custom-CAP (Santa Clara, Calif) for decentered treatment, therapeutic (off label) use of wavefront-driven custom treatment, and topography-driven custom treatment. Unstable corneas with changing refractive error due to ectasia or incisional trauma may require Intacs (Addition Technology, Sunnyvale, Calif) placement or keratoplasty. What follows is a selection of cases to illustrate these points.

Case I

A 19-year-old female presented for LASIK evaluation. She desired to improve her vision and be free of the contacts "required to keep her eyes straight." She had a history of strabismus surgery for correction of an intermittent esotropia OD, which left her slightly exotropic and diplopic only when tired. Her manifest refraction found +1.75 +0.50 x 25 (20/40 due to amblyopia) OD and +0.75 (20/25) OS. However, cycloplegia revealed significant latent hyperopia: +4.25 OD, +1.50 OS. After a strabismus consult to ensure stable fusion, she elected to pursue LASIK for correction of her hyperopia. The planned LASIK correction was +2.75 +1.00 x 30 OD, and +1.00 OS. Her femtosecond-laser assisted LASIK was uneventful, and 3 months postoperatively, she was pleased with her vision, then 20/30 OD, 20/25 OS.

Seventeen months later, however, she presented reporting a loss of uncorrected vision OD. Without correction, she now read 20/50 OD and 20/25 OS, and refracted to +1.50 +1.25 x 180 (20/30) OD and +0.50 DS (20/20) OS. Upon cycloplegic refraction, she refracted to +3.00 +1.25 x 180 OD. She elected to undergo an enhancement OD, with a planned treatment of +1.50 +1.25 x 180. At her 1-month follow-up visit, she reported feeling "unbalanced." Her postoperative maps are shown in Figure 22-7.

Her autorefraction revealed significant hyperopia of +1.50 +0.50 x 50. Over time, her refraction remained stable. However, her manifest refraction consistently found -1.50 DS, which failed to subjectively improve her vision from her unaided 20/60. Interestingly, wavefront refraction found hyperopia. Her refractions are listed in Table 22-2. Despite attempts at correction using soft contacts and glasses, she continued to complain of reduced vision and "feeling unbalanced." The central elevation noted in Figure 22-7B causes her to appreciate the myopia found in the central 2 mm of her cornea and resulted in a multifocal effect that is not corrected by spectacles or hydrogel contacts. She could not tolerate gas perm lenses. Her symptoms improved 25% using Restasis (Allergan, Irvine, Calif) BID, but her loss of vision quality requires custom correction currently unavailable in the United States.

Case II

A 55-year-old female presented for further correction of her vision following repeated LASIK surgery. She had previously undergone myopic LASIK OU followed by an enhancement of the left eye 5 months later. At the time of the initial evaluation, her refractive error was -2.00 +1.00 x 100, which increased her uncorrected vision of 20/80 to 20/50. Her curvature and elevation maps are shown in Figure 22-8A. Gas permeable contact lens overrefraction found greater than 2 lines of improvement in her acuity, and a custom-contoured ablation pattern (CAP) treatment for a superior ablation was discussed. She underwent the

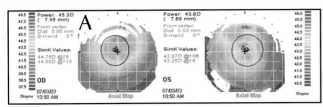

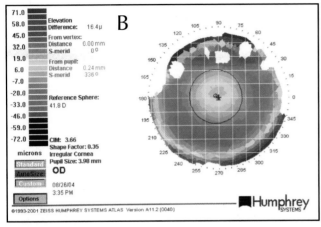

Figure 22-7. (A) Axial maps of both eyes 18 months S/P hyperopic LASIK. Vision was satisfactory OS but problematic OD. (B) The right eye viewed as an elevation map. Note the small central elevation secondary to the hyperopic treatment. (C) The wavefront map using ray-tracing technology of the same eye. (D) The wavefront map using Hartmann-Shack technology of the same eye.

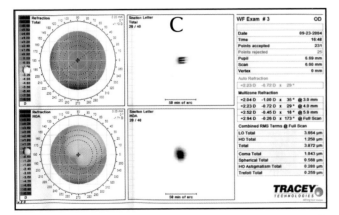

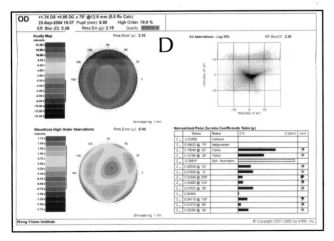

Table 22-2

Refractions As Measured Using Various Techniques

Method	Refraction
WaveScan	+1.74 +0.85 x 75 (5.0 mm)
I-Trace	+2..07 +.045 x 118 (5.0 mm)
Autorefractor	+1.75
Manifest	-1.50 +0.75 x 75

Figure 22-8. (A) Elevation and curvature mapping of a patient with a BSCVA of 20/50 due to decentration and irregular astigmatism. (B) Custom-CAP ablation plan for the same eye.

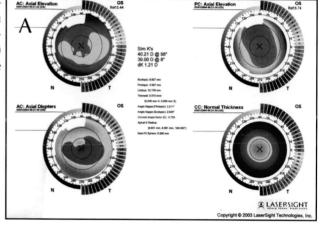

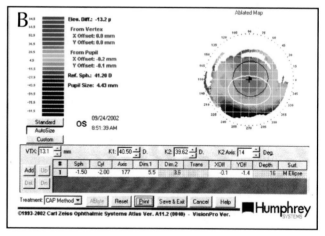

treatment according to the plan shown in Figure 22-8B. Her postoperative maps are shown in Figure 22-8C and show a significant improvement in the ablation zone size and location.

Despite a more regular corneal topographic map, the vision was less than satisfactory. Her resultant refraction was -3.75+1.25 x 90, with vision limited to 20/50. Gas perm and soft toric lens fits failed to improve her vision. What is interesting about the patient's astigmatism was the change in refraction with gas perm over-refraction. With a gas perm lens, her astigmatism flipped to plano +3.00 x 180, suggesting nonanterior corneal surface changes. Note the increased higher-order aberrations (Figure 22-8D) and regular posterior floats images OS

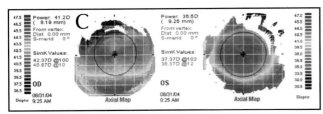

Figure 22-8 (cont). (C) S/P Custom Cap OS. Note the improvement in the shape of the ablation zone over the pupil. Despite the improvement, vision failed to significantly improve. (D) Waveprint S/P custom-CAP showing increased higher-order aberrations. There is not a predominance of coma due to the custom-CAP procedure, but rather a "mixed bag" of coma, spherical aberration, and trefoil. It was concluded the patient's visual problems were not primarily due to the anterior cornea. (E) The Orbscan of the same eye. Note the astigmatism on the posterior surface that manifested with gas perm over-refraction as significant astigmatism 90 degrees away from that found using manifest refraction.

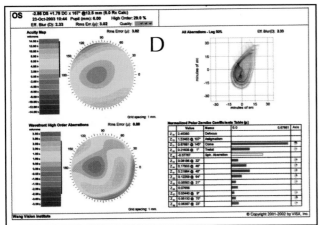

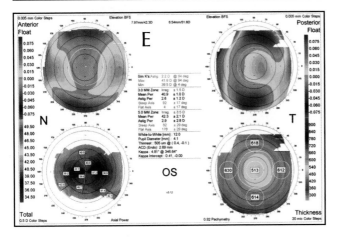

(Figure 22-8E). A hydrogel bifocal contact lens fitting OU was successful and allowed her to read 20/25 OU at distance with J3 vision while reading.

Case III

A 59-year-old male presented for correction of residual myopia following LASIK 6 years prior. His manifest refraction at initial evaluation was -1.00 OD (20/20) and -1.50 +0.50 x 165 OS (20/20). A demonstration of surgical enhancement OD to increase his distance vision while preserving his near vision was preferred by the patient, and he elected to undergo an enhancement OD. Due to a slightly irregular ablation zone as shown in Figure 22-9A, we performed CustomVue LASIK (VISX).

Day 1 he was 20/40 due to edema, and the flap was well-placed and free of debris. However, he presented 1 month later complaining of double vision. His topographic map

Figure 22-9. (A) Curvature map 1 month after his relift enhancement. Note the plateau at 3 o'clock OD due to a large patch of epithelial ingrowth. (B) The axial and elevation map showing a slight decentration. Patient was correctable to 20/20 pre-enhancement. (C) Slit lamp view of the ingrowth corresponding to these maps.

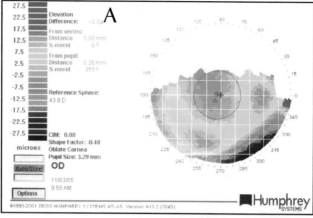

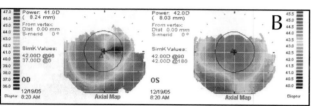

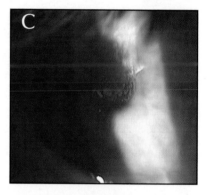

Table 22-3

Case IV Preoperative Information

	Manifest Refraction	Keratometry	Pachymetry
OD	-7.00 -0.350 x 135 DS, 20/20	43.37/45.12	537 (Avg)
OS	-9.00 +1.00 x 75, 20/20	43.87/46.12	576 (Avg)

is seen in Figure 22-9B and shows significant central irregularity. The patient had developed epithelial ingrowth along the horizontal meridian, shown in Figure 22-9C, which induced 2.75 D of astigmatism. The flap was relifted and cleaned and the patient experienced a full recovery of vision and normal topographic pattern.

Case IV

A 35-year-old male presented for LASIK evaluation. Comprehensive examination revealed no ocular health issues. His pertinent ocular findings are listed in Table 22-3.

He underwent femtosecond laser-assisted LASIK OU. His postoperative day 1 unaided acuities were 20/25 in each eye. At 3 months postoperatively, his vision was 20/30 OD, 20/40+ OS unaided with 1.00 D of astigmatism in each eye. He was instructed to aggressively treat his dry eye using Restasis BID and Alrex QID (Bausch & Lomb, Rochester, NY).

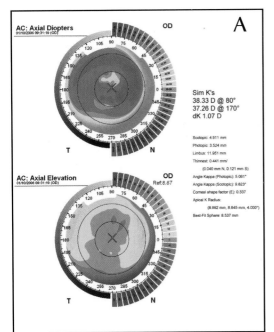

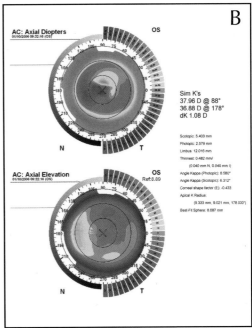

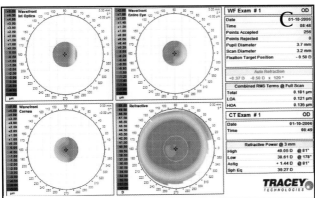

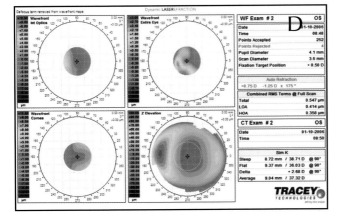

Figure 22-10. (A) Axial and elevation maps for the right eye of a patient with an oblate cornea following LASIK for high myopia. (B) Axial and elevation maps for the left eye of a patient with an oblate cornea following LASIK for high myopia. (C) Corneal wavefront maps for the right eye of the same patient. (D) Corneal wavefront maps for the left eye of the same patient.

Figure 22-11. (A) Axial maps in a patient S/P LASIK 4 years earlier. The preoperative maps were normal with no sign of FFKC. (B) Slit scanning images of the right eye of the same patient.

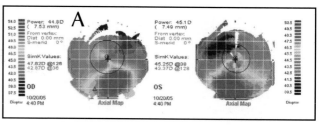

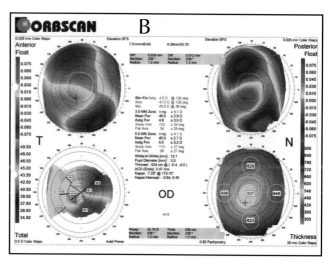

Over the next year, his unaided acuity improved to 20/20 OD, OS. However, he complained bitterly of glare and halos that failed to respond to brimonidine 1% drops prescribed for a miotic effect. The postoperative axial and elevation maps are shown in Figures 22-10 A and B. Note the red ring around the axial map of the left eye corresponding to the edge of the ablation. His wavefront maps can be seen in Figures 22-10 C and D. This is an excellent example of how the loss of the natural prolate shape leads to higher-order aberration, particularly spherical aberration, and subjective loss of vision when the patient's refraction is essentially plano in each eye, and unaided acuity is 20/20. The patient needs custom treatment to surgically restore a more prolate shape while maintaining the refractive status.

Case V

A 45-year-old male presented for evaluation 4 years after myopic LASIK in each eye followed by astigmatic keratectomy OS. He reported requiring glasses 1 year after surgery and needed to wear them full time. Unaided, he read 20/30 OD and 20/400 OS. Refraction of -6.00 +4.50 x 130 corrected the vision OD to 20/25, and -3.75 DS corrected the left eye to 20/30. Ultrasound pachymetry found 567 μm OD, 533 OS (average). The axial maps can be seen in Figure 22-11A.

We followed him for 2 years to find the corneas stable as measured by topography. Over this period, however, the myopia OS increased to -5.25 with a BSCVA of 20/25. The slit scanning maps can be seen in Figures 22-11B and C. Note the posterior elevation and irregular astigmatism. This irregular astigmatism on the axial map is manifested as smeared vision, which the patient reported was "remarkably similar" to the PSF shown in Figures 22-11D and E and the Snellen letter examples in Figures 22-11F and G. Due to the lack of refractive stability, surgery was not recommended.

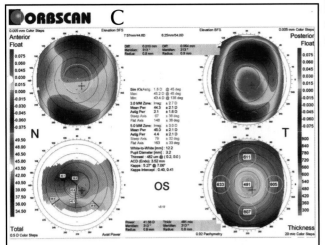

Figure 22-11 (cont). (C) Slit scanning images of the left eye of the same patient.

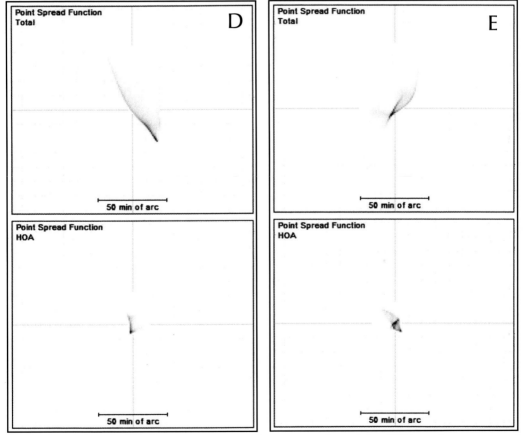

Figure 22-11 (cont). (D) Computer-generated representation of the PSF based on measured higher-order aberrations for the right eye. (E) Computer-generated representation of the point-spread function based on measured higher-order aberrations for the left eye.

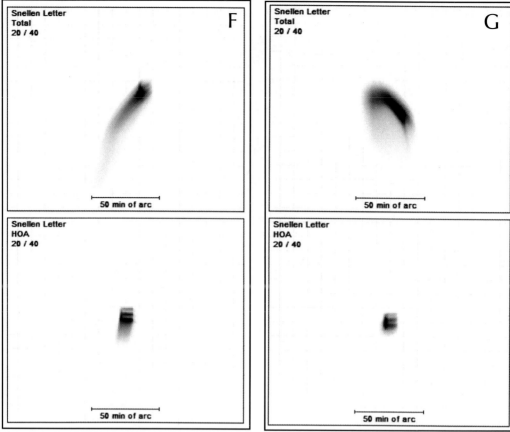

Figure 22-11 (cont). (F) Computer-generated representation of a Snellen letter based on measured higher-order aberrations for the right eye. (G) Computer-generated representation of a Snellen letter based on measured higher-order aberrations for the left eye.

CONCLUSION

These cases are unfortunate examples of how refractive surgery can result in severe irregularities on both topography and aberrometry. The use of corneal wavefront may be easier for clinicians less familiar with topography to understand the effects of changes in corneal shape upon the eye's optics. When significant, these irregularities may prohibit successful topographic and aberrometry mapping and require custom treatments for successful surgical management.

KEY POINTS

1. Topographically, irregular astigmatism, defined as astigmatism in which the principle meridians are not 90 degrees apart and associated with decreased BSCVA, represents one of the most serious and frequent complications of corneal refractive surgery.

2. Simulated keratometry (SimK) provides the power and axis of the steepest and flattest meridian similar to values provided by the keratometer.

3. The majority of the eye's refraction occurs where the tear film meets the cornea's anterior surface. Corneal distortion always significantly affects the total ocular wavefront aberration.

4. Just as topographers exhibit difficulty capturing irregular corneal surfaces, aberrometers falter on irregular wavefronts.

5. Elevation mapping, an improvement over curvature mapping for surgical correction of loss of visual quality following refractive surgery, made surgical planning using corneal topography a reality. Unfortunately, irregular surfaces cause data capture failure, and algorithms may be less accurate for highly irregular surfaces.

REFERENCES

1. Alessio G, Boscia F, La Tegola MG, Sborgia C. Topography-driven excimer laser for the retreatment of decentralized myopic photorefractive keratectomy. *Ophthalmology.* 2001;108(9):1695-1703.

2. Alessio G, Boscia F, La Tegola MG, Sborgia C. Corneal interactive programmed topographic ablation customized photorefractive keratectomy for correction of postkeratoplasty astigmatism. *Ophthalmology.* 2001;108(11):2029-2037.

3. Smolek MK, Klyce SD. Zernicke polynomial fitting fials to represent all visual signficant corneal aberrations. *Invest Ophthalmol Vis Sci.* 2003;44:4676-4681.

CUSTOMIZED LASIK AFTER PREVIOUS REFRACTIVE SURGERY

Roberto Pinelli, MD; Patrizia Portesi, OT; and
Cristian Bacchi, OD

INTRODUCTION

Laser assisted in-situ keratomileusis (LASIK) represents one of the most interesting and flexible techniques in the field of corneal surgery. In fact, it is very effective either in primary refractive strategies or in order to fix refractive problems after previous corneal or intraocular approaches.[1]

THE MEANING OF "CUSTOMIZED"

According to our opinion and to our personal experience, the word *customized* not necessarily means an approach involving the wavefront technology or the aberrations analysis. Most of the time, we define a traditional surgical approach as customized simply because it will help the patient A's problem. Patient B, even with a visual situation very similar to A, will not benefit from solution A because it was thought and planned exclusively for A. Surely, there are patients that can be better helped through a different approach that involves the wavefront technology, especially in those cases in which the problem seems to be related to the quality of vision than refractive.[2,3]

PATIENT EXAMPLE 1

Low Hyperopia and Presbyopia: LASIK After Conductive Keratoplasty

A 47-year-old woman came to our institute asking for refractive surgery to fix her low amount of hyperopia. In particular, she presented:
- RE far UCVA 20/25; BCVA 20/20 sph. +1; near BCVA J1 sph. +2.50
- LE far UCVA 20/25; BCVA 20/20 sph. +1; near BCVA J1 sph. +2.50

Eight spots conductive keratoplasty (CK) (normal pressure) were performed in both eyes. The patient was satisfied with near vision (she could read J1 bilaterally), but she referred some difficulties in her far vision; in fact, the left eye showed an overcorrection. Her visual situation after conductive keratoplasty in both eyes was as follows:

- RE far UCVA 20/20
- LE far UCVA 20/70; BCVA 20/20 sph –1.00 cyl –0.75 axis 160 degrees

Twelve months after CK, we opted for LASIK in the left eye to improve the patient's far vision. Because the LE was nondominant, we decided to correct myopia for half of its amount and the astigmatism completely (monovision).

The LASIK procedure after CK was successful. The patient was very satisfied and presented UCVA of 20/20 and J2 bilaterally.

In this example, LASIK balanced the far vision in both eyes, still maintaining the prolate shape of the cornea after CK.

PATIENT EXAMPLE 2

High Myopia: LASIK After Phakic Intraocular Lenses

A 43-year-old woman came to the institute asking for refractive surgery in order to fix a very high myopia in both eyes. She presented:

- RE far UCVA 20/1000; BCVA 20/40 sph –24.00
- LE far UCVA 20/1000; BCVA 20/40 sph –24.00.

The central pachymetry of the cornea was 560 μm in the RE, 550 μm in the LE.

Since the ACD of both eyes was 3.4 mm, a Verisyse phakic intraocular lens (IOL) implantation was planned and performed in both eyes.

The patient was informed that completely correcting such a high defect was really a challenging issue.

In fact, her visual situation after the IOL intervention was:

- RE far UCVA 20/70; BCVA 20/50 sph –4.00 cyl –1.50 axis 75 degrees
- LE far UCVA 20/70; BCVA 20/50 sph –4.00 cyl –1.50 axis 95 degrees

Three months after IOL procedure, we opted for LASIK in both eyes in order to eliminate the residual myopia and the astigmatism. After LASIK, the patient presented an unusual difference between the 2 eyes:

- RE far UCVA 20/50
- LE far UCVA 20/200; BCVA 20/50 sph –3.50 cyl –1.50 axis 115 degrees

After 3 more months, a LASIK enhancement was performed in the left eye.

Finally, after the LASIK enhancement the patient was able to see 20/30 bilaterally, showing a plano refraction. This extreme case of bioptics illustrates the tremendous impact of LASIK and LASIK enhancement for the complete success of the surgical strategy (Figure 23-1).

PATIENT EXAMPLE 3

Myopia and High Astigmatism: LASIK After Penetrating Keratoplasty

A 44-year-old man was referred to the institute for refractive surgery after penetrating keratoplasty (PK) in both eyes (RE in 1989, LE in 1992). The patient presented with:

- RE far UCVA 20/1000; BCVA 20/40 cyl –10.00 axis 90 degrees; pachymetry 601 μm
- LE far UCVA 20/1000; BCVA 20/25 sph –4.00 cyl –1.00 axis 130 degrees; pachymetry 552 μm

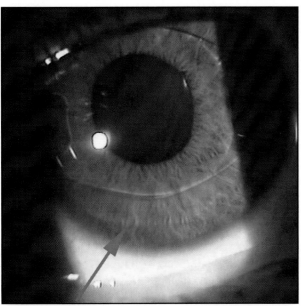

Figure 23-1. LASIK after Verisyse phakic IOL. Note the flap border.

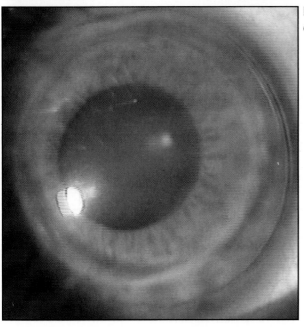

Figure 23-2. Slit lamp image of the left eye (LASIK).

The LASIK procedure was performed after discussing the following surgical strategy with the patient: emmetropia was the goal for the left eye while the correction of 7.00 D of astigmatism was planned for the right eye.

After the LASIK intervention, the patient presented with the following situation:

- RE far UCVA 20/200; BCVA 20/100 cyl –3.00 axis 95 degrees; pachymetry 511 μm
- LE far UCVA 20/25; pachymetry 506 μm

The patient was very satisfied (Figure 23-2).

PATIENT EXAMPLE 4

Hyperopia After RK: LASIK After RK

A 55-year-old man was referred to our center to improve his vision in his right eye, especially for near; 4 years before, an RK for 5.00 D of myopia was performed in another center in both eyes.

The RK procedure was successful in the left eye. In the right eye (the nondominant one), he reported the following situation:

- RE far UCVA 20/200; BCVA 20/25 sph +3.50 cyl +0.50 axis 25 degrees
- Near UCVA J10; pachymetry 570 µm (16 radial cuts)

An hyperopic LASIK procedure was performed. The flap showed a mild "pizza pie" complication and was smoothly replaced after the laser ablation. No contact lens was used.

At day 1 after surgery, the patient showed:

- RE far UCVA 20/30; BCVA 20/25 sph –1.00; UCVA near J2-3.

In this case, the LASIK procedure was very effective for improving the UCVA for far and near.

PATIENT EXAMPLE 5

Hyperopic Regression After PRK: LASIK After PRK

A 56-year-old woman asked us to surgically improve her vision after previous PRK in both eyes (2001).

She had the following situation:

- RE far UCVA 20/40; BCVA 20/20 sph +1.50; pachymetry 520 µm
- LE far UCVA 20/40; BCVA 20/20 sph +1.50; pachymetry 511 µm

A hyperopic LASIK procedure was performed.

In the left eye, the flap presented a mild epithelial shift, probably due also to the previous PRK intervention.

In fact, it's quite common when we perform LASIK after PRK to find an unusual response of the epithelium to the cut.

At day 3 postop, the epithelium of the left eye presented a regular situation and the patient was showing a visual improvement in far and near vision. This case shows us that LASIK can help also after a previous PRK, if the pachymetry allows it.

PATIENT EXAMPLE 6

Decentration After PRK: LASIK After PRK

A 42-year-old man presented with bad vision in the left eye after a monolateral PRK (performed at another center). The topography showed an important decentration. The right eye was emmetropic.

The manifest refraction of the LE showed a low negative sphere and a low but irregular astigmatism due to the decentered ablation done.

The LASIK procedure was performed in order to eliminate the low negative sphere. The main difficulty encountered during the treatment was to solving the coma induced. The result was a high reduction of the coma as the optical zone was more regular in its own extension and shape.

The patient was very satisfied with the new visual condition of his left eye.

KEY POINTS

1. LASIK represents one of the most interesting and flexible techniques in the field of corneal surgery and is very effective either in primary refractive strategies or in order to fix refractive problems after previous corneal or intraocular approaches.
2. One can use wavefront technology to help treat patients with refractive nightmares.
3. One good example of treatment is for decentered ablations. These cases can be treated well with customized laser treatment.
4. Understanding the topography and aberrometry in patients is crucial.

REFERENCES

1. Gimbel H, Anderson Penno A. *LASIK complications: Prevention and Management.* Thorofare, NJ: SLACK Incorporated; 2001:139-148.
2. Wang M. *Cornea Topography in the Wavefront Era: A Guide for Clinical Application.* Thorofare, NJ: SLACK Incorporated; 2006:113-118.
3. Agarwal S, Agarwal A, Agarwal A. *Dr. Agarwals' Textbook on Corneal Topography.* New Delhi, India: Jaypee Brothers; 2006.

IV

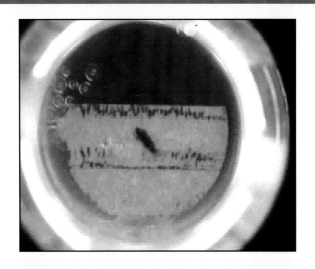

Lens-Based Refractive Surgery

Chapter 24

Accurate Biometry and Intraocular Lens Power Calculations

Noel Alpins, FRACS, FRCOphth, FACS and
Gemma Walsh, B Optom

Introduction

Technology employed in small incision cataract surgery is constantly evolving and continues to improve upon outcomes that already exceed acceptable standards. The modern surgical cataract goal has become more refractive in nature, which is highlighted by the widespread use of presbyopic multifocal and accommodative intraocular lenses (IOLs). Patients are informed and have high expectations for their visual result following surgery. This demands a high level of precision in biometry measurements. The ability to accurately predict the postoperative refraction is required more critically now than ever.

There are several factors that contribute to the final refractive outcome. These include biometry measurements, IOL power formulas, and surgical technique. Surgical technique is not covered in this chapter as it is obviously an intrinsic property of each surgeon, but may still influence the final result. For example, when the capsulorrhexis is larger than the optic of the IOL, a postoperative myopic shift may occur as the capsular bag contracts and displaces the IOL anteriorly. A retrospective analysis of the results for each surgeon will allow customization of the IOL power formula to account for these differences in surgical technique.

Causes of Unexpected Outcomes

Of all the components required to determine IOL power, inaccurate measurement of the axial length (AL) of the eye is the most frequent factor causing unexpected outcomes.[1,2] An AL measurement that is erroneous by only 100 µm translates into a 0.28-D error in the postoperative refraction.[2] Though inaccurate corneal power measurements account for a much smaller percentage of unexpected outcomes,[1] careful attention should always be paid to keratometry. It is best to designate one keratometer that is regularly calibrated for all biometry measurements.

The remaining error may be attributed to inaccurate calculation of the final IOL position within the eye.[1] This is the predicted depth of the power plane of the IOL optic after surgery and is sometimes referred to as the postoperative anterior chamber depth (ACD). It is more

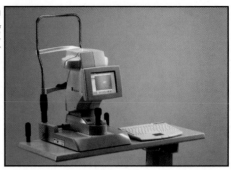

Figure 24-1. IOLMaster. (Reprinted with permission from Agarwal A. *Phaco Nightmares: Conquering Cataract Catastrophes.* Thorofare, NJ: SLACK Incorporated; 2006.)

accurately termed the effective thin-lens position (ELP). The final position of the IOL in the capsular bag can have an effect on the final refraction. A lens that sits more posteriorly than expected will lead to postoperative hyperopia and vice versa.[3] Considering the crystalline lens is approximately 5 mm thick and an IOL averages about 1 mm in thickness, there is a significant margin for potential error. The final ELP is naturally dependent to a certain extent on surgical technique but is also a predicted value within the IOL power formulas. Thus, while accurate determination of AL and corneal power are critical, the use of an appropriate IOL power formula is also of great importance.

BIOMETRY TECHNIQUES FOR MEASURING AXIAL LENGTH

Regardless of the biometry technique employed, it is important to check the results of the scan for inconsistencies. Biometrists need to be trained in detecting unusual measurements that should raise an alarm. For instance, if there is a significant difference in AL or keratometry between eyes, the measurements should be examined more closely. If there is more than 1.00 D difference in IOL power between eyes, this also needs to be confirmed. The predicted IOL power and AL should correlate with the refraction; if the results indicate a 15.00-D IOL for a +6.00-D hyperope, then an error has occurred somewhere. Of course, both eyes should have biometry measurements prior to the first surgery as standard practice to allow a comparison between eyes.

Applanation ultrasound A-scan is the most common technique employed for the measurement of axial length,[2,4] though a trend to move toward the highly accurate partial coherence laser interferometry (PCLI), otherwise known as optical biometry, is emerging. Sixty-one percent of ophthalmology departments in the United Kingdom now employ this method.[5] Immersion ultrasound biometry is the least commonly used method.

Partial Coherence Laser Interferometry

This technique of optical biometry measures the axial length of the eye from the anterior cornea to the retinal pigment epithelium along the visual axis using a coaxial dual beam.[6] It is highly accurate as the resolution is greater than that with ultrasound (0.012 mm compared to 0.10 to 0.12 mm).[5] This results in an outstanding accuracy of 15 to 20 μm, significantly greater than that of applanation ultrasound technique.[2] The measured AL with PCLI is approximately 0.30 mm longer than immersion ultrasound, and up to 0.96 mm longer than in applanation ultrasound.[6]

PCLI technology is commercially available as the Zeiss IOLMaster (Dublin, Calif) (Figure 24-1). The retinal endpoint of the AL measurement is different with PCLI compared to ultrasound A-scans (retinal pigment epithelium compared to internal limiting membrane), and

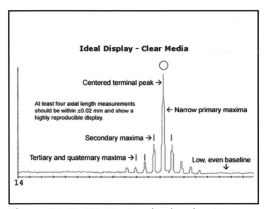
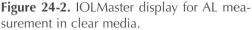

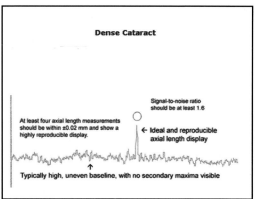

Figure 24-2. IOLMaster display for AL measurement in clear media.

Figure 24-3. IOLMaster display for AL measurement in dense cataract.

as such, the PCLI software has built in correction factors to allow for this (Figures 24-2 and 24-3). Despite this, different constants for the same IOL must be used for the 2 different biometry techniques.[5]

The measurement of the preoperative ACD with the IOLMaster is done using a photographic technique rather than with PCLI. The corneal power is measured with automatic keratometry, which has been shown to correlate well with manual readings over an average power range.[7] However, automatic keratometry may be an unreliable technique for measuring the magnitude and meridian of astigmatism, particularly when the magnitude is small. It is therefore recommended that the measurements are cross-checked with manual readings for accuracy.

The test is fairly comfortable as it is noncontact and performed in a sitting position rather than supine. It is essentially operator independent with results reproducible to 0.02 mm, even when technicians have minimal experience.[2,5] There can be no confusion between measuring right and left eyes as the machine automatically detects and records this.

Another advantage over ultrasonography is the ability to accurately measure the AL in an eye filled with silicone oil following vitreoretinal surgery.[8] The software does this by changing the mean refractive index to account for the silicone oil. Ultrasonography may also be used to measure through the silicone oil, but it is more challenging because oil droplets may create artifacts, resulting in the absence of a retinal peak. This is particularly the case for immersion ultrasonography where the patient is lying down. The PCLI software also allows easy measurement through phakic IOLs, a problem that will become more widespread as implantation of these devices gains popularity.

PCLI does require adequate fixation, and this may be a source of difficulty in patients with poor cooperation or reduced visual acuity. It also will not take measurements through dense cataracts. Consequently, the test may be rendered ineffective in approximately 10% to 20% of cases.[2,4,7] Therefore, proficiency in the other methods of measuring AL is still required.

Immersion Ultrasound A-Scan

Though the resolution with ultrasonography is not as great as with PCLI, this is still a highly-accurate technique and is useful particularly in cases in which a measurement cannot be obtained with optical biometry. This might include patients with poor fixation from maculopathy, nystagmus, or dense cataracts. Although the results are comparable with PCLI,[7] the immersion technique is not widely utilized. This is likely due, in part, to the use of the

Figure 24-4. Immersion A-scan ultrasonography.

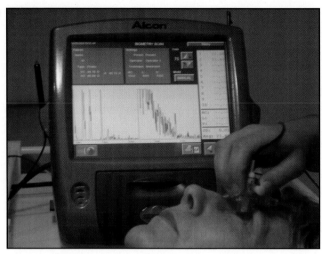

water and the scleral shell that renders this test more uncomfortable for the patient. Due to physical constraints, it is not always feasible for the patient to lay flat for the measurement either (Figure 24-4).

In contrast to optical biometry, the axial length is measured from the anterior cornea to the inner limiting membrane (ILM).[6] This may account for slight differences in results between ultrasonography and PCLI as the ILM is more variable in thickness compared to the retinal pigment epithelium. However, as previously mentioned, the PCLI software has been calibrated against results from immersion biometry to account for this to some extent.

One disadvantage with ultrasonography is that small misalignments may occur with the transducer probe, and the ultrasonic beam may not be perpendicular to the intraocular surfaces. This results in a jagged retinal peak or the absence of a posterior lens peak on the A-scan. However, 2 corneal peaks (anterior and posterior cornea) are seen with an immersion ultrasound scan compared to a single peak with the applanation method. These 2 peaks may be aligned to judge whether the measurement has been taken on the optical axis.[5]

In ultrasonography A-scans, the AL measurements are made along the optical axis rather than the visual axis, which can lead to erroneous results in long eyes. For instance, the AL measured along the optical axis in an eye with a posterior staphyloma may be overestimated by 3.0 mm, resulting in an unwanted refractive error of up to +8.00 D.[4] In cases of high myopia, a combination A/B-scan may be more accurate.

Combination Immersion A/B-Scan

A high proportion of highly myopic eyes with an AL of greater than 30.0 mm have a posterior staphyloma temporal to the fovea.[9] This often leads to erroneously long measurements of AL and subsequent postoperative hyperopia. In these cases, an immersion A/B-scan may be appropriate.[9,10] A horizontal immersion B-scan with simultaneous vector A-scan is taken. The B-scan allows visualization of the fovea so the retinal peak of the A-scan may be aligned more exactly with it to avoid measurement of a staphyloma. This technique also allows precise centration of the corneal peak. The main disadvantage of this technique is that it requires an experienced operator who is familiar with B-scan technology because the fovea is not always easy to identify.[9]

Applanation Ultrasound A-Scan

Despite being one of the most widely performed techniques, this method has the lowest accuracy.[2] The main disadvantage of this method is applanation of the cornea, resulting in corneal compression of between 0.14 to 0.47 mm, depending on the experience of the biometrist.[2,5,11] An A-scan that has indented the cornea will still appear acceptable to view on the screen, but it could result in an unwanted error of the calculated IOL power of more than 1.00 D.[12] This technique is highly operator dependent. If one technician performs all A-scans within a clinic, a retrospective analysis may be performed to allow for the applanation within the IOL power formula. However, as the amount of compression is likely to vary with the level of intraocular pressure, errors may still occur.[12]

INTRAOCULAR LENS POWER FORMULAS

It has been shown that the modern third- and fourth-generation theoretical IOL power formulas are more accurate than the earlier empirical formulas such as the SRK I, SRK II, and Binkhorst.[13,14] There are 5 well-known theoretical IOL power formulas: Holladay 1 and 2, Hoffer-Q, SRK/T, and Haigis. All are based on thin lens optics and utilise the refractive vergence formula in the calculation of IOL power, which has 6 variables and 2 constants.[15] The formulas differ in how they estimate the final ELP.

The 3 third-generation formulas (Holladay 1, Hoffer-Q, and SRK/T) predict the ELP based on 2 variables: net corneal power and AL. This makes a number of broad assumptions about the eye, including that the anterior and posterior segments are roughly proportional. The 2 fourth-generation formulas (Holladay 2 and Haigis) utilize more variables when calculating the ELP. These formulas address the variable relationship between the ACD and length of the posterior segment, and as such have a higher rate of accuracy over a wider range of ALs. The Holladay 2 formula is widely considered to be very accurate, though it has the disadvantage of requiring the measurement of 7 variables. The Haigis formula has a similar level of accuracy if properly customized (see later) and has the advantage of requiring only 3 variables (AL, corneal power, and ACD).[14]

Customizing Intraocular Lens Formula Constants to Improve Accuracy

Each formula has a "constant" associated with predicting the ELP. The Holladay 1 formula uses a "surgeon factor" that is the distance between the iris plane and the power plane of the IOL, where the distance from the cornea to the iris plane is calculated as the dome height of the cornea.[16] The Hoffer-Q formula uses the "ACD-constant" which is the average distance between the power plane of the cornea and the IOL.[16] The SRK/T formula uses the "A-constant" supplied by the manufacturer of the IOL. The Holladay 2 formula also uses an "ACD-constant."[16] The Haigis formula uses 3 constants: a0, a1, and a2. The a0 constant works in a similar manner as the constants for the other formulas. The a1 constant relates to the measured ACD, and the a2 constant to the measured AL.[14]

It is recommended that these constants be customized through retrospective analysis for the individual surgeon and IOL type to further increase accuracy in IOL power calculations.[5,16,17] In the case of the Haigis formula, all 3 constants may be customized, though at present this regression analysis is only carried out by either Dr. Wolfgang Haigis himself or his colleague Dr. Warren Hill.[14] The IOLMaster also includes software to track outcomes and personalize the A-constant for the SRK/T formula. However, even with personalized constants, there are still errors with predicting IOL power in high ametropia.[16]

Table 24-1

Preferred Intraocular Lens Power Formulas for Differing Axial Length[5]

Short eyes <22.0 mm	Hoffer-Q, Holladay 2
Medium eyes 22.0 to 24.5 mm	Holladay 1 or 2, Hoffer-Q, SRK/T, Haigis
Medium long eyes 24.6 to 26.0	Holladay 1 or 2
Long eyes >26.0 mm	SRK/T, Haigis*, Holladay 2

*Customized to the surgeon and type of IOL

INTRAOCULAR LENS POWER FORMULAS
FOR EXTREME AMETROPIA

Accuracy in IOL calculations for extreme ametropia has always been challenging, even with personalized modern IOL power formulas. It has been shown that the different formulas perform differently depending on the AL of the eye.[18] This is summarized in Table 24-1. For an eye of average length (22.0 to 26.0), any modern formula performs well.[18] For very short eyes (<22.0 mm) the Hoffer-Q or Holladay 2 formula is the most accurate.[5,18] For very long eyes (>26.0 mm), the SRK/T formula gives the best results,[5,9,18] though it still has a tendency to predict an IOL power that is too great.[9]

Accurate prediction of IOL power in patients with extreme axial hyperopia is relatively easy; accurately obtaining the AL is easier, and the Hoffer-Q or Holladay 2 formula predicts the IOL power with a high degree of accuracy. By contrast, accurately predicting the IOL power for extremely high axial myopia is more challenging even using the SRK/T and fourth-generation formulas.

In patients with extreme myopia, the required IOL is one of a low positive power, zero power, or a low negative power. Implantation of a zero power IOL is more beneficial than leaving the eye aphakic because it provides a barrier function to reduce the rate of posterior capsule opacification.[10,19] The IOL also stabilizes the vitreous base if a YAG capsulotomy is required, potentially reducing the incidence of retinal detachment. When an IOL of low positive power is predicted, the results are more accurate than if a negative-powered IOL is predicted.[9,19] If the calculated IOL power is between –1.00 to –4.00 D, postoperative hyperopia is more often seen.

This could be due in part to inaccurate estimation of AL in these highly myopic patients. As discussed earlier, PCLI with the IOLMaster and immersion A/B-scans are the 2 most accurate methods of biometry in long eyes. However, while these techniques of biometry have been shown to improve accuracy of the SRK/T formula, it is still not uncommon for a post-operative refraction of approximately +1.00 D to occur.[19] It has been suggested that transforming the AL scale to a population mean AL of 24.00 mm may help reduce the error in the Holladay 1, Hoffer-Q, and SRK/T IOL power formulas in cases of extreme ametropia.[16]

The answer to predicting IOL power in extreme myopia remains elusive. In patients whose predicted IOL is of a negative power, it is worthwhile considering the possibility of an overcorrection and factoring this into the final selection of IOL for implantation by choosing a lens of less negative power.

SUMMARY

There are many factors that contribute to the final refractive outcome of small incision cataract surgery. These include the measurement of axial length, corneal power, and selection of the appropriate IOL power formula. Though some occur more commonly than others in unexpected outcomes, they all have equal importance in preventing a postoperative surprise. The method employed to measure axial length should be considered, and keratometry readings should be cross-checked for accuracy. A single IOL power formula should not be used across the board for all calculations, especially in cases of extreme ametropia. The appropriate formula must be considered for the individual case, and for greater accuracy it should be personalized for the surgeon and type of IOL.

KEY POINTS

1. The modern surgical cataract goal has become more refractive in nature, which is highlighted by the widespread use of presbyopic multifocal and accommodative IOLs.
2. Of all the components required to determine IOL power, inaccurate measurement of the axial length (AL) of the eye is the most frequent factor causing unexpected outcomes.
3. The final position of the IOL in the capsular bag can have an effect on the final refraction.
4. The retinal endpoint of the axial length measurement is different with partial coherence laser interferometry (PCLI) compared to ultrasound A-scans (retinal pigment epithelium compared to ILM.
5. For an eye of average length (22.0 to 26.0) any modern formula performs well. For very short eyes (<22.0 mm), the Hoffer-Q or Holladay 2 formula is the most accurate. For very long eyes (>26.0 mm), the SRK/T formula gives the best result.

REFERENCES

1. Olsen T. Sources of error in intraocular lens calculation. *J Cataract Refract Surg.* 1992;18:125-129.

2. Findl O, Kriechbaum K, Sacu S. Influence of operator experience on the performance of ultrasound biometry compared to optical biometry before cataract surgery. *J Cataract Refract Surg.* 2003;29:1950-1955.

3. Elder MJ. Predicting the refractive outcome after cataract surgery: the comparison of different IOLs and SRK-II v SRK-T. *British Journal Ophthal.* 2002;86:620-622.

4. Tehrani M, Krummenauer F, Kumar R et al. Comparison of biometric measurements using partial coherence interferometry and applanation ultrasound. *J Cataract Refract Surg.* 2003;29:747-752.

5. Gale RP, Saha N, Johnston RL. National biometry audit II. *Eye.* 2006;20:25-28.

6. Kielhorn I, Rajan M, Tesha P. Clinical assessment of the IOLMaster. *J Cataract Refract Surg.* 2003;29:518-522.

7. Mamalis N. Intraocular lens power accuracy: how are we doing? *J Cataract Refract Surg.* 2003;29:1-3.

8. Dietlein T, Roessier G, Luke C et al. Signal quality of biometry in silicone oil-filled eyes using partial coherence interferometry. *J Cataract Refract Surg.* 2005;31:1006-1010.

9. Zaldivar R, Schultz M, Davidorf J. Inraocular lens power calculations in patients with extreme myopia. *J Cataract Refract Surg.* 2000;26:668-674.

10. Huber C. Effectiveness of intraocular lens calculation in high ametropia. *J Cataract Refract Surg.* 1989; 15:667-671.

11. Hennesy MP, Franzco, Chan DG. Contact versus immersion biometry of axial length before cataract surgery. *J Cataract Refract Surg.* 2003;29:2195-2198.

12. Schroff NM, Ray S, Kumar K, et al. A practical device to aid in immersion a-scan biometry. *J Cataract Refract Surg.* 2004;30:1386-1387.

13. Olsen T, Thim K, Corydon L. Accuracy of the newer generation intraocular lens power calculation formulas in long and short eyes. *J Cataract Refract Surg.* 1991;17:187-193.

14. Hill W. Highly accurate IOL calculations. *Cataract and Refractive Surgery Today.* 2005;March:67-70.

15. Basu S. Comparison of IOL power calculations by the IOLMaster vs theoretical calculations. *Eye.* 2006; 20:90-97.

16. Norrby S, Lydahl E, Koranyi G, et al. Reduction of trend errors in power calculation by linear transformation of measured axial lengths. *J Cataract Refract Surg.* 2003;29:100-105.

17. Zuidervaart W, Luyten G. A retrospective analysis of five intraocular lenses and the predictive value of six different intraocular lens power calculation formulas. *Ophthalmologica.* 2005;219:390-393.

18. Hoffer KJ. Clinical results using the Holladay 2 intraocular lens power formula. *J Catract Refract Surg.* 2000;26:1233-1237.

19. MacLaren RE, Sagoo MS, Restori M. Biometry accuracy using zero and negative powered intraocular lenses. *J Cataract Refract Surg.* 2005;31:280-290.

**Please see Cataract After Radial Keratotomy
video on enclosed CD-ROM.**

Chapter 25

MIRLEX

Amar Agarwal, MS, FRCS, FRCOphth;
Mahipal S. Sachdev, MD; and Clement K. Chan, MD, FACS

HISTORY

On August 15, 1998, Dr. Agarwal performed a 1-mm cataract surgery with a technique called Phakonit[1-6] (phacoemulsification performed with needle incision technology). Dr. Jorge Alió in Spain coined the term microincision cataract surgery (MICS) for all surgeries, including laser cataract surgery and phakonit. Dr. Randall Olson of USA first used a 0.8-mm phaco needle and a 21-gauge irrigating chopper and called it microphaco. These techniques are also known internationally as bimanual phaco. If the technique is used for clear lenses, it is known as microincisional refractive lens exchange (MIRLEX).

On May 21, 2005, Dr. Agarwal used a 0.7-mm phaco needle tip and a 0.7-mm irrigating chopper through sub-1.0 mm microincisions to remove cataracts for the first time. He named this microsurgical technique, microphakonit.

The novice phakonit surgeon may encounter more complications[1-5] since it is associated with a steeper learning curve in comparison to other methods. The term *phakonit* has been coined to signify the performance of phacoemulsification (phako) via a needle-induced (N) microsurgical incision (I) with the phako tip (T). Thus, it is phacoemulsification with the so-called needle incision technology (NIT).

PHAKONIT

The following paragraphs describe the detailed surgical techniques associated with phakonit for cataracts and clear lens exchange (MIRLEX).

Anesthesia

The technique of phakonit can be performed with a variety of anesthesia. The microincisional nature of this technique vastly reduces the requirements of anesthesia. Dr. Agarwal has even performed this technique without any topical, periocular, or intracameral anesthesia (no-anesthesia cataract surgery) with good surgical outcome and patient comfort. He found minimal differences between topical anesthesia and no-anesthesia cataract surgery. For a difficult case, he employs a peribulbar block.

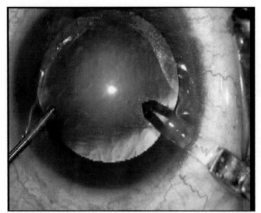

Figure 25-1. Clear corneal incision made with a special knife from MST. Note the left hand has a globe stabilization rod to stabilize the eye. This knife can create an incision from sub-1 mm to 1.2 mm.

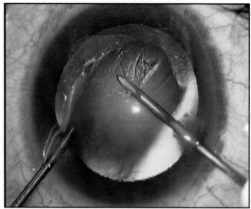

Figure 25-2. Rhexis started with a needle.

Incision

A 26-gauge needle is used to make a limbal incision for the side port and inject viscoelastic into the anterior chamber. The viscoelastic will deepen the anterior chamber so that a clear temporal corneal incision can be more easily made. A special knife (1.2 mm) can be used for this purpose (Figure 25-1). Note that in Figure 25-1, the surgeon's left hand holds a globe stabilization rod (Geuder, Heidelberg, Germany) to stabilize the eye while he or she creates the clear corneal incision. He or she holds the knife with his dominant hand. This knife, designed by Dr. Mateen Amin, creates an incision of either sub-1 mm or 1.2 mm, depending on the size of the knife that the surgeon chooses. For a knife creating a sub-1 mm incision, one should use a 21-gauge irrigating chopper and a 0.8-mm phaco needle. The microsurgical instruments for phakonit are manufactured by Huco (Geneva, Switzerland), Geuder (Heidelberg, Germany), and Microsurgical Technology Incorporated (Redmond, Wash).

Rhexis

The surgeon then performs a 5- to 6-mm rhexis with a 26-gauge needle. He or she uses his or her nondominant hand to stabilize the eye with the globe-stabilizing rod, while he or she creates the rhexis with the dominant hand (Figure 25-2). The globe stabilization rod allows improved control and stability, particularly in cases with minimal to no anesthesia. Microsurgical Technology Incorporated has manufactured a pair of rhexis forceps that goes through a 1-mm incision for achieving rhexis as an alternative to the needle during phakonit.

Hydrodissection

Next, hydrodissection is performed and the fluid waves passing under the nucleus are checked. The surgeon should also carefully inspect for rotation of the nucleus.

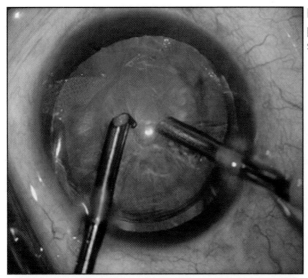

Figure 25-3. Phakonit irrigating chopper and phako probe without the sleeve inside the eye.

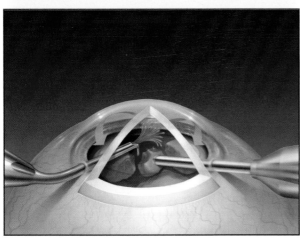

Figure 25-4. Phakonit done. Notice the irrigating chopper with an end opening. (Courtesy of Larry Laks, MST.)

Phakonit

After enlarging the side port, the surgeon inserts into the anterior chamber a 20- or 21-gauge irrigating chopper connected to the infusion line of the phaco machine with the foot pedal control on Position 1. There are various irrigating choppers, including the Agarwal irrigating chopper specially designed by Larry Laks, available through Microsurgical Technology Incorporated. This feature has been incorporated in the Duet phacoemulsification system.

The phaco probe connected to the aspiration line with a tip without an infusion sleeve is then introduced through the main clear corneal incision (Figures 25-3 and 25-4). The surgeon first employs moderate ultrasonic power to embed the phaco tip toward the central nucleus starting from the superior edge of the rhexis by directing the probe in an oblique and downward direction. The setting at this stage is 50% phaco power, flow rate of 24 mL/min, and vacuum of 110 mmHg (Alcon Universal II, Fort Worth, Tex). When nearly half of the central nucleus is embedded, Position 2 of the foot pedal is activated to firmly grasp the nucleus with the probe due to vacuum rise. To avoid undue pressure on the posterior lenticular capsule, the surgeon uses his or her nondominant hand to slightly lift the nucleus

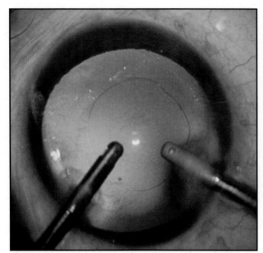

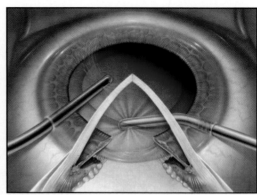

Figure 25-6. Soft tip I/A from MST. (Courtesy of Larry Laks, MST.)

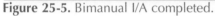

Figure 25-5. Bimanual I/A completed.

with the irrigating chopper inserted via the side port for nuclear chopping. The surgeon then performs chopping in a straight downward motion, starting from the right inner edge of the rhexis to the center of the nucleus, and then toward the left portion of the nucleus in the form of a laterally reversed L. Once a nuclear crack is created, the nucleus is split at the center. The nucleus is then rotated 180 degrees and cracked again, so that it is completely split.

The nucleus is then rotated 90 degrees and the probe is directed horizontally to embed half of the nucleus. Following the manner of the previously described maneuvers, 3 pie-shaped quadrants are created in one-half of the nucleus. Similarly, 3 pie-shaped fragments are created in the other half of the nucleus. With a short burst of ultrasonic energy at pulse mode, each pie-shaped fragment is lifted and brought anteriorly to the level of iris, where it is further emulsified and aspirated sequentially. After completion of nuclear removal, cortical clean-up is performed with the bimanual irrigation-aspiration (I/A) technique (Figure 25-5). Microsurgical Technology has also manufactured a soft irrigation-aspiration tip that allows safe polishing of the posterior lens capsule (Figure 25-6).

Phakonit With Cut Sleeve

The splashing of irrigating fluid at the base of the phaco needle outside the incision is another problem that occurs during phacoemulsification with the phakonit technique. This problem is related to the release of fluid droplets during emulsification of the lens. The splashing fluid droplets may deposit on the objective lens of the microscope and hamper the view of the surgeon. To prevent the splashing of fluid during emulsification from the base of the phaco needle, we fashion a cut sleeve around the base of the phaco needle to seal the outer margin of the limbal wound. We cut the sleeve in such a manner that it covers only the base of the phaco needle without entering the eye.

A constant flow of fluid to the wound is needed to cool the wound and prevent wound burns during phacoemulsification. The constant outward leak of fluid through the main non-watertight surgical wound surrounding the "naked" phaco needle without a plastic sleeve allows proper cooling of the wound. The inward fluid infusion is generated by the irrigating chopper via the surgical side port. Positive pressure irrigation or gas-forced infusion (GFI) through this irrigating chopper connected to the fluid bottle is generated by an air pump specially devised for this purpose.

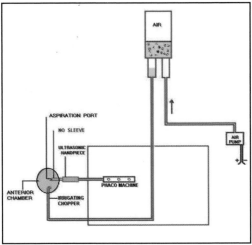

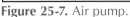

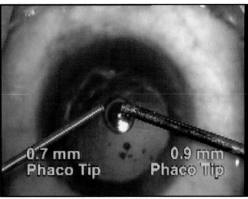

Figure 25-8. 0.7-mm phaco tip (micropha-konit) as compared to a 0.9-mm phaco tip (phakonit).

Figure 25-7. Air pump.

As noted above, fluid is constantly leaking from the eye's main entry wound during pha-konit, as the incision around the phaco needle without a plastic sleeve is not watertight. This fluid is coming from the irrigating chopper connected to the air injector. If we were to connect another fluid irrigating line to the phaco needle with cut sleeve, fluid would travel from the base of the phaco needle toward the entry wound from the outside. The meeting of this stream of fluid with the stream of fluid from the inside of the eye at the corneal entry wound would create turbulence and fluid collection in the operating field, reducing visibility for the surgeon during surgery. In addition, the internal cooling of the wound by the outward leaking irrigating fluid obviates this second irrigation line. More importantly, constant fluid irrigation associated with a second irrigating line is redundant because fluid irrigation is only needed during the emulsification process. Hence, the authors advocate judicious intermittent manual irrigation of the cornea and surgical wounds by a surgical assistant during phakonit. This maneuver, otherwise known as phakonit with cut sleeve without irrigation, reduces the tendency for fluid splashing and improves the surgeon's visibility during phakonit.

AIR PUMP

An important problem encountered in phakonit is destabilization of the anterior cham-ber and fluid surge during surgery. The use of an 18-gauge irrigating chopper reduces this problem. In addition, Dr. Sunita Agarwal developed an anti-chamber collapser[4,5] that injects air into the infusion bottle to enhance fluid infusion into the eye via an air pump (Figure 25-7). This enhanced-positive pressure infusion technique deepens the anterior chamber sufficiently during the entire surgery and particularly prevents fluid surge even in the event of high vacuum settings. This technique increases the safety of emulsification during both phakonit and conventional phacoemulsification.

MICROPHAKONIT

The advantages of a sub-1-mm microincision associated with microphakonit are coun-ter-balanced by the reduction in delivery of ultrasonic energy and fluid flow through the smaller-diameter needle. The actual diameter of the inner lumen of the needle regulates the

Figure 25-9. Microphakonit started. A 0.7-mm irrigating chopper and 0.7-mm phaco tip without the sleeve inside the eye. All instruments are made by MST. The assistant continuously irrigates the phaco probe area from outside to prevent corneal burns.

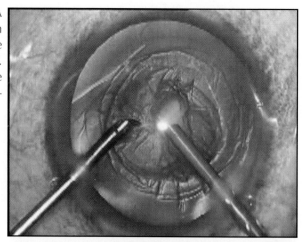

Figure 25-10. Bimanual I/A completed with the 700-μm set.

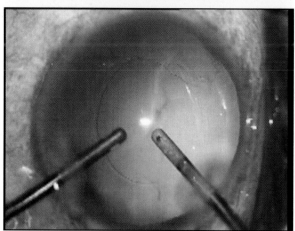

aspiration flow rate of the phaco needle. Larry Laks of Microsurgical Technologies solved the latter problems by reducing the thickness of the needle wall in order to increase the effective inner diameter of the 0.7-mm needle (Figure 25-8). The enlarged lumen of the modified 0.7-mm phaco needle makes the aspiration flow rate closer to but not the same as a 0.9-mm phaco tip. Subsequent modification of the phaco tip with a 30-degree beveled needle further improves the flow rate. When combined with the use of positive-pressure fluid flow or GFI through an irrigating chopper via the side port, this modified phaco tip allows greater speed and efficiency for microphakonit similar to the level achieved with phakonit, otherwise not possible without such modifications.

To maximize fluid flow into the eye, we decided to use an end-opening irrigating chopper. The enhanced fluid infusion with this type of chopper improves the fluidics, and dovetails with the need for a proper balance between inward and outward fluid flow for optimal emulsification and visibility for the surgeon during microphakonit (Figure 25-9).

Bimanual I/A is performed with bimanual I/A instruments. These instruments are also manufactured by Microsurgical Technology. Previously, we used a 0.9-mm I/A set. Currently, we use a new 0.7-mm bimanual I/A set that obviates the enlargement of the entry wound during nuclear removal (Figure 25-10).

Table 25-1 outlines the differences between the 2 techniques.

Table 25-1
Differences Between Phakonit and Microphakonit

Features	Phakonit	Microphakonit
Irrigating chopper	0.9 mm	0.7 mm
Phaco needle	0.9 mm	0.7 mm
Control in surgery	Good	Better control
Valve construction	Extremely important	Not very important as incision is much smaller
Iris prolapse	Can occur if valve is bad	Very rare
Intraoperative floppy iris syndrome	Can be managed	Much easier to manage because incision is much smaller and there is better control
Hydrodissection	Possible via either incision	To be carefully performed due to minimal space for escape of fluid
Air pump with GFI	Enhances efficiency of procedure	Mandatory for 0.7 mm irrigating choppers with positive pressure infusion
Flow rate	Any value	Avoid high flow rate. Maintain at 20 to 24 mL/min
Bimanual I/A	0.9 mm	0.7 mm

WOUND CONSTRUCTION

The importance of a perfectly constructed wound in phakonit cannot be overstated. A well-constructed wound is the key to achieving a flawless self-sealing wound that requires no sutures. A well-constructed wound can be closed by any method with good results. A poorly constructed wound can be a continuous source of astigmatism, leakage, irritation, hemorrhage, and corneal trauma despite a satisfactory wound closure.

COMPLICATIONS RELATED TO NUCLEUS (EMULSIFICATION TECHNIQUE)

While manipulating the nucleus for its emulsification, great care should be taken not to sink the instrument too deeply into the soft nucleus that might rupture the posterior capsule. The ultrasonic energy must be substantially reduced when lens fragments are small, in order to reduce erratic movements of the fragments on the phaco tip when the power is activated.

When removing the nuclear chips, it is advisable to employ pulsed mode to reduce the "chattering" of the chips. Moreover, the posterior capsule is covered by the outer nucleus, that acts as a thick layer of foam rubber separating the firm inner nucleus from the capsular bag during the entire emulsification process.

Figure 25-11. Capsular phimosis. One can see the anterior capsular rim in the central pupillary zone. The treatment of this complication is enlargement of the opening with the YAG laser. (Courtesy of Dr. Prakash, DP.)

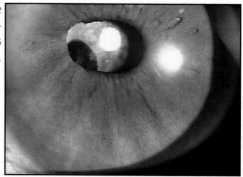

If the phaco tip does not emulsify the nucleus properly, correction of one or more of the following responsible conditions is required:

- The titanium needle is not tightly screwed to the handpiece
- The aspiration system is partially blocked by a piece of nucleus
- The ultrasound setting is too low for a particular piece of nuclear fragment

Moreover, the handpiece temperature should be monitored at all times, and it should not be allowed to become too warm. After cortical aspiration, meticulous anterior capsular vacuuming should be performed to eliminate residual equatorial lenticular epithelial cells that could lead to capsular phimosis (Figure 25-11).

CORNEAL COMPLICATIONS

Many corneal complications may develop especially for the novice phakonit surgeon. They are summarized in Table 25-2.

Transient postoperative superior corneal edema is usually present in cases of phakonit for beginners (Figure 25-12). Moreover, adequate incision construction, proper instrumentation, and avoidance of false passages reduce the occurrence and hasten the resolution of corneal edema. Incisional burns can be averted by minimizing the phaco time and avoiding an incision that is too tight by using cold balanced salt solution (BSS) (4°C) as irrigating fluid.

Moreover, diffuse corneal haze (Figure 25-13) or loss of corneal clarity is a common problem encountered during phakonit for beginners. Topical medications should be used judiciously, as their prolonged and frequent instillation may induce superficial punctate and striate keratopathy.

Descemet's detachment and tears may also develop occasionally. The anterior tip of the incision should be lifted when the instruments are inserted. Descemet's tears can also be prevented by using appropriately sharp instruments. The probe tip should be inserted with the bevel down. The side port entry should also be made with a bevelled instrument in a similar fashion. Any mechanical damage to the Descemet's membrane should be avoided.

Corneal endothelium damage can be further prevented by decreasing the effective emulsification time and confining emulsification to the nucleus with the lowest-required ultrasonic energy in the posterior chamber. Only high-quality ophthalmic fluids (ie, BSS, sodium hyaluronate, similar viscoelastics, etc) should be used.

In the event of postoperative corneal decompensation, anti-inflammatory and cycloplegic agents should be applied to counteract the associated inflammation and achieve cycloplegia, respectively. Hyperosmotics may also be useful for decongesting microcystic corneal edema. In the event of irreversible corneal endothelial damages, however, penetrating keratoplasty may be required.

Table 25-2

Corneal Complications of Phakonit

1.	Epithelial	Abrasion
		Filamentary keratitis
		Toxic keratopathy
2.	Corneal burns	Due to dehydration
		Associated with cautery
		Due to excessive phaco power
3.	Infection	Bacterial wound infection
		Fungal wound infection
		Herpetic keratitis
4.	Sterile corneal ulceration and stromal melting	Rheumatoid arthritis
		Collagen vascular disease
		Keratoconjunctivitis sicca
5.	Descemet's membrane damages	Blunt blade injury
		Oblique instrument insertion
		Incomplete insertion of instruments
		Injection of viscoelastic, air, or irrigation fluids into the wrong space
6.	Corneal endothelial damage	Poor preoperative endothelial cell count or quality
		Intraocular mechanical damage
		Anterior chamber collapse
		Instrument/endothelial contact
		Irrigating fluid disturbances
		Anterior chamber emulsification
		Lenticular nuclear fragment/endothelial touch
		IOL/endothelial touch
		Foreign object/endothelial contact
		Toxicity
		Irrigating solutions
		Povidone iodine
		Drug or chemical toxicity
		Chronic endothelial touch
		IOL
		Vitreous
		Faulty IOL
		Closed loop anterior chamber IOL
		Iris supported IOL
		Poorly coated surfaces
		Ingrowth of cells:
		- epithelial
		- fibrous
7.	Corneal complications—postoperative	Endothelial decompensation
		Striate keratopathy
		Bullous keratopathy

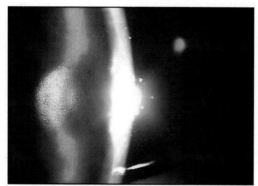

Figure 25-12. Corneal edema. (Courtesy of Dr. Prakash, DP.)

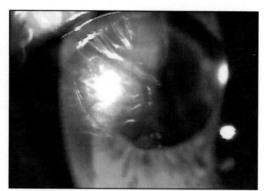

Figure 25-13. Striate keratopathy. (Courtesy of Dr. Prakash, DP.)

Iris Injury

Injury to both the superior and inferior portions of the iris may occur during phakonit. Iris fluttering should always be prevented during phacoemulsification. While performing phacoemulsification, the bevel of the phaco needle should be pointed upwards and maintained parallel to the iris plane throughout the process.

Vitreous Loss

The closed system inherent with the microincisional wound of phakonit limits vitreous loss and enhances the surgeon's ability to perform an adequate vitrectomy. The constant pressure in the anterior chamber due to the closed system associated with phakonit reduces the tendency of anterior vitreous prolapse. The small incision also limits the amount of vitreous extrusion from the eye. Zonular dehiscense may occur if an attempt is made to rotate the nucleus after an inadequate hydrodissection, partially due to the lack of capsular flexibility upon stress.

Unplanned posterior capsulotomy that violates the anterior vitreous hyaloid face tends to induce vitreous loss. Factors that inhibit early recognition of a posterior capsular rent by the surgeon (ie, obstruction of view by a large and opaque nuclear fragment) may increase the tendency for vitreous loss.

In the event of a posterior capsular rent with no vitreous loss, vitrectomy may not be required. Nevertheless, the flow rate and infusion should be decreased to avoid subsequent anterior vitreous herniation. However, a vitrectomy is mandatory when vitreous loss is confirmed. A single vitrectomy probe with a coaxial cannula should generally be avoided in favor of a bimanual vitrectomy technique using separate infusion cannula and a vitrectomy probe (Figure 25-14). A coaxial infusion probe may require enlargement of the original incisional wound. Coaxial infusion also tends to open the posterior capsular flap and hydrate the vitreous more than a separate infusion cannula, thus promoting anterior vitreous prolapse. With the bimanual technique, a limited anterior vitrectomy is performed and the main body of the posterior vitreous is not disturbed. During the procedure, vitreous removal should generally be performed posterior to the plane of the posterior lens capsule. Irrigation should be gentle and limited to the anterior chamber. Following vitrectomy, a posterior IOL may be inserted in front of the anterior capsule in the ciliary sulcus if an adequate capsular rim is present. Vitreous loss can be prevented or minimized by avoiding phacoemulsification on

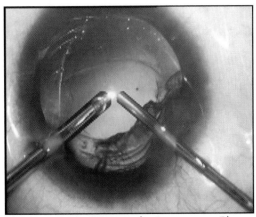

Figure 25-14. Bimanual vitrectomy. Please note separate vitrectomy probe and infusion cannula.

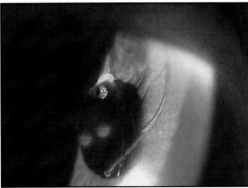

Figure 25-15. Haptic of an IOL in the anterior chamber. (Courtesy of Dr. Prakash, DP.)

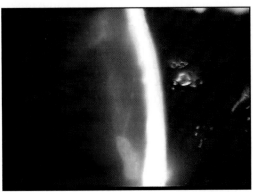

Figure 25-16. Severe inflammatory reaction in the anterior chamber. (Courtesy of Dr. Prakash, DP.)

the posterior surface of the nucleus. Improper vitrectomy can result in postoperative malpositioning of the IOL (Figure 25-15) and severe intraocular inflammation (Figure 25-16).

EXPULSIVE HEMORRHAGE

Expulsive suprachoroidal hemorrhage rarely occurs in conjunction with a 1-mm incision associated with phakonit. This small beveled incision is self-sealing and, therefore, usually prevents extrusion of intraocular contents associated with the suprachoroidal hemorrhage. In the event of a hemorrhagic choroidal detachment, the performance of a posterior sclerotomy to allow release of the suprachoroidal hemorrhage and a rapid closure of the surgical wounds minimize the chance of an expulsive hemorrhage.

CONVERSION TO EXTRACAPSULAR CATARACT EXTRACTION

Upon the first sign of excessive corneal clouding or anterior vitreous prolapse, the surgeon should consider converting phakonit to extracapsular cataract extraction (ECCE) in order to enhance the likelihood of good functional visual outcome. Conversion should be undertaken preferably before the development of excessive corneal endothelial damages and capsular rupture.

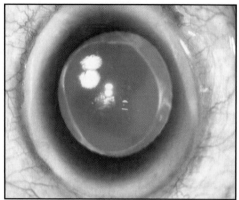

Figure 25-17. IOL opacification.

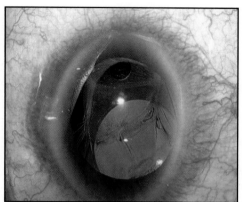

Figure 25-18. IOL decentration.

Planned conversion to ECCE is better than forced conversion. The surgeon should enlarge the limbal wound for extracapsular delivery of the nucleus from the posterior chamber upon the first sign of anterior vitreous herniation. A lens loop or equivalent instrument may be inserted under the nucleus for its expression out of the eye. After the nucleus is out, an irrigation-aspiration handpiece with a 0.5-mm tip is employed with low vacuum for lenticular cortical clean-up. However, lens fragments dislocated into the vitreous cavity are left alone for subsequent management with vitreoretinal techniques. The cataract surgeon unfamiliar with vitreoretinal techniques should refer the patient to a vitreoretinal surgeon. Attempts in removing posteriorly dislocated lens fragments without proper vitreoretinal techniques tend to cause retinal complications. In the event of vitreous loss, cortical aspiration may be difficult, and a vitrectomy probe is usually a better tool for completing the cortical clean-up.

Miscellaneous Intraocular Lens Problems

A number of problems may be associated with the IOL itself. For instance, defective IOL due to improper manufacturing may cause increased tendency for opacification of the IOL (Figure 25-17). The IOL may also decenter, tilt, or extrude (Figures 25-18 and 25-19).

Nuclear Dislocation

If the posterior capsular rent is large, the nucleus may migrate into the posterior vitreous cavity. Since an exposed nucleus is strongly antigenic and may cause a severe ocular phacoanaphylactic or phacotoxic reaction, its removal is mandatory. A soft nucleus can be removed with a vitrectomy probe alone, but a hard one requires posterior phacofragmentation, usually via a pars plana approach. An alternative method for removing a large and hard nuclear fragment is floating it anteriorly with perfluorocarbon liquids (PFCL) after a posterior vitrectomy. The anteriorly displaced lens fragment can then be delivered out of an enlarged corneal-scleral limbal wound. One can also use the FAVIT technique for removing dropped nuclear pieces.[6]

FAVIT was introduced by Agarwal et al. FAVIT stands for FAllen and VITreous, meaning a technique to remove fragments fallen into the vitreous.[6] First, an infusion cannula is fixated through the first port. An endoilluminator is then inserted through the second port, and a vitrectomy probe without an infusion sleeve is inserted through the third port. Once vitrectomy is completed, a phaco needle is exchanged for the vitrectomy probe subsequently. One

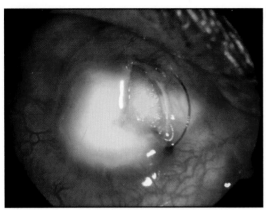

Figure 25-19. IOL extrusion.

may use an air pump to drive the irrigation through the infusion cannula so that no collapse of the eye occurs while removing the nucleus, and a precise intraocular pressure level is maintained at all times. The better method now is to use the microphakonit needle (phaco needle of 0.7 mm) to embed the nucleus and then remove it.

If one uses a Chandelier illumination system, in which the light source is connected to the infusion cannula, then one can do FAVIT as a proper bimanual vitrectomy. Preservative free triamcinolone is first injected and the vitrectomy is then done, which will help one know that the whole vitreous has been removed. One can do proper bimanual vitrectomy because one hand can hold the vitrectomy probe and the other the phaco needle probe (Figure 25-20). Any adhesions of the vitreous can be cut with the vitrectomy probe while removing the nucleus. Then the phaco needle embeds the nucleus and it is then brought anteriorly.

One can use a combination of perflurocarbon liquids and FAVIT also (Figure 25-21). Once vitrectomy is done, PFCL is injected to raise the nuclear fragments from the retinal level. Then using the phaco needle, they are removed. Retinal breaks and peripheral retinal detachment discovered during the inspection are then promptly treated with the appropriate modality (eg, laser, cryotherapy, scleral buckling, fluid-air or gas exchange). Residual PFCL is removed before closure. The postoperative therapy includes the application of topical steroidal or nonsteroidal anti-inflammatory medications, antibiotics, and cycloplegics.

Intraocular Lens Drop

Disturbing visual symptoms such as diplopia, metamorphopsia, and hazy images are associated with a dislocated IOL. Contemporaneous with advances in phakonit microsurgical techniques for treating cataracts, a number of highly effective surgical methods have been developed for managing a dislocated IOL. They include IOL manipulation with PFCL, scleral loop fixation, use of a snare, employing 25-gauge IOL forceps, temporary haptic externalization, as well as managing the single plate implant and 2 simultaneous intraocular implants. One excellent method is the use of the diamond-tipped forceps to grasp the malpositioned IOL during a vitrectomy for its explantation or repositioning. The primary aim of such methods is to reposition the dislocated IOL close to the original site of the crystalline lens in an expeditious manner and with minimal morbidity in order to optimize the visual outcome.

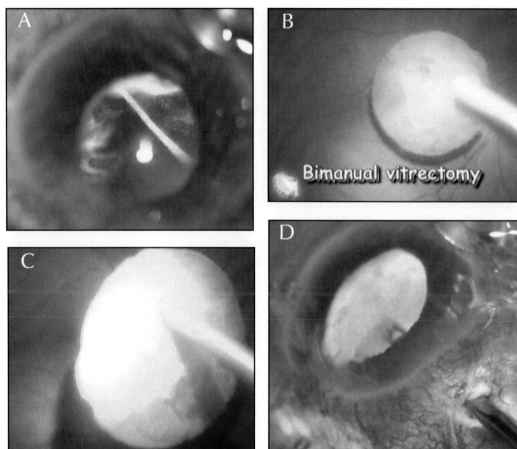

Figure 25-20. Dropped nucleus removed by FAVIT and Chandelier illumination. (A) Triamcinolone injection. (B) Nucleus lying on the retina. Illumination is through the Chandelier illumination system. Bimanual vitrectomy being done. In the right hand is the microphakonit 0.7-mm phaco needle. In the left hand is the vitrectomy probe. Note no endoilluminator in the hand. A wide field contact lens is used for visualization so that the entire retina is seen. (C) Nucleus embedded by the microphakonit needle. (D) Nucleus brought anteriorly and then removed.

CHANDELIER ILLUMINATION

The introduction of Chandelier illumination supplemented with xenon lighting markedly enhances the surgical versatility of the ophthalmic surgeon for performing complex surgical maneuvers (Figure 25-22). This lighting system provides high-quality and diffuse illumination over a wide surgical field for the surgeon's viewing without the need of an endoilluminating fiber-optic probe. With this system, both hands of the surgeon are available for performing surgical tasks. For instance, he or she may use one hand to excise vitreous adhesions with a vitrectomy probe and his other hand to grasp the dislocated IOL with diamond-tipped forceps. He may also perform bimanual manipulation of the dislocated IOL with separate forceps (hand-shake technique) for its removal or repositioning. For optimal viewing quality, special fiber-optic light sources providing high intensity and diffuse lighting are required for chandelier illumination (eg, PHOTON Light Source [Synergetics, O'Fallon, Mo] and Alcon Xenon Light Source).

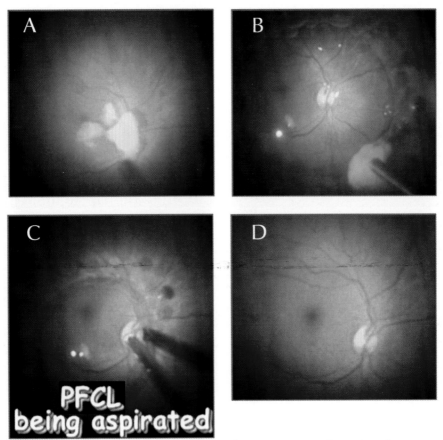

Figure 25-21. Combination of PFCL and FAVIT. (A) Small nuclear fragments are lying on the retina. (B) Perfluorocarbon liquid is injected once vitrectomy is done. Then using the phaco needle the nuclear pieces are removed. (C) The PFCL is then aspirated. (D) The retina as seen once the case is completed.

WIDE-ANGLE VIEWING SYSTEM

Modern panoramic viewing systems provide superior wide-angle viewing during a vitrectomy, previously not obtainable with conventional contact lenses. There are 2 different types of commercially available wide-angle viewing system, namely the noncontact and contact viewing systems. Both types of viewing systems have distinct advantages and disadvantages, and both have their proponents and detractors.

Noncontact Wide-Angle Viewing System

The SDI/BIOM noncontact wide-field viewing system manufactured by OCULUS Optikgeraete GmBH (Wetzlar, Germany) is the most common example of the first type of viewing system. With this system, a reduction lens and high-powered wide-angle front lenses (60 degrees, 90 degrees, or 120 degrees) mounted on a metallic extension are attached to the bottom of the operating microscope and then positioned over the surgical eye during a vitrectomy. Since wide-field indirect (inverted) images are provided by this viewing system, a reinverting box (Stereoscopic Diagnostic Inverter) inserted within the optical path of the microscope is required for converting the inverted images to direct (upright) images for the

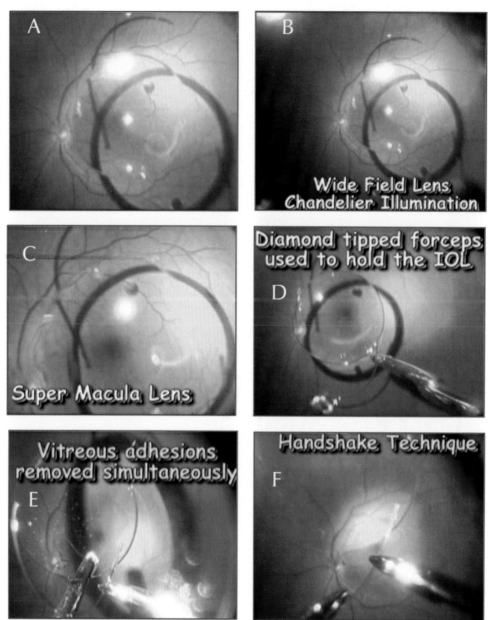

Figure 25-22. Views of chandelier illumination for removal of a dislocated IOL. (A) View of a dislocated IOL on the retinal surface. (B) View of an IOL on the macular surface. Notice the wide-field retinal image provided by a special panoramic contact lens with lighting via chandelier illumination. (C) View with the super-macula Volk lens that provides stereoscopic macular images. (D) View of diamond-tipped forceps lifting a looped IOL from the retinal surface after performance of a vitrectomy. (E) View of bimanual technique in manipulating a dislocated IOL, whereby the surgeon uses one hand to grasp the dislocated IOL with forceps and his or her other hand to cut vitreous adhesion with a vitrectomy probe. Appropriate lighting for this bimanual technique is achieved through chandelier illumination. (F) Handshake technique using 2 intraocular forceps to grasp the IOL.

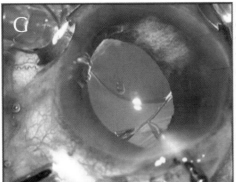

Figure 25-22 (cont). (G) View of explantation of a dislocated IOL through a limbal incision. Notice the presence of separate infusion cannulas at both the upper right and upper left corners of the surgical field. One cannula is for fluid infusion whereas the other is for chandelier illumination. Fluid infusion and chandelier illumination can also be achieved through the same specially manufactured dual-function cannula.

surgeon during a vitrectomy. The surgeon can activate the reinverting mechanism either via a foot switch or a button mounted on the microscope. Autoclavable or disposable lenses are available.

In recent years, Möller-Wedel (Möller-Wedel GmbH, Wedel, Germany) introduced a non-contact wide-angle viewing system that provides erect images for the surgeon without the need of a reinverting box. Similar to the SDI/BIOM system, this system (known as the Erect Indirect Binocular Ophthalmic System [EIBOS]) is also mounted on the bottom of the microscope.

The most important advantage of the noncontact viewing system is the lack of requirement of expensive contact lenses and the aid of highly skillful surgical assistants to stabilize those lenses on the cornea during a vitrectomy. However, there is a relatively steep learning curve in achieving optimal viewing of both the posterior and the peripheral fundus with the noncontact system.

Contact Wide-Angle Viewing System

The second type is the contact panoramic viewing system. Wide-angle viewing contact lenses constructed with special material are positioned on the cornea of the surgical eye to provide panoramic viewing during a vitrectomy. These lenses are attached with handles for the surgical assistants to stabilize and manipulate them on the surgical eye. One of the first contact wide-angle viewing systems (AVI Panoramic Viewing System [Advanced Visual Instruments, New York, NY]) was developed by Avi Grinblat under the guidance of Stanley Chang, MD in 1989. It consists of a stereoscopic image inverter, wide-field indirect aspheric contact lenses, lens handles, lens retaining ring, and fiber-optic chandelier illumination that fits through a single 20-gauge sclerotomy. The Volk Reinverting Operating Lens System (ROLS or ROLS plus [Volk Optical Inc, Mentor, Ohio]) with single-element prism design is another example of a high-quality stereoscopic wide-angle viewing system. A series of wide-angle contact lenses are used with this system (eg, Super-Macula lens for macular viewing, the Mini Quad, and Mini Quad XL lenses for the peripheral fundus [up to 127 degrees and 134 degrees, respectively], Dyna View 156 degrees [full field fundus viewing], etc) Wide-angle contact lenses with special high-index material manufactured by OCULUS Optikgeraete GmBH (Wetzlar, Germany) and Ocular Instruments (Ocular Instruments, Bellevue, Wash) are also available for panoramic viewing during a vitrectomy (eg, OWIV-HM [100 degrees], OLIV-EQ-2 [131 degrees], and OLIV-WF [146 degrees]). All such systems provide panoramic viewing via special wide-angle contact lenses for the posterior fundus, including the macula, the equator, and beyond, as well as the far peripheral fundus. Depending on the lenticular and refractive status of the surgical eye, viewing of the peripheral fundus may reach as far as the ora serrata with specific wide-angle lenses for certain eyes. Similar to the SDI/BIOM noncontact viewing system (OCULUS Optikgeraete GmBH, Wetzlar, Germany), the contact viewing systems also require the incorporation of a reinverting box along the optical pathway of the microscope to convert inverted images to erect images for the surgeon. Sterilization of these lenses may require ethylene oxide, steam sterilization, Steris (Mentor, Ohio), or Sterrad (Miami, Fla) system, depending on the product specification.

The most valuable aspect of various contact panoramic viewing systems is the availability of both posterior and peripheral panoramic fundus images with unparalleled resolution via specially designed contact lenses. However, careful maintenance of expensive contact lenses and skillful stabilization of the contact lenses on the cornea are required.

Endophthalmitis

Highly effective therapy is available for treating infectious endophthalmitis in the 21st century. Aqueous and vitreous specimens may be obtained in an office setting or at the time of a vitrectomy. In the former situation, careful administration of local anesthesia (topical, subconjunctival, peribulbar, or retrobulbar) and sterile prepping with 5% povidone-iodine solution are recommended. A small volume of aqueous specimen (0.1 to 0.2 mL) is then carefully withdrawn via a 27- or 30-gauge needle at the limbus into a tuberculin syringe. The vitreous specimen may be obtained with 1 of the following 2 methods:

1. Needle tap: A 22- to 27-gauge needle attached to a tuberculin syringe is inserted through the pars plana into the vitreous cavity for gentle aspiration of 0.1 to 0.3 mL of liquid vitreous. Excessive force must be avoided to prevent vitreoretinal traction. A "dry tap" requires the conversion to a mechanized biopsy.

2. Mechanized vitreous biopsy: A 1-, 2-, or 3-port pars plana vitrectomy with a mechanized 20-gauge vitrectomy probe is employed for the biopsy. A small volume of undiluted specimen (up to 0.3 mL) from the anterior vitreous is collected into a sterile syringe connected to the aspiration line of the vitrectomy probe through gentle manual suction by a surgical assistant during the vitrectomy.

Diluted specimens collected into a larger syringe or into a vitrectomy cassette may also be concentrated either with the suction-filtered technique or the centrifuged method (Figure 25-23). The former involves passing the diluted specimens in an upper sterile chamber through a membrane filter with 0.45-μm pores into a lower chamber connected to suction. With the aid of sterile forceps and scissors or knives, the membrane filter containing the concentrated specimens is then cut into small pieces for direct inoculation on solid and into liquid media for cultures. Concentrated specimens scraped off the surface of the membrane filter are also applied on slides for preparation of various stains. The alternative centrifuged method requires the transfer of the diluted specimens into a sterile centrifuge tube for high-speed centrifuge. The sediments from the centrifuged tube are then processed for microbiological stains and cultures.

Empiric intravitreal antimicrobial regimens in a "shot gun" approach constitute the first line of therapy with a proven track record in treating most forms of endophthalmitis. New advances in antimicrobial therapy allow consistent control of infections induced by a broad spectrum of organisms. Vitrectomy is required in certain cases. A 3-port pars plana vitrectomy using standard 20-gauge instruments and concentrating on the "core" vitreous is usually recommended, although a 1- or 2-port approach may be sufficient for a limited vitreous biopsy.

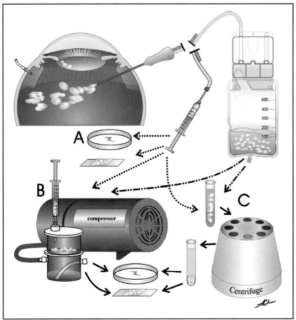

Figure 25-23. Methods of collecting specimens. (A) Undiluted aqueous and vitreous specimens may be directly inoculated onto culture media and used for smear preparation. (B) Diluted vitreous specimen collected into a syringe or a cassette is either first concentrated by vacuuming the diluted fluid in a sterile upper chamber through a 0.45-µm membrane filter into a lower sterile chamber (suction filter method). (C) Concentrated in a sterile centrifuge tube after performing high-speed centrifuge (centrifuge method). Small cut segments of the membrane filter with the concentrated specimens or the sediments from the centrifuged tube are innoculated into culture media and applied on slides for smear preparation.

KEY POINTS

1. A poorly constructed wound can be a source of astigmatism, filtration, irritation, hemorrhage, and corneal trauma despite a satisfactory wound closure.

2. The handpiece temperature should be monitored at all times, and it should not be allowed to become too warm.

3. In the event of a postoperative corneal decompensation, anti-inflammatory and cycloplegic agents should be applied to counteract the associated inflammation and achieve cycloplegia, respectively. Hyperosmotics may also be useful for decongesting microcystic corneal edema. In the event of irreversible corneal endothelial damages, however, penetrating keratoplasty may be undertaken.

4. A single vitrectomy probe with a coaxial cannula should generally be avoided in favor of a bimanual vitrectomy technique using separate infusion cannula and a vitrectomy probe.

5. A true expulsive suprachoroidal hemorrhage through the 1-mm incision associated with phakonit is rare.

REFERENCES

1. Agarwal A, Agarwal S, Agarwal A. Phakonit: lens removal through a 0.9 mm incision. In: Agarwal A. *Phacoemulsification, Laser Cataract Surgery and Foldable IOLs*. New Delhi, India: Jaypee Brothers; 1998.

2. Agarwal A, Agarwal A, Agarwal S. No anesthesia cataract surgery. In: Agarwal A. *Phacoemulsification, Laser Cataract Surgery and Foldable IOLs*. 2nd ed. New Delhi, India: Jaypee Brothers; 2000.

3. Chang S. Perfluorocarbon liquids in vitreo-retinal surgery. *Int Ophthalmol Clin*. 1992;32(2):153-163.

4. Chan CK. An improved technique for management of dislocated posterior chamber implants. *Ophthalmology*. 1992;99:51-57.

5. Chan CK, Agarwal A, Agarwal S, Agarwal A. Management of dislocated intraocular implants. *Ophthalmol Clin North Am*. 2001;14:681-693.

6. Agarwal A, Siraj AA. FAVIT—a new method to remove dropped nuclei. In: Agarwal S, Agarwal A, Sachdev MS, et al, eds. *Phacoemulsification, Laser Cataract Surgery and Foldable IOLs*. 2nd ed. New Delhi, India: Jaypee Brothers; 2000:538-544.

Please see Perfecting Your Curves: Mastering Bimanual Phacoemulsification video on enclosed CD-ROM.

Chapter 26

REFRACTIVE SHIFT AFTER PEDIATRIC CATARACT SURGERY

Rupal H. Trivedi, MD, MSCR and M. Edward Wilson, Jr, MD

INTRODUCTION

A process known as emmetropization regulates the growth of different components of the eye. Pediatric cataract surgery results in loss of the natural crystalline lens before completion of this complex process. In phakic eyes, as the eye size increases (average 17 to 24 mm), compensatory changes occur in the curvature of the crystalline lens (from 34.4 to 18.8 D). As a result, the refractive error in most children changes little despite marked increase in the length and size of the eye. After the crystalline lens is removed surgically, every millimeter of axial growth of the globe changes the refractive error of the eye by more than 2.50 D. This results in a shift of refraction toward myopia (Figure 26-1). Note, that this is a refractive shift toward myopia and not a myopic refraction. In other words, eventually, postoperative refraction is mainly based on how much initial refraction there was after the cataract surgery. In aphakic eyes, the shift averages 10.00 D from infancy to adulthood, compared with 0.90 D in normal phakic eyes.[1-4] In pseudophakic eyes, it mainly depends on initial refraction while selecting an intraocular lens (IOL) power.

FACTORS AFFECTING MYOPIC SHIFT OF REFRACTION

Age of the Child at the Time of Cataract Surgery

The younger the age at the time of cataract surgery, the greater the myopic shift. In general, myopic shift follows the axial growth of normal human eyes. Extensive growth of normal phakic infant eyes has been well documented in the literature.[5,6] Larsen[5] reported a rapid postnatal growth phase, with an increase in axial length (AL) of 3.7 to 3.8 mm in the first 1.5 years of life, followed by a slower infantile growth phase from the second to the fifth year of life, with an increase in AL of 1.1 to 1.2 mm; and, finally, by a slow juvenile growth phase lasting until the age of 13 years, with an increase of 1.3 to 1.4 mm. We have noted eye growth in our patients all the way to age 20. Gordon and Donzis[6] noted that the AL increases from an average of 16.8 mm at birth to 23.6 mm in adult life. It is reasonable to believe that eyes with cataracts follow a similar triphasic curve before surgery as well as

Figure 26-1. The shift of refraction toward myopia.

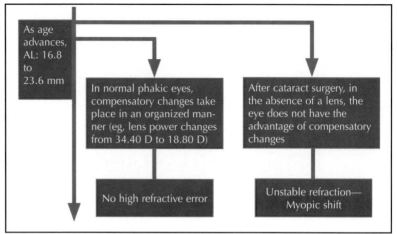

after surgery. However, we have noted that the mean AL of our patients' cataractous eyes is different (20.6 ± 2.9 mm) from that of the noncataractous eyes in Gordon and Donzis's data (21.9 ±1.6 mm).[7] Not only did the mean values differ, but more importantly, the standard deviation was 2 to 3 times that of the normal population. Also, the younger the age at the time of measurement, the more variability existed.

Several studies performed on animal and human eyes report the effect of age at the time of lens removal on future growth of the eye and later shift of refraction. Lambert[8] reported that age at the time of lensectomy appears to be a critical factor in determining later axial growth in monkeys. Moore[9] noted that the refractive error of the aphakic eye of patients treated for unilateral congenital cataracts decreases most rapidly during infancy and less rapidly during the next few years of childhood. McClatchey and Parks[4] reported that the average refraction follows a logarithmic decline with age. The average rate of myopic shift (not quantity) was −5.50 D. The authors performed a stepwise regression and inferred that age at surgery had a small, but significant, effect on the rate of growth.[4] Much of the observed myopic shift in aphakic eyes is because of the normal growth of the eye. McClatchey and Parks[3] used aphakic refraction at the last follow-up to calculate the final pseudophakic refraction, and these values were compared with the prediction of a logarithmic model of myopic shift. They reported median calculated pseudophakic refraction at last follow-up of −6.60 D, with a range of −36.30 to +2.90 D. Children who underwent surgery in the first 2 years of life had a substantially greater myopic shift (11.90 D) than older children (4.70 D) and a larger variance in this myopic shift. The logarithmic model accurately predicated the final refraction within 3.00 D in 24% of eyes undergoing surgery before 2 years old and in 77% of eyes undergoing surgery after this age. Dahan and Drusedau[10] reported an average elongation of 19% for ages <18 months and 3.4% for ages >18 months. Enyedi and colleagues[11] reported that children operated on at years 0 to 2, 2 to 6, 6 to 8, and >8 had refractive shifts of −3.00, −1.50, −1.80, and −0.40 D, respectively. The authors noted a statistically significant difference in the average total change in refraction between the youngest age group (0 to 2 years) and the oldest age group (>8 years). Flitcroft and colleagues[12] reported a mean increase in AL of 3.4 mm in congenital cataract (patient <1 year of age), versus 0.4 mm in developmental cataracts (patient >1 year of age). Plager and associates[13] reported that children operated on at ages 2 to 3, 6 to 7, 8 to 9, and 10 to 15 years had mean myopic shifts of −4.60, −2.70, −1.30, and −0.60 D, respectively. Crouch and colleagues[14] reported that children operated on at years 1 to 3, 3 to 4, 5 to 6, 7 to 8, 9 to 10, 11 to 14, and 15 to 18 years had mean myopic shifts of −6.00, −3.70, −3.40, −2.00, −1.90, −1.00, and −0.40 D, respectively, with an average follow-up of 5.5 years. Vasavada and coauthors[15] noted that the rate of axial growth (RAG) in children when operated at ≤1-year of age (23.5%) was significantly higher than in those operated between 1 to 3 years (4.8%; $P < 0.001$, confidence interval [CI] 1.05 to 3.2), and 3 to 10 years old (4.3%; $P < 0.001$, CI 1.3 to 3.1). In children operated at ≤1-year of age, the temporal profile of RAG was higher in the first 2 years after surgery.

Gender

Sex-linked differences in AL have been reported in the literature on normal phakic eyes. Larsen[5] reported that AL values in girls were, on average, 0.3 to 0.4 mm shorter than in boys. Gwiazda and colleagues[16] also noted a sex-linked difference in AL. In eyes with cataracts, we have noted that, overall, girls have a significantly shorter AL than boys (23.9 versus 24.4 mm). However, in the first year of life, males have a shorter AL than females.[7]

McClatchey and Parks[4] noted that gender had no effect on the rate of myopic shift in pediatric aphakic eyes. Further prospective studies of large sample size are required to answer a question if myopic shift of refraction is influenced by gender.

Ethnicity

Several studies in normal phakic eyes have reported racial differences with respect to axial and refractive status. The prevalence of myopia is 37% among Chinese school-children vs only 7.5% among American school-children.[17,18] Gwiazda and colleagues[16] noted that they did not find a difference in axial dimensions in different ethnic groups. In our cataractous population, we noted significantly longer eyes in African-American patients than in Caucasian patients (21.8 vs 20.1 mm).[7] We are not aware of any study showing the pattern of growth and its relation to ethnicity.

Heredity

Any hereditary form of refractive error may superimpose on refractive shift. Parental refractive error has also been shown to be an important predictor for the refractive errors of their children. For example, if both parents are myopic, 30% to 40% of their children become myopic, whereas if only 1 parent is myopic, 20% to 25% of their children will become myopic. If neither parent is myopic, fewer than 10% of their children will become myopic.[19]

Moore[9] noted that 2 of 42 patients were highly myopic in their phakic eyes but were less hyperopic in their aphakic eyes than the group mean. Both of these patients had a father with high bilateral myopia and can be presumed to have a hereditary form of myopia superimposed on their unilateral congenital cataract. Plager and associates[13] noted an unexpectedly large myopic shift in a genetically predisposed patient, with moderate myopia in both parents.

Unilateral Versus Bilateral Cataract

Eyes with a unilateral cataract have been shown to have a longer AL than eyes with bilateral cataracts (21.0 vs 20.4 mm), even before cataract surgery, secondary to deprivation amblyopia.[7] In eyes with a unilateral cataract, axial elongation and myopic shift relative to the unaffected eye have been well described in aphakic and pseudophakic eyes.

Rasooly and BenEzra[20] reported that in cases of unilateral aphakia, the aphakic eye was consistently longer than the normal fellow eye. In their prospective study of children with congenital cataract, Lorenz and associates[21] reported that the mean decrease in refraction was 15.00 D in unilateral cataracts and 10.00 D in bilateral cataracts. In older children, Kora and coauthors[22] reported a longer AL in operated eyes than in normal fellow eyes. Eyes with unilateral cataracts have a higher rate of myopic shift than eyes with bilateral cataracts; this effect was statistically significant among eyes with cataract removal after the age of 6 months. Hutchinson and coworkers[23] reported a series of children <2 years old with IOL implantation. The authors reported that in eyes with a unilateral cataract, the operated eye grew an average of 0.4 mm more than the fellow noncataractous eye (calculation was done from data in reference,[23] but only 9 eyes with a unilateral cataract were included here for analysis). Operated eyes grew 1.5 mm (SD, 0.8) on average, while unoperated eyes grew 1.1 mm (SD, 0.9). Griener and coauthors[24] concluded from their retrospective study that there was a reduction in axial growth in unilateral pseudophakic eyes compared to fellow normal eyes. The authors noted that in 7 patients receiving unilateral IOL implantation between 2 and 4 months of age, the mean AL was 0.5 mm less in the pseudophakic eye than in the fellow eye (range, 0.2 to 0.7 mm).[24] Crouch and coworkers[14] noted that there was a small myopic shift difference in patients with binocular implants, suggesting that both eyes grew similarly. In the unilateral case, they noted that the pseudophakic eye showed a larger myopic shift than the unoperated fellow eye. Weakley and colleagues[25] noted that the difference in refractive rate of growth between good- and poor-seeing eyes was less in eyes with bilateral cataracts than in eyes with unilateral cataracts. Vasavada and colleagues[15] noted that in children operated at ≤1 year of age, RAG in unilateral pseudophakia was 25.5% compared with 18.5% in bilateral pseudophakia ($P = 0.001$, CI −13.00 to −0.20). In children operated at >1 year of age, the corresponding RAG was 4.2% and 4.5% ($P = 0.8$, CI −2.6 to −3.3). In children >1 year of age, laterality had no significant effect on RAG.

Interocular Axial Length Difference

We have recently reported the influence of axial length of the fellow eye on the growth of an eye.[26] Interocular axial length difference (IALD) was defined as the AL of the study eye minus the AL of the fellow eye. Two groups were compared: short eyes with an IALD <0 and long eyes with an IALD >0. Average age at surgery between these 2 groups was similar ($P = 0.246$) as was age at follow-up ($P = 0.834$). The difference in IALD was significant when short eyes were compared to long eyes (0.28 ± 0.70 mm vs -0.14 ± 0.59 mm, $P = 0.007$). The average rate of AL growth was more in eyes with shorter preoperative IALD when compared with longer preoperative IALD (3.07 mm vs 1.89 mm, $P = 0.050$). We concluded that eyes with a shorter AL than the fellow eye showed faster axial growth postoperatively, while a longer AL than the fellow eye showed slower axial growth.

Aphakia Versus Pseudophakia

Several studies have reported that aphakic eyes grow more than pseudophakic eyes.[15,27,28] We propose that several reasons contribute to this retardation of growth in pseudophakic eyes and elongation of aphakic eyes.
- Aphakic eyes may have a poorer visual outcome compared to pseudophakic eyes, which in turn leads to axial elongation from form vision deprivation.
- Optical reasons may have an impact on emmetropization and thus axial growth.
- Aphakic eyes may be shorter to start with, so to "catch up" they grow more.
- In addition, longer follow-up of most studies for aphakic eyes, as compared with pseudophakic eyes, may have contributed more axial elongation in the aphakic cohort.

Sinskey and associates[27] reported the case of an 18-year old patient who had developmental cataracts treated at 7 years of age with bilateral cataract extraction and implantation of an IOL in 1 eye only. The AL increased in the eye with a contact lens compared with the eye with the IOL. Overall, pseudophakic eyes showed a lower rate of refractive growth than aphakic eyes (−4.60 vs −5.70 D; *P* = 0.03).[27] Superstein and associates[28] inferred that pseudophakic eyes show less postoperative myopic shift than aphakic eyes.

Intraocular Lens Size and Power

Animal studies have shown that inappropriate IOL size can adversely influence ocular growth.[29] Implanting a standard adult-sized IOL in a newborn rabbit eye retards eye growth. The mathematical analysis by McClatchey and Parks[3] showed that choosing an IOL to give initial moderate hyperopia results in less myopic shift as the eye grows than choosing an IOL to give initial emmetropia for optical reasons alone. High-power IOLs result in a greater myopic shift for the same increase in AL.

Glaucoma

Excessive eye elongation may be a presenting sign of aphakic glaucoma.[30,31] However, controlled glaucoma has been shown to have no effect on the rate of growth.[4] A marked and rapid shift of refraction in an infantile eye alerts the physician to check for evidence of glaucoma.

Visual Axis Opacification

It is reasonable to assume that, in the amblyogenic age group, visual axis opacification may lead to elongation of the eye if the opacification is not treated promptly. However, it is difficult to document the exact onset of visual axis opacification. When it is noticed, the tendency is to clear it as soon as possible. Thus, it is not surprising that one study did not find this to be a significant factor.[32]

Visual Acuity and Amblyopia Status

Emmetropization of the eye may be affected by visual experience. Excessive eye elongation may be induced in experimental animals by lid suturing, corneal opacification, or opaque contact lenses. These conditions resulted in axial elongation, whereas lesser degrees of visual deprivation were shown to retard axial growth. Poor vision seems to influence the evolution of ocular growth away from emmetropization. In humans, however, this is not always predictable. With cataracts in children, 2 main reasons predict the preoperative AL. Developmental anomalies may lead to microphthalmos and a shorter AL, while deprivation amblyopia may lead to axial elongation. In a case report of identical twins, Johnson and colleagues[33] reported that the AL of the visually deprived eye was 2 mm longer than the fellow eye. The authors noted a statistically significant increase in AL in the fixating eye of patients with hypermetropia compared with the amblyopic eye. In patients with myopia, less of an increase in AL was found in the fixating eye compared with the amblyopic eye. Several investigators have examined the association between visual acuity outcome and myopic shift or axial elongation in both aphakic and pseudophakic eyes. McClatchey and Parks[4] noted that best-corrected visual acuity (BCVA) had no significant effect on rate of myopic shift in their cohort. Weakley and colleagues,[25] however, noted that the rate of growth was significantly lower in eyes with better acuity.

Excessive Near-Work and Optical Correction of Refractive Error During Childhood

Near-work may increase the risk of myopia. Optical correction of refractive error during childhood may disturb the process of emmetropization. In the phakic state, a higher percentage of children with moderate or high hyperopia remain hyperopic if their hyperopia is cor-

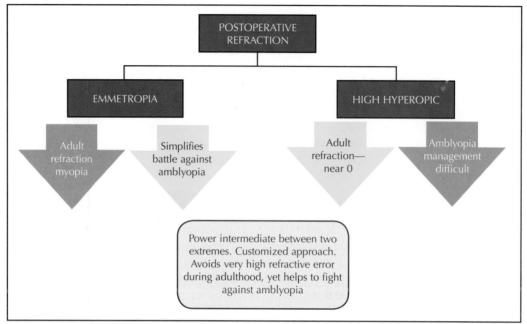

Figure 26-2. Three major approaches have been used for IOL power calculation in children.

rected with spectacles during infancy. Emmetropization occurs more rapidly in the presence of high refractive errors. Thus, if we leave behind high residual refractive error, these eyes may grow more.

As can be seen above, refractive shift after pediatric cataract surgery is a result of several cumulative reasons. Studies reporting a longer follow-up will show more myopic shift than studies reporting a shorter follow-up. Crouch and colleagues observed a myopic shift that ranged from plano to -2.25 D. With a longer follow-up of 5.5 years, the same authors observed a more significant myopic shift.[14] As long-term follow-up of these children becomes available, we may come across more refractive surprises in these children. Refractive shift may be minimum after age 13 years; however, it may continue until age 20. Most studies show no sharp cutoff point when axial growth (and subsequently refractive shift) stabilizes.

PREVENTION

Eyes with cataract surgery without IOL implantation will result in refractive shift based on causes that are generally not modifiable. However, eyes with cataract surgery and IOL implantation will result in refractive error that is based on residual refractive error (in general, hyperopia) at the time of that surgery. This residual refractive error is based on selection of an IOL power. Historically 3 major approaches have been used for IOL power calculation in children (Figure 26-2):

1. *Initial hyperopia*: Several studies reported before 1995 recommended using a standard adult IOL power. However, as the pediatric eye is not yet fully grown, an IOL with a typical adult power will result in hyperopia initially. This hyperopia will improve as the axial growth increases. As a result, the adult refraction may turn out to be at or near plano, unless the eye started out microphthalmic from developmental arrest or axially elongated from visual deprivation. In addition, uncorrected hyperopic refractive error in children may cause or worsen amblyopia.

Table 26-1	
Age of the Patient at Cataract Surgery and **Residual Refraction (Reflecting Our 2006 Recommendations** **If Late Myopia Is To Be Minimized)***	
Age at Surgery	*Residual Refraction at the Time of Surgery**
First month	+ 12
2 to 3 months	+ 9
4 to 6 months	+ 8
6 to 12 months	+ 7
1 to 2 years	+ 6
2 to 4 years	+ 5
4 to 5 years	+ 4
5 to 6 years	+ 3
6 to 7 years	+ 2
7 to 8 years	+1.5
8 to 10 years	+ 1
10 to 14 years	+ 0.5
>14 years	Plano

*Other factors described in the chapter must be considered before IOL power—fellow eye status, degree of amblyopia, assumed compliance, and parental refractive error.

2. *Initial emmetropia*: To minimize the amblyogenic effect, some surgeons prefer to correct children to emmetropia regardless of the age at surgery. Using this approach, no spectacles or contact lenses are needed initially for distance viewing. Thus, it is thought to simplify the battle against amblyopia. However, optimal near visual acuity will still not be achieved without glasses. In addition, significant late myopia will be more and more common as the years pass since young children's eyes continue to grow. This is especially true if an IOL is implanted during the first 2 years of life.

3. *Customized approach*: Both of the above approaches have advantages and disadvantages. The best solution probably lies in finding a compromise between these 2 extremes. Appropriate undercorrection can be used based on age at surgery. Table 26-1 describes our recommendation based on age at surgery, if late myopia is to be lessened. We recently analyzed our data to see how much we actually undercorrect our pediatric eyes,[7] and found that typically we do less undercorrection than is described in Table 26-1. This reflects our tendency to look at multiple reasons while selecting the IOL power for a child (eg, laterality of cataract, visual acuity, parental refractive error).

TREATMENT

As time passes, more and more children will present for treatment with significant pseudophakic myopia. For aphakic eyes, treatment choices include secondary IOL implantation (if enough capsule support exists) and corneal refractive surgery. For pseudophakic eyes, choices include IOL exchange, implantation of a piggyback IOL, or corneal refractive surgery.

Hutchinson[34] has reviewed refractive surgery outcomes in children. The ideal procedure for children would be one that is painless, needs little cooperation, has precise refractive predictability that is stable over time, a low risk for loss of BCVA, and is adjustable (or can be advanced). In addition, it must withstand the rigors of the normally traumatic development of a child into an adult. This ideal procedure does not exist. Each of the currently available procedures has advantages and disadvantages when pediatric use is expected. LASIK allows faster visual rehabilitation and needs a shorter course of postoperative medications. The corneal flap, however, may be vulnerable to childhood trauma. PRK would hold up much better to trauma but has a slower healing and needs a longer course of postoperative medications. LASEK has been used in children as a variation in the PRK procedure, but more data are needed before its role in pediatric refractive surgery can be defined. Each of these procedures could be used for the moderate degree of myopia that will develop in most pseudophakic children and young adults. If high myopia develops, an IOL exchange would likely be chosen over laser refractive surgery. Based on the literature available, Hutchinson[34] implied that pediatric refractive outcomes are less predictable and are likely to be less stable than in adults. As more data are collected, nomograms designed specifically for children, perhaps even specific to pseudophakic children, will be developed. After cataract surgery, children will most likely need laser refractive surgery at the end of their growing years. At that age, predictability and stability may approach that found in adults.

Summary

The surgeon who performs pediatric cataract surgery must be prepared for a wide variation in long-term myopic shift. Both the magnitude of and the variance in this myopic shift are likely to be greater among children who undergo cataract surgery in the first few years of life. Much of the myopic shift can be attributed to normal eye growth; however, other causes, including age at surgery, visual input, presence or absence of an IOL, and laterality, also play a role in this process. Anticipation of this myopic shift and appropriate correction or compensation will help achieve better anatomical and functional outcomes of young eyes undergoing cataract surgery.

The authors have no financial or proprietary interest in any product mentioned herein.

Supported in part by the NIH/NEI grant EY-014793, the Grady Lyman Fund of the MUSC Health Sciences Foundation, and an unrestricted grant to MUSC-SEI from Research to Prevent Blindness Inc, New York, NY.

KEY POINTS

1. The growth of different components of the eye is regulated by a process known as emmetropization. Pediatric cataract surgery results in loss of the natural crystalline lens before completion of this complex process.

2. The younger the age at the time of cataract surgery, the greater the myopic shift. In general, myopic shift follows the axial growth of normal human eyes.

3. Eyes with cataract surgery without IOL implantation will result in refractive shift based on causes that are generally not modifiable. However, eyes with cataract surgery and IOL implantation will result in refractive error that is based on residual refractive error (in general, hypermetropia) at the time of that surgery.

4. As time passes, more and more children will present for treatment with significant pseudophakic myopia.

5. The surgeon who performs pediatric cataract surgery must be prepared for a wide variation in long-term myopic shift. Both the magnitude of and the variance in this myopic shift are likely to be greater among children who undergo cataract surgery in the first few years of life.

REFERENCES

1. McClatchey SK. Intraocular lens calculator for childhood cataract. *J Cataract Refract Surg*. 1998;24(8): 1125-1129.

2. McClatchey SK, Dahan E, Maselli E, et al. A comparison of the rate of refractive growth in pediatric aphakic and pseudophakic eyes. *Ophthalmology*. 2000;107(1):118-122.

3. McClatchey SK, Parks MM. Theoretic refractive changes after lens implantation in childhood. *Ophthalmology*. 1997;104(11):1744-1751.

4. McClatchey SK, Parks MM. Myopic shift after cataract removal in childhood. *J Pediatr Ophthalmol Strabismus*. 1997;34(2):88-95.

5. Larsen JS. The sagittal growth of the eye. IV. Ultrasonic measurement of the axial length of the eye from birth to puberty. *Acta Ophthalmologica*. 1971;49(6):873-886.

6. Gordon RA, Donzis PB. Refractive development of the human eye. *Arch Ophthalmol*. 1985;103(6):785-789.

7. Trivedi RH, Wilson ME, et al. AL and keratometry in eyes with pediatric cataract. Poster presented at ASCRS; October, 2002; Philadelphia, Pa.

8. Lambert SR. The effect of age on the retardation of axial elongation following a lensectomy in infant monkeys. *Arch Ophthalmol*. 1998;116(6):781-784.

9. Moore BD. Changes in the aphakic refraction of children with unilateral congenital cataracts. *J Pediatr Ophthalmol Strabismus*. 1989;26(6):290-295.

10. Dahan E, Drusedau MU. Choice of lens and dioptric power in pediatric pseudophakia. *J Cataract Refract Surg*. 1997;23(Suppl 1):618-623.

11. Enyedi LB, Peterseim MW, Freedman SF, Buckley EG. Refractive changes after pediatric intraocular lens implantation. *Am J Ophthalmol*. 1998;126(6):772-781.

12. Flitcroft DI, Knight-Nanan D, Bowell R, Lanigan B, O'Keefe M. Intraocular lenses in children: changes in axial length, corneal curvature, and refraction. *Br J Ophthalmol*. 1999;83(3):265-269.

13. Plager DA, Kipfer H, Sprunger DT, Sondhi N, Neely DE. Refractive change in pediatric pseudophakia: 6-year follow-up. *J Cataract Refract Surg*. 2002;28(5):810-815.

14. Crouch ER, Crouch ER, Jr, Pressman SH. Prospective analysis of pediatric pseudophakia: myopic shift and postoperative outcomes. *J AAPOS*. 2002;6(5):277-282.

15. Vasavada AR, Raj SM, Nihalani B. Rate of axial growth after congenital cataract surgery. *Am J Ophthalmol.* 2004;138(6):915-924.

16. Gwiazda J, Marsh-Tootle WL, Hyman L, Hussein M, Norton TT, Group CS. Baseline refractive and ocular component measures of children enrolled in the correction of myopia evaluation trial (COMET). *Invest Ophthalmo Vis Sci.* 2002;43(2):314-321.

17. Chung KM, Mohidin N, Yeow PT, Tan LL, O'Leary D. Prevalence of visual disorders in Chinese school-children. *Optom Vis Sci.* 1996;73(11):695-700.

18. Zadnik K, Satariano WA, Mutti DO, Sholtz RI, Adams AJ. The effect of parental history of myopia on children's eye size. *JAMA.* 1994;271(17):1323-1327.

19. Lambert SR. Ocular growth in early childhood: implications for pediatric cataract surgery. *Op Techn Cataract Refract Surg.* 1998;1:159-164.

20. Rasooly R, BenEzra D. Congenital and traumatic cataract. The effect on ocular axial length. *Arch Ophthalmol.* 1988;106(8):1066-1068.

21. Lorenz B, Worle J, Friedl N, Hasenfratz G. Ocular growth in infant aphakia. Bilateral versus unilateral congenital cataracts. *Ophthalmic Paediatrics Genetics.* 1993;14(4):177-188.

22. Kora Y, Shimizu K, Inatomi M, Fukado Y, Ozawa T. Eye growth after cataract extraction and intraocular lens implantation in children. *Ophthalmic Surgery.* 1993;24(7):467-475.

23. Hutchinson AK, Wilson ME, Saunders RA. Outcomes and ocular growth rates after intraocular lens implantation in the first 2 years of life. *J Cataract Refract Surg.* 1998;24(6):846-852.

24. Griener ED, Dahan E, Lambert SR. Effect of age at time of cataract surgery on subsequent axial length growth in infant eyes. *J Cataract Refract Surg.* 1999;25(9):1209-1213.

25. Weakley DR, Birch E, McClatchey SK, et al. The association between myopic shift and visual acuity outcome in pediatric aphakia. *J AAPOS.* 2003;7(2):86-90.

26. Trivedi RH, Wilson ME. Interocular axial length difference: does it change after pediatric cataract-intraocular lens implantation surgery? *J AAPOS* (in press).

27. Sinskey RM, Stoppel JO, Amin PA. Ocular axial length changes in a pediatric patient with aphakia and pseudophakia. *J Cataract Refract Surg.* 1993;19(6):787-788.

28. Superstein R, Archer SM, Del Monte MA. Minimal myopic shift in pseudophakic versus aphakic pediatric cataract patients. *J AAPOS.* 2002;6(5):271-276.

29. Kugelberg U, Zetterstrom C, Lundgren B, Syren-Nordqvist S. Ocular growth in newborn rabbit eyes implanted with a poly(methyl methacrylate) or silicone intraocular lens. *J Cataract Refract Surg.* 1997;23 Suppl 1:629-634.

30. Dietlein TS, Jacobi PC, Krieglstein GK. Assessment of diagnostic criteria in management of infantile glaucoma. An analysis of tonometry, optic disc cup, corneal diameter and axial length. *Int Ophthalmol.* 1996;20(1-3):21-27.

31. Egbert JE, Kushner BJ. Excessive loss of hyperopia. A presenting sign of juvenile aphakic glaucoma. *Arch Ophthalmol.* 1990;108(9):1257-1259.

32. Wilson ME Jr, Trivedi RH. Eye growth after pediatric cataract surgery. *Am J Ophthalmol.* 2004;138(6):1039-1040.

33. Johnson CA, Post RB, Chalupa LM, Lee TJ. Monocular deprivation in humans: a study of identical twins. *Invest Ophthalmol Vis Sci.* 1982;23(1):135-138.

34. Hutchinson AK. Pediatric refractive surgery. *Curr Opin Ophthalmol.* 2003;14(5):267-275.

VITREORETINAL COMPLICATIONS ASSOCIATED WITH REFRACTIVE SURGERY

Clement K. Chan, MD, FACS; Steven G. Lin, MD; and
Astha S. D. Nuthi, DO

INTRODUCTION

Photorefractive keratectomy (PRK) and laser in situ keratomileusis (LASIK) are 2 of the most common refractive procedures performed in the modern era of refractive surgery. In recent years, LASIK has become an increasingly prevalent refractive procedure.[1-20] Its generally consistent and precise outcome achieved in a rapid manner and with less discomfort in comparison to PRK has established its dominant role in the world of refractive surgery.[13,19] Previously, Leaming estimated in his American Society of Cataract and Refractive Surgery's Practice Styles and Preferences Survey that there were close to 170,000 cases of LASIK performed in the United States in 1997,[20] 440,000 cases in 1998,[21] and close to a million cases by 2000.[22] More recently, phakic intraocular lens implantation and refractive lensectomy have gained popularity as viable refractive procedures.[23-28] Uncommon anterior segment complications associated with LASIK include flap slippage, flap wrinkles or folds, decentered ablation, under- or overcorrections, residual astigmatism, epithelial ingrowth, diffuse lamellar keratitis (DLK), infection, corneal ectasia, etc.[13,19,29-33] Vitreoretinal complications after refractive surgery are rare but may induce an unfavorable visual outcome. There have been a number of reports in the literature on vitreoretinal complications after PRK and LASIK.[34-100] The most common reports of postrefractive surgical vitreoretinal complications included retinal breaks and retinal detachment.[35-56, 63-68, 72-75] Other rare reports of posterior segment complications after refractive surgery include formation of a macular hole,[77-82] premacular subhyaloid hemorrhage,[83] submacular lacquer cracks,[95] submacular hemorrhage and choroidal neovascularization,[84-94,96-98] retinal vascular occlusion,[99] and cystoid macular edema.[100]

Though uncommon, the large volume of refractive surgeries and high expectation of refractive patients make any vitreoretinal complications with poor visual outcome after refractive surgery highly important.

RETINAL BREAKS AND DETACHMENT

Photorefractive Keratectomy

The development of retinal detachment (RD) after PRK was first reported by Treister and Charteris in 1997.[34,35] Treister et al described RD in an eye with -7.00 D of myopia 6 months after PRK.[35] Charteris et al also presented 11 myopic eyes with RD.[35,36] In 1999, Vilaplana reported development of giant retinal tears in 2 highly myopic patients at 2 and 3 months after PRK respectively.[37] In 2000, Ruiz-Moreno et al reported 5 cases in 5936 myopic eyes of 3184 patients (0.08%) after PRK.[38] The spherical equivalents of those 5 cases were all more than -9.00 D. Buch et al described an additional case of RD 5 months after PRK in a highly myopic eye (-12.50 D spherical equivalent) in 2000.[39] With the exception of 3 of the 11 cases reported by Charteris et al, the common feature among all of the eyes with RD in the above reports was high myopia.[68]

Laser In Situ Keratomileusis

Case reports on retinal breaks and detachment after LASIK first appeared in the literature in the 1990s. Ozdamar et al first reported a single case of bilateral giant retinal-tear detachment in a highly myopic eye 2 months after LASIK in 1998.[40] In their prospective study in 1999 on the complications of 1062 myopic eyes in 574 patients undergoing LASIK, Stulting et al presented 1 highly myopic eye (-22.50 D) that developed RD (0.09%).[41] In their retrospective study in 1999, Ruiz-Moreno et al reported 4 of 1554 myopic eyes (0.25%) that developed RD within 2 to 19 months after LASIK.[42] The degree of myopia was -8.00 to -27.50 D for those eyes.[42] In 2000, Aras et al presented 10 eyes in 10 patients with myopia (between -6.37 to -17.00 D) that developed RD within 2 to 9 months after LASIK.[43] Farah et al also reported RD in 4 highly myopic eyes (range -13.00 to -19.00 D) from 30 to 80 days after LASIK.[44] Two of those four RD were associated with a giant retinal tear. In 2000, Arevalo et al reported a retrospective study of 13 eyes in 12 patients that developed rhegmatogenous retinal detachments after LASIK between 1 and 36 months (mean 12.6 months) after LASIK for myopia.[45] The degree of myopia of the affected eyes ranged from -1.50 to -16.00 D (mean = -6.95 D). All affected eyes were successfully managed with vitrectomy, cryoretinopexy, scleral buckling, argon laser retinopexy, or pneumatic retinopexy.

In another retrospective report in 2000, Arevalo et al presented 14 eyes that developed RD (Figure 27-1) and 4 eyes that developed retinal tears without RD within 1.5 to 36 months after LASIK performed on 29.916 eyes (0.06%).[46] In Arevalo's latter report, 83.2% eyes were myopic (range of -0.75 to -29.00 D), and 16.8% eyes were hyperopic (range of +1.00 to +6.00 D). Similar to their other report, the eyes with retinal tears were treated with laser or cryotherapy, and those with RD were treated with vitrectomy, cryopexy, pneumatic retinopexy, or scleral buckling. In 2001, Arevalo et al presented additional myopic eyes with rhegmatogenous RD after LASIK.[47] In 2001, Tsai and coworkers reported a case report of RD associated with a giant retinal tear in an eye with -10.00 D of myopia 9 months after LASIK.[48] It was successfully repaired with scleral buckling, vitrectomy, and fluid-gas exchange. In 2002, Vakili et al also reported a case report of retinal tear in an eye with -7.75 D of myopia 1 month after LASIK enhancement.[49] The retinal tear responded well to laser therapy via laser indirect ophthalmoscopy. In 2002, Arevalo et al reported 33 myopic eyes (range -.075 to 129.0 D) that developed rhegmatogenous RD (0.08%) within 12 days to 60 months after LASIK (mean, 26.3 months).[50] In that series, the mean myopia for eyes with RD was -8.75 D. Most of the RDs (71.1%) were found in the temporal quadrants.[51] In 2003, Hernáez-Ortega and coauthor reported bilateral RD associated with giant retinal tears

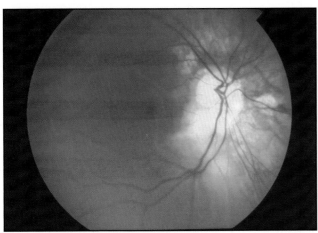

Figure 27-1. Fundus photograph of a subtotal inferotemporal retinal detachment with macular involvement after laser in situ keratomileusis, right eye. (Courtesy of JF Arevalo.)

in eyes with -14.00 D of myopia 2 months after LASIK.[51] Both eyes were successfully treated with scleral buckling, vitrectomy, and perfluorocarbon liquid with good responses.

In 2004, Chan et al reported the characteristics of 60 myopic eyes that developed post-LASIK vitreoretinal complications despite pre-LASIK retinal examinations.[52] The vitreoretinal complications included retinal breaks and retinal detachment. This retrospective study involved a worldwide survey of 424 vitreoretinal surgeons on their experience in managing tertiary referral of vitreoretinal complications after LASIK. Thirty-five (8.3%) reported managing retinal breaks or detachment after LASIK. There was an average of 2.3 breaks per eye, corresponding to a total of 140 breaks in the 60 eyes (Table 27-1). Twenty of the 60 eyes had only retinal breaks, whereas 40 eyes had both retinal breaks and detachment. Substantial myopia was present in large percentages of the affected eyes (mean myopia of -9.50 ± 5.80 D, with a range of -1.50 to -28.00 D.)

Prevalence of Post-LASIK Retinal Breaks in Temporal Quadrants

In their study, Chan et al reported that the retinal breaks were distributed evenly between the superior and inferior quadrants ($P = 0.82$, χ^2). However, there were significantly more temporal than nasal retinal breaks (breaks, $p < 0.001$; tears, $p < 0.001$, χ^2), (Table 27-2).[52] The study by Arevalo et al also pointed out a greater distribution of post-LASIK retinal breaks and RD in the temporal than nasal quadrants.[45-47,50,53] They speculated that the location of the temporal handle of the microkeratome could have created extra pressure on the temporal side of the eye undergoing LASIK.[45-47,50,53] However, Chan et al noted that previous studies on older adult patients (older than 40 years of age) not involved with LASIK also found more retinal breaks on the temporal than nasal fundus.[52] For instance, Menezo et al reported 67.2% of retinal tears in the temporal quadrants versus 30% of retinal tears in the nasal quadrants in their series of non-LASIK myopic eyes with RDs.[54] Although the precise reasons for the predominance of the temporal quadrants for retinal breaks and RDs for both LASIK and non-LASIK eyes are unknown, there are several viable explanations. One possibility is that the longer chord length of the temporal fundus may make the temporal globe more vulnerable to vitreoretinal traction.[52] However, the most likely reason for the increased vulnerability of the temporal globe is related to the basic anatomy of the vitreous base, previously elucidated by the studies of Glasgow et al.[55] Their studies showed an average width of 3.2 mm for the vitreous base, which is shorter in the temporal than the nasal quadrants on account of the more anterior location of the temporal posterior vitreous base. Therefore, the temporal posterior vitreous base is located closer to the thinner anterior retina. In addition,

Table 27-1

Retinal Conditions of 60 LASIK Eyes in 51 Patients

# With Bilateral Condition (%)	# of Breaks Only (%)	# of Retinal Detachment (%)	# of Total Breaks	# of Tears (% B)	# of Holes (% B)	# With Dialysis (%)
9 pts (17.7%): 4RD/RD; 4 B/B; 1 RD/B 18 eyes (30.0%)E	20 (33.3%)	40 (66.7%)	140	71 (50.7%)	69 (49.3%)	3 (2.1% B) (5.0% E)

# of Macular Holes (%)	# of Giant Tears (%)	# of Proliferative Vitreoretinopathy (%)	# B ≥2 (%)	# B ≥3 (%)	Mean B Per Eye	# Total RD(%)
1 (0.7%) B (1.7%) E	4 (2.9%) B (6.7%) E	5 (8.3%)	32 (53.3%)	16 (26.7%)	2.3	5 (8.3%)

B, breaks; RD, retinal detachment; E, eyes; Tears, flap tears, dialysis, and giant tears; Holes, peripheral and macular holes. Adapted from *Retina*, Volume 24, Chan CK, Arevalo JF, Akbatur HH, Sengün A, et al. Characteristics of sixty myopic eyes with pre-laser in situ keratomileusis retinal examination and post-laser in situ keratomileusis retinal lesions, page 709, 2004, with permission from Lippincott Williams & Wilkins.

Table 27-2
Distribution of Retinal Tears, Holes, Lattice Degeneration, and Retinal Detachment of 60 Eyes With Pre-LASIK Retinal Examination

Condition	Location by Quadrant				
	ST	SN	IT	IN	Macula
Retinal tears	28.83 (40.6%)	10.83 (15.3%)	22.5 (31.7%)	8.83 (12.4%)	NA
Retinal holes	17.0 (24.6%)	11.5 (16.7%)	24.5 (35.5%)	15.0 (21.7%)	1 (1.5%)
Lattice	10.5 (40.4%)	8.0 (30.8%)	6.5 (25.0%)	1 (3.8%)	NA
RD	26 (65.0%)	22 (55.0%)	29 (72.5%)	29 (72.5%)	24(60.0%)

Each retinal tear or hole located at 12-, 3-, 6-, or 9 o'clock is assigned a 0.5 value for each of the 2 overlapping quadrants. A giant retinal tear extending throughout 3 quadrants is assigned a 0.33 value for each of the 3 quadrants. A lattice lesion spanning 2 quadrants is assigned a 0.5 value for each quadrant. Total RD = 40 eyes (16 macula-on and 24 macula-off); total percentages of RD >100% due to the overlapping involvement of multiple quadrants for most of the RD. There was a lack of statistical significance for distribution of retinal breaks (P=0.82), tears (P=0.32), and holes (P=0.18), χ^2, between the superior and inferior quadrants, but a significant difference between the temporal and nasal quadrants (P < 0.001 for breaks, and P < 0.001 for tears, χ^2). ST, superior temporal; SN, superior nasal; IT, inferior temporal; IN, inferior nasal; NA, not applicable; RD, retinal detachment.

potentially risky vitreoretinal lesions (ie, lattice degeneration and retinal holes) are located closer to the more anteriorly located temporal posterior vitreous base and further away from the nasal posterior vitreous basis (Figure 27-2). Thus, the vitreous base anatomy explains why vitreoretinal stress induced at the posterior vitreous base during a posterior vitreous detachment will more likely lead to retinal breaks and RDs on the temporal than the nasal fundus, irrespective of any refractive surgery.

Mechanisms of Retinal Breaks and Detachment After Refractive Surgery

The reasons for retinal breaks after refractive surgery are not known. There is lack of irrefutable evidence that substantiates a causal relationship between refractive surgery and vitreoretinal complications. Some have stated that most eyes undergoing refractive surgery are myopic and, therefore, have greater inherent risk for retinal breaks and detachment, irrespective of refractive surgery.[53,56] However, multiple investigators have proposed potential mechanisms of vitreoretinal complications after refractive surgery.[35-38,40,42-47,50,52] For instance, Aras et al and Seiler et al speculated that shock waves generated by the excimer laser may play a role in the development or amplification of vitreoretinal pathology (Figure 27-3).[43,57,58] In their experimental study, Gobbi et al found that intraocular changes induced by the excimer photoablation of the cornea oscillate between positive pressure up to 90 bars

Figure 27-2. The vitreous base anatomy explains the greater vulnerability of the temporal vitreous base to vitreoretinal complications. The width of the temporal vitreous base (B to B[1]) is shorter than the nasal vitreous base (A to A[1]) because the temporal posterior vitreous base is located more anteriorly, closer to the inner retina. More risky retinal lesions (eg, lattice degeneration and holes) are also located closer to the temporal posterior vitreous base and further away from the nasal posterior vitreous bases; thus, the temporal retina is more vulnerable for retinal complications during a posterior vitreous detachment. (Reprinted from Chan CK, Arevalo JF, Akbatur HH, Sengün A, et al. Characteristics of sixty myopic eyes with pre-laser in situ keratomileusis retinal examination and post-laser in situ keratomileusis retinal lesions *Retina*. 2004; 24:711 with permission from Lippincott Williams & Wilkins.)

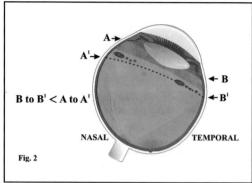

Figure 27-3. Diagram of eye showing propagation of acoustic shock waves generated by the excimer laser through ocular tissues. (Courtesy of CA Chan, Inc.)

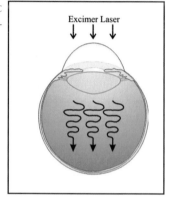

and negative pressure of up to -40 bars.[59] Kermani et al found that at clinically relevant laser energy densities (200 mJ/cm² and 500 mJ/cm²) generated by application of a 193-nm ArF excimer laser pulse (20 nanoseconds) for corneal photoablation, the resultant shock waves reach 80 bars and 150 bars, respectively[60] On the other hand, Krueger et al measured the decrease of stress wave amplitudes to less than 10 Atmosphere (ATM) at the retina associated with little potential harm, despite the generation of stress wave amplitudes by the excimer laser of up to 100 ATM at the posterior lens and anterior vitreous cavity in enucleated porcine and human eyes during photoablation.[61,62] All of the above studies point to the potential association of photoacoustic shock waves with vitreoretinal complications.

Certain investigators have also speculated that the acute and severe intraocular pressure changes associated with the application of the microkeratome suction ring during LASIK may induce vitreoretinal traction.[40,42-47,50,52] Previously, Alió et al reported increased tendency for posterior vitreous detachment (PVD) resulting from changes in intraocular pressure.[63] The sudden globe compression by the microkeratome ring at 2 to 4 mm posterior to the limbus may exert acute intraocular pressure rise to above 60 mmHg and induce anterior-posterior elongation and horizontal contraction of the globe. The subsequent decompression of the suction ring may also cause equatorial elongation and anterior-posterior contraction (Figure 27-4).[40,42-47,50,52] Such rapid and drastic changes of the globe provide the potential mechanism for vitreoretinal stress on the vitreous base, possibly aggravating pre-existing

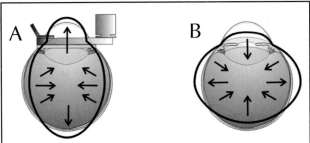

Figure 27-4. Diagrams showing abrupt (A) vertical elongation and (B) horizontal widening of the globe during application of the microkeratome ring for LASIK. (Courtesy of CA Chan, Inc.)

vitreoretinal pathology. Luna et al showed acute PVD after LASIK in their experimental study with porcine eyes.[64] The associated diminished electroretinographic recordings noted in their study also suggested transient choroidal circulatory abnormalities. In addition, they reported clinical evidence of vitreoretinal changes after LASIK.[64] Smith and coauthors presented a case of bilateral complete PVD immediately after LASIK.[65] In 2004, Flaxel et al studied the effects of the microkeratome suction ring on 8 human eye bank eyes.[66] They found a mean axial length increase of 1.125 mm ($P = 0.02$) with anterior displacement of the vitreous base during compression of the microkeratome. Their study found no significant difference in the anterior chamber depth ($P = 0.98$) associated with the microkeratome application. They speculated that such globe deformation may predispose susceptible eyes to anterior retinal breaks during and after LASIK. In 2005, Mirshahi and coworkers reported the incidence of PVD after LASIK in a prospective study.[67] They performed B-scan ultrasonography immediately before and one week after LASIK on 103 myopic or myopic-astigmatic eyes (mean spherical equivalent of -4.85 D and mean axial length of 25.13 mm). They found that 92.2% of study eyes had no preoperative PVD, and only 9 eyes (9.5%) developed an incomplete PVD after LASIK. They also found that 8 eyes (7.8%) had a partial preoperative PVD, but only 1 of those eyes developed extension of the partial PVD after LASIK. Their conclusion of the rare tendency of LASIK in inducing PVD is hard to interpret because their performance of ultrasonography was limited to only 1 month after LASIK. It is not known whether serial ultrasonography over a more extended period of time would show different results.

Another proposed mechanism for vitreoretinal complications after refractive surgery involves postsurgical intraocular inflammation. Ruiz-Moreno et al cited previous studies showing increased frequency of age-related maculopathy in surgical in comparison to nonsurgical eyes and changes in choroidal hemodynamics leading to leakage in surgical eyes.[68-71]

Despite all of the previously proposed mechanisms for vitreoretinal complications associated with refractive surgery, there is no definitive proof of a direct causal relationship between refractive surgery and vitreoretinal complications. However, it is prudent to conduct close vitreoretinal monitoring before and after refractive surgery, particularly for eyes predisposed to vitreoretinal complications.

Relation of Pre- and Post-LASIK Retinal Lesions

In 2003, Lin et al reported a prospective study on the safety and efficacy of pre-LASIK prophylactic laser for retinal breaks in myopic eyes.[72] They examined a total of 1931 eyes in 1006 patients before LASIK and found and treated retinal breaks in 39 eyes (2.02%) of 32 patients (3.2%). The preoperative spherical equivalent was -7.55 ± 3.72 D (range of -1.87 to -34.50 D). They found a significantly higher preoperative spherical equivalent in eyes with retinal breaks in comparison to those without (-9.41 ± 4.15 D versus -7.52 ± 3.71 D, respectively, $P = 0.017$). Although none of the treated eyes developed post-LASIK vitreoretinal complications, the mean follow-up time was only 19 months.

In 2005, Chan and coauthors retrospectively analyzed 67 highly myopic eyes (mean myopia of –11.00 D) in 56 patients with vitreoretinal complications that also had pre-LASIK vitreoretinal pathology (lattice degeneration, retinal breaks).[73] They found that 17 of the 67 eyes (25.4%) had pre-LASIK vitreoretinal pathology. Prophylactic retinal treatment on 10 of those 17 eyes did not prevent subsequent vitreoretinal complications. They found that post-LASIK vitreoretinal lesions developed adjacent to pre-LASIK lesions for 88.2% of eyes and outside of quadrant(s) of pre-LASIK eyes for 29.4% of eyes. Their conclusion was that pre-LASIK retinal examination may predict the locations of certain post-LASIK retinal lesions that may develop in highly myopic eyes with pre-LASIK vitreoretinal pathology, but may not prevent all post-LASIK vitreoretinal complications.[73]

Phakic Intraocular Lens and Refractive Lensectomy

Multiple investigators have reported retinal breaks and retinal detachment following phakic intraocular lens and refractive lensectomy.[23-28,74,75] Previously, Alió et al reported 3 cases,[63] Fechner et al reported 1 case,[24] Pesando et al reported 1 case (5.26%),[24] Zaldivar et al reported 1 case (0.8%),[25] Panozzo et al reported 4 cases,[74] and Ruiz-Moreno et al reported 8 cases of RD (4.8%) following phakic intraocular lens insertion.[75] Ruiz-Moreno et al noted that some of the above incidences of RD are higher than the incidences of RD in myopic eyes with more than -6.00 D reported in the literature (3.1%).[68,75,76] However, many eyes that underwent phakic intraocular lens implantation and developed RD were highly myopic (eg, more than –10.00 D). Ruiz-Moreno et al also reported a highly variable lapse time between the insertion of phakic intraocular lens and onset of RD (1 to 52 months).[68,75] Such a highly variable range makes the relationship between the 2 unclear. In a similar fashion, refractive lensectomy also involves highly myopic eyes. Ruiz-Moreno et al[68] noted that the incidences of RD after refractive lensectomy varied from 6.1% for a series of eyes with a mean spherical equivalent of -19.50 D[26] to 4% for eyes with a spherical equivalent of more than –12.00 D,[27] and 1.9% for eyes with more than -12.00 D of myopia.[28] More studies are needed to elucidate the relationship between phakic intraocular lens implantation and refractive lensectomy with RD.

MACULAR HOLE

In 2001, Chan and Lawrence first published 2 cases of macular hole formation after LASIK, and 1 case of macular hole after PRK.[77] The macular hole formed between 4 and 7 weeks after LASIK in 1 eye of a 48-year old woman with -6.50 D of myopia, and within 2 months after LASIK in 1 eye of a 36-year old woman with -8.50 D of myopia. A 45-year old man with -7.00 D of myopia also developed a macular hole in 1 eye 9 months after PRK.[77] Ruiz-Moreno et al reported the formation of a macular hole in 1 eye of a 53-year old woman with -6.75 D of myopia 12 months after LASIK.[78] In 2004, Arevalo et al reported unilateral macular hole formation in 10 eyes from 1 to 30 months (mean of 9.1 months) after bilateral LASIK.[79] The mean age of the patients was 42.5 years, and 90% of patients were female and myopic. PVD was not present before but documented after LASIK in 80% of eyes.[79] In 2005, Arevalo et al reported on 14 eyes in 13 patients that developed a macular hole at an average of 13 months (range of 1 to 83 months) after bilateral LASIK (Figure 27-5).[80] The mean myopia was -8.40 D (range of -0.50 to -19.75 D). With the exception of 1 set of bilateral macular holes, the rest were unilateral macular holes. Most of the macular holes (50%) were stage 4, and most lacked yellow deposits on the underlying retinal pigment epithelium and

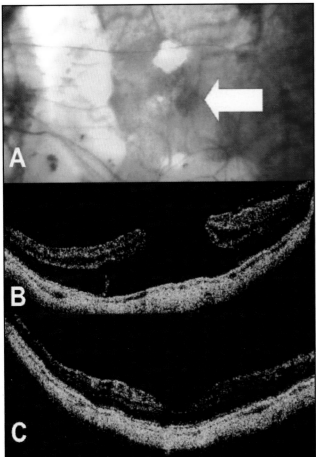

Figure 27-5. (A) Preoperative fundus photograph shows a stage 4 macular hole (arrow) associated with a macular detachment. (B) OCT before surgery shows both macular detachment and macular schisis of same eye. (C) OCT after vitrectomy shows closure of the macular hole. VA improved from counting fingers to 20/150 after successful macular hole closure. (Courtesy of JF Arevalo; Reprinted from *Br J Ophthalmol*, Volume 89, Arevalo JF, Rodriguez FJ, Rosales-Meneses JL, Dessouki A, et al, Vitreoretinal surgery for macular hole after laser assisted in situ keratomileusis for the correction of myopia, page 1425, 2005, with permission from BMJ Publishing Group Ltd.)

surrounding epiretinal membranes. Most of those macular holes also were centric and had associated subretinal fluid. The average diameter of the macular holes was 385.3 μm (range 200 to 750 μm). PVD was not present before but was documented after LASIK for 42.8% of eyes. A vitrectomy closed the macular hole in 92.8% of the eyes. In 2005, Arevalo et al also reported formation of a macular hole in 20 eyes of 19 patients.[81] The macular hole formed within 6 months after LASIK for 60% of eyes, and equal to or greater than 1 year after LASIK for 30% of eyes. The mean myopia was -8.90 D (range of -0.50 to -19.75 D). PVD was not present before but was documented after LASIK in 55% of eyes. A vitrectomy closed the macular hole in 14 eyes that underwent surgical management, and visual improvement was achieved in 13 of the 14 eyes (92.8%).

The rare complication of macular hole formation after refractive surgery is not limited to myopic eyes. In 2006, Arevalo et al reported 2 hyperopic eyes that developed a unilateral macular hole in 15 and 38 months after bilateral LASIK, respectively.[82] The cause of macular hole in these 2 eyes is unknown, particularly in light of the lack of tendency of most hyperopic eyes for macular hole formation. However, age-related changes could be a contributing factor in this situation.

Although unproven, vitreoretinal interface changes after LASIK may have been responsible for the macular hole formation in eyes after refractive surgery.[77-82] Similar to retinal breaks and detachment after refractive surgery, photoacoustic shock waves generated by the excimer laser and acute intraocular pressure changes associated with application of the microkeratome ring are speculated to be contributing factors. However, a causal relationship has not been substantiated.

PREMACULAR SUBHYALOID HEMORRHAGE

In 2000, Mansour et al reported a case of premacular subhyaloid hemorrhage that developed on the second postoperative day after unilateral LASIK, with a visual acuity of finger-counting at 1 meter on account of the large subhyaloid hemorrhage covering the macula in the operated eye.[83] Subsequent Nd:YAG laser posterior hyaloidotomy led to progressive clearance of the subhyaloid hemorrhage. There was recovery of her visual acuity to 10/20 for the operated eye 11 months later. Neto et al presented a similar case of premacular hemorrhage after LASIK in 1 eye of an 18-year old woman with -3.00 D of myopia after uneventful bilateral LASIK (Scientific Poster 339, American Academy of Ophthalmology, Orlando, Florida, October 1999).[68] The visual acuity improved from 5/400 to 20/20 5 days after Nd:YAG laser posterior hyaloidotomy for the affected eye. Mansour et al noted that subhyaloid hemorrhage is induced by a sudden increase or decrease in venous pressure within the eye, leading to rupture of superficial peripapillary and perifoveal retinal capillaries, as in the case of valsalva retinopathy.[83] Thus, they speculated that the acute intraocular pressure changes from over 65 mmHg to zero associated with the sudden release of the vacuum pump for the microkeratome might have contributed to the subhyaloid hemorrhage. The temporal correlation of the hemorrhage in the operated eye within 2 days after LASIK made spontaneous etiology of the hemorrhage unlikely.

SUBMACULAR LACQUER CRACKS, SUBMACULAR HEMORRHAGE, AND CHOROIDAL NEOVASCULARIZATION

Submacular hemorrhage associated with choroidal neovascularization after PRK was first described by Brancato et al in 1993.[84] Subsequently, Kim in 1994,[85] Toda et al in 1996,[86] Loewenstein and coworkers in 1997,[87,88] and Ruiz-Moreno in 2000 reported submacular hemorrhage with or without choroidal neovascularization after PRK.[89] Salah et al,[7] Kim et al,[15] and Pallikaris et al[17] reported a total of 4 cases of submacular hemorrhage after LASIK. One of those cases showed lacquer cracks only, whereas two cases showed choroidal neovascularization on fluorescein angiography. Knorz et al[14] also reported subretinal hemorrhages after LASIK. The first report of bilateral submacular hemorrhage was made by Luna et al on a 31-year-old man 17 days after bilateral LASIK in 1999.[90] Fundus examination showed multiple patches of posterior subretinal hemorrhage, including the macula. Fluorescein angiography showed macular defects consistent with lacquer cracks. In 2000, Ellies and coauthors reported 2 women with -12.00 and -18.00 D of myopia, respectively, that developed bilateral submacular hemorrhage within 1 and 4 days after LASIK, respectively in 2000.[91,92] Fluorescein angiography showed macular lacquer cracks without choroidal neovascularization at the site of hemorrhage in 1 eye 1 month later. However, fluorescein angiography showed a submacular choroidal neovascular process measuring 300 μm in diameter on a previous site of posterior pigmented Fuch's spot on the day after the hemorrhage for the other eye. In his report of 20 eyes with vitreoretinal pathologic conditions in 2001, Arevalo et al described 1 eye with a juxtafoveal choroidal neovascular membrane surrounded by a ring of hemorrhage and cystoid macular edema.[46] This patient underwent a vitrectomy and removal of the choroidal neovascular membrane. In 2001, Ruiz-Moreno et al also reported on eyes with choroidal neovascularization following LASIK.[93] In 2001, Chen and coauthors published on submacular hemorrhage 2 weeks after bilateral LASIK in both eyes of a 32-year-old high myope (> -13.00 D).[94] Submacular hemorrhage recurred at week 7 and again at week 22 in both eyes. Bilateral choroidal neovascularization was detected on fluorescein angiography on week 24. In 2003, Ruiz-Moreno described submacular lacquer crack formation and hemorrhage in a myopic eye that underwent a phakic intraocular anterior chamber lens implantation in August 2001, followed by uncomplicated LASIK on December 11, 2001.[95] Fluorescein angiography failed to show a choroidal neovascular process associated with the large lacquer crack. For this case, the macular lesion formed on the same day as the LASIK. Maturi et al also reported a patient with severe myopia (-16.00 D) that developed multiple posterior lacquer cracks in the right eye 1 day after uncomplicated bilateral LASIK in 2003.[96] An elevated subfoveal choroidal neovascular process with a ring of hemorrhage formed in the same eye 2 months later. Likewise in 2004, Spraul et al reported a case of subretinal choroidal neovascularization in a 33-year-old patient.[97] In 2004, Principe and coauthors reported a case of submacular hemorrhage in the left eye of a 36-year-old woman with moderate myopia (-5.00 D OD, and -6.00 D OS) 1 day after undergoing bilateral LASIK. For that case, the corneal flap was created with the IntraLase femtosecond laser associated with a much lower rise in intraocular pressure in comparison to the microkeratomes.[99] The submacular hemorrhage cleared 2 months later, and the best-corrected visual acuity (BCVA) was recovered to 20/25 for the affected eye 6 months later.

The mechanism of lacquer crack formation and associated submacular hemorrhage is unknown (Figure 27-6). Maturi et al pointed out that the eye wall tension (T) increases proportional to the increase in axial length, according to LaPlace's Law (T= PR/2), (Radius R = ½ axial length).[96] Thus, the wall tension of a myopic eye with a high axial length is substantially greater than the wall tension found in a normal eye. They speculated that the increase in wall tension leads to a break in Bruch's membrane and the subsequent hemorrhage and predisposes choroidal neovascular formation. Similar to the formation of retinal breaks and detachment after LASIK, the acoustic shock waves created by the excimer laser and the acute intraocular pressure changes associated with application of the microkeratome ring are implicated in the development of submacular lacquer cracks, hemorrhage, and choroidal neovascularization.[84-98] However, a causal relationship has not been definitively established. For instance, the case of submacular hemorrhage described by Principe et al was associated with the femtosecond laser instead of a microkeratome for creation of a corneal flap during LASIK.[98] For that case, there was lack of extreme intraocular pressure changes during LASIK. Yet, the submacular hemorrhage still formed. Further studies are needed on this subject.

OTHER POSTERIOR SEGMENT LESIONS

Vascular occlusion (ie, branch retinal vein occlusion)[99] and cystoid macular edema[100] have developed after refractive surgery. However, the etiologies of these lesions are unknown. Ruiz-Moreno et al has pointed out that their association with refractive surgery could be coincidental.[68]

Figure 27-7. (A) Fundus photograph shows prominent posterior lacquer cracks in a highly myopic eye. (B) Fundus photograph and (C) corresponding fundus angiography show hemorrhage associated with lacquer cracks after refractive surgery for another highly myopic eye after refractive surgery. (Courtesy of JF Arevalo).

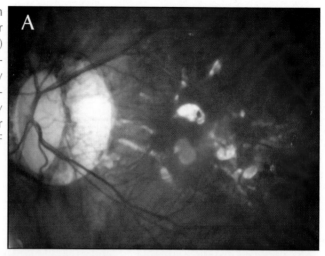

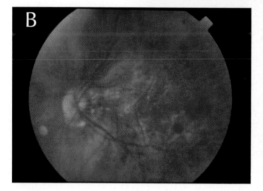

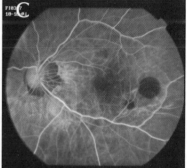

CONCLUSION

Although the occurrence of posterior segment pathology after refractive surgery is uncommon, the sheer volume of refractive surgery and the high expectation of the refractive patients tend to magnify the importance of any posterior segment complications, which are frequently sight threatening. Each individual refractive surgeon may encounter only a small number of cases of vitreoretinal complications. However, the cumulative numbers of such complications could be substantial. For instance, an incidence of 0.01% would yield 100 cases, and an incidence of 0.1% would yield 1000 cases of vitreoretinal complications for close a million cases of LASIK performed each year in the United States alone. Most eyes undergoing refractive surgery are myopic and are at inherent risk for vitreoretinal complications irrespective of the refractive surgery. Although the acoustic shock waves generated by the excimer laser and the acute intraocular pressure fluctuation induced by the microkeratome ring have been implicated as contributing factors to the vitreoretinal complications, a direct causal relationship has not been substantiated. Only a prospective study can establish an accurate incidence of such complications. Further investigation on this subject is needed. Meanwhile, vulnerable eyes intended for refractive surgery should undergo careful preoperative and repeated postoperative retinal monitoring.

KEY POINTS

1. The most common reports of postrefractive surgical vitreoretinal complications include retinal breaks and retinal detachment.
2. Other reports of posterior segment complications after refractive surgery include formation of a macular hole, premacular subhyaloid hemorrhage, submacular lacquer cracks, submacular hemorrhage, choroidal neovascularization, retinal vascular occlusion, and cystoid macular edema.
3. There is a greater distribution of post-LASIK retinal breaks and RD in the temporal than nasal quadrants.
4. Shock waves generated by the excimer laser may play a role in the development or amplification of vitreoretinal pathology.
5. The acute and severe intraocular pressure changes associated with the application of the microkeratome suction ring during LASIK may induce vitreoretinal traction.

REFERENCES

1. Pallikaris IG, Papatzanaki ME, Stathi EZ, et al. Laser in situ keratomileusis. *Lasers Surg Med.* 1990;10:463-468.
2. Pallikaris IG, Papatzanaki ME, Siganos DS, Tsilimbaris MK. A corneal flap technique for laser in situ keratomileusis. Human studies. *Arch Ophthalmol.* 1991;109:1699-1702.
3. Brint SF, Ostrick DM, Fisher C, et al. Six-month results of the multicenter phase I study of excimer laser myopic keratomileusis. *J Cataract Refract Surg.* 1994;20:610-615.
4. Kremer FB, Dufek M. Excimer laser in situ keratomileusis. *J Refract Surg.* 1995;11(3 Suppl):S244-S247.
5. Fiander DC, Tayfour F. Excimer laser in situ keratomileusis in 124 myopic eyes. *J Refract Surg.* 1995;11(3 Suppl):S234-S238.
6. Salah T, Waring GO III, el-Maghraby A, et al. Excimer laser in-situ keratomileusis (LASIK) under a corneal flap for myopia 2 to 20 D. *Trans Am Ophthalmol Soc.* 1995;93:163-183.
7. Salah T, Waring GO III, El Maghraby A, et al. Excimer laser in situ keratomileusis under a corneal flap for myopia of 2 to 20 diopters. *Am J Ophthalmol.* 1996;121:143-155.
8. Kohlhaas M, Lerche RCC, Draeger J, et al. Keratomileusis mit einem lamellären Mikrokeratom und einem Excimer-Laser. *Ophthalmologe.* 1995;92:499-502.
9. Bas AM, Onnis R. Excimer laser in situ keratomileusis for myopia. *J Refract Surg.* 1995;11(3 Suppl);S229-S233.
10. Guell JL, Muller A. Laser in situ keratomileusis (LASIK) for myopia from -7 to -18 diopters. *J Refract Surg.* 1996;12:222-228.
11. Marinho A, Pinto MC, Pinto R, et al. LASIK for high myopia: one year experience. *Ophthalmic Surg Lasers.* 1996;27(5 Suppl):S517-S520.
12. Helmy SA, Salah A, Badawy TT, Sidky AN. Photorefractive keratectomy and laser in situ keratomileusis for myopia between 6:00 and 10:00 diopters. *J Refract Surg.* 1996;12:417-421.
13. Gimbel HV, Basti S, Kaye GB, Ferensowicz M. Experience during the learning curve of laser in situ keratomileusis. *J Cataract Refract Surg.* 1996;22:542-550.
14. Knorz MC, Liermann A, Seiberth V, et al. Laser in situ keratomileusis to correct myopia of -6.00 to -29.00 diopters. *J Refract Surg.* 1996;12:575-584.
15. Kim HM, Jung HR. Laser assisted in situ keratomileusis for high myopia. *Ophthalmic Surg Lasers.* 1996;27(5 Suppl):S508-S511.
16. Condon PI, Mulhern M, Fulcher T, et al. Laser intrastromal keratomileusis for high myopia and myopic astigmatism. *Br J Ophthalmol.* 1997;81:199-206.

17. Pallikaris IG, Siganos DS. Laser in situ keratomileusis to treat myopia: early experience. *J Cataract Refract Surg.* 1997;23:39-49.

18. Danasoury MA, Waring GO III, El Maghraby A, Mehrez K. Excimer laser in situ keratomileusis to correct compound myopic astigmatism. *J Refract Surg.* 1997;13:511-520.

19. Wang Z, Chen J, Yang B. Comparison of laser in situ keratomileusis and photorefractive keratectomy to correct myopia from -1.25 to -6.00 diopters. *J Refract Surg.* 1997;13:528-534.

20. Leaming DV. Practice styles and preferences of ASCRS members—1998 survey. *J Cataract Refract Surg.* 1999;25:851-859.

21. Leaming DV. Practice styles and preferences of ASCRS members—1999 survey. *J Cataract Refract Surg.* 2000;26:913-921.

22. Leaming DV. Practice styles and preferences of ASCRS members—2000 survey. American Society of Cataract and Refractive Surgery. *J Cataract Refract Surg.* 2001;27:948-955.

23. Fechner PU, Strobel J, Wicchmann W. Correction of myopia by implantation of a Concave Worst-iris claw lens into phakic eyes. *Refract Corneal Surg.* 1991;7:286-298.

24. Pesando PM, Ghiringhello MP, Tagliavacche P. Posterior chamber collamer Phakic intraocular lens for myopia and hyperopia. *J Refract Surg.* 1999;15:415-423.

25. Zaldivar R, Davidorf JM, Oscherow S. Posterior chamber phakic intraocular lenses for myopia of -8 to -19 diopters. *J Refract Surg.* 1998;14:294-305.

26. Chastang P, Ruellan YM, Rozenbaum JP, et al. Phacoemulsification for visual refraction on the clear lens. A propos of 33 severely myopic eyes. *J Fr Ophtalmol.* 1998;21:560-566.

27. Pucci V. Morselli S, Romanelli F, et al. Clear lens phacoemulsification for correction of high myopia. *J Cataract Refract Surg.* 2001;27:896-900.

28. Colin J, Robinet A. Clear lensectomy and implantation of a low-power posterior chamber intraocular lens for correction of high myopia: a four-year follow-up. *Ophthalmology.* 1997;104:73-77.

29. McLeod SD, Mather R, Hwang DG, Margolis TP. Uveitis-associated flap edema and lamellar interface fluid collection after LASIK. *Am J Ophthalmol.* 2006;141:232.

30. Schwartz GS, Park DH, Schloff S, Lane SS. Traumatic flap displacement and subsequent diffuse lamellar keratitis after laser in situ keratomileusis. *J Cataract Refract Surg.* 2001;27:781-783.

31. Lin RT, Maloney RK. Flap complications associated with lamellar refractive surgery. *Am J Ophthalmol.* 1999;127:129-136.

32. Wang MY, Maloney RK. Epithelial ingrowth after laser in situ keratomileusis. *Am J Ophthalmol.* 2000; 129:746-751.

33. Twa MD, Nichols JJ, Joslin CE, et al. Characteristics of corneal ectasia after LASIK for myopia. *Cornea.* 2004;23:447-457.

34. Treister G, Harel O, Kremer I. Discoid corneal oedema and high intraocular pressure following PRK. *Br J Ophthalmol.* 1997;81:708-709.

35. Charteris DG, Cooling RG, Laving MJ, McLeod D. Retinal detachment following excimer laser. *Br J Ophthalmol.* 1997;81:759-761.

36. Charteris DG. Retinal detachment associated with excimer laser. *Curr Opin Ophthalmol.* 1999;10:173-176.

37. Vilaplana D, Guinot A, Escoto R. Giant retinal tears after photorefractive keratectomy. *Retina.* 1999; 19:342-343.

38. Ruiz-Moreno JM, Artola A, Alió JL. Retinal detachment in myopic eyes after photorefractive keratectomy. *J Cataract Refract Surg.* 2000;26:340-344.

39. Buch H, Vesti, Neilsen N. Keratopathy and pachymetric changes after photorefractive keratectomy and vitrectomy with silicone oil injection. *J Cataract Refract Surg.* 2002;26:1078-1081.

40. Ozdamar A, Aras C, Sener B, et al. Bilateral retinal detachment associated with giant retinal tear after laser-assisted in situ keratomileusis. *Retina.* 1998;18:176-177.

41. Stulting RD, Carr JD, Thompson KP, et al. Complications of laser in situ keratomileusis for the correction of myopia. *Ophthalmology.* 1999;106:13-20.

42. Ruiz-Moreno JM, Perez-Santonja JJ, Alió JL. Retinal detachment in myopic eyes after laser in situ keratomileusis. *Am J Ophthalmol.* 1999;128:588-594.

43. Aras C, Ozdamar A, Karacorlu M, et al. Retinal detachment following laser in situ keratomileusis. *Ophthalmic Surg Lasers*. 2000;31:121-125.

44. Farah ME, Höfling-Lima AL, Nascimento E. Early rhegmatogenous retinal detachment following laser in situ keratomileusis for high myopia. *J Refract Surg*. 2000;16:739-743.

45. Arevalo JF, Ramirez E, Suarez E, et al. Rhegmatogenous retinal detachment after laser-assisted in situ keratomileusis (LASIK) for the correction of myopia. *Retina*. 2000;20:338-341.

46. Arevalo JF, Ramirez E, Suarez E, et al. Incidence of vitreoretinal pathologic conditions within 24 months after laser in situ keratomileusis. *Ophthalmology*. 2000;107:258-226.

47. Arevalo JF, Ramirez E, Suarez E, et al. Rhegmatogenous retinal detachment in myopic eyes after laser in situ keratomileusis. Frequency, characteristics, and mechanism. *J Cataract Refract Surg*. 2001;27:674-680.

48. Tsai YY, Lin JM, Tsai SC. Giant tear retinal detachment after laser in situ keratomileusis—a case report. *Kaohsiung J Med Sci*. 2001;17:586-589.

49. Vakili R, Tauber S, Lim ES. Successful management of retinal tear post-laser in situ keratomileusis retreatment. *Yale J Biology Med*. 2002;75:55-57.

50. Arevalo JF, Ramirez E, Suarez E, et al. Retinal detachment in myopic eyes after laser in situ keratomileusis. *J Refract Surg*. 2002;18:708-714.

51. Hernáez-Ortega MC, Soto-Pedre E. Bilateral retinal detachment associated with giant retinal tear following LASIK. *J Refract Surg*. 2003;19:611.

52. Chan CK, Arevalo JF, Akbatur HH, et al. Characteristics of sixty myopic eyes with pre-laser in situ keratomileusis retinal examination and post-laser in situ keratomileusis retinal lesions. *Retina*. 2004;24:706-713.

53. Mackool RJ. Cause of post-LASIK retinal detachment [letter]. *J Cataract Refract Surg*. 2001;27:1708-1709. Arevalo FJ. [reply]. *J Cataract Refract Surg*. 2001:27:1709.

54. Menezo JL, Suarez-Reynolds R, Francés J, et al. Shape, number and localization of retinal tears in myopic over 8 D, aphakic and traumatic cases of retinal detachment, an experience report. *Ophthalmologica*. 1977;175:10-18.

55. Glasgow BJ, Foos RY, Yoshizumi MO, Straatsma BR. Degenerative diseases of the peripheral retina. In: Tasman W, Jaeger EA, eds. *Duane's Clinical Ophthalmology*. Vol 3. Philadelphia, Pa: Lippincott-Raven; 1996:1-30.

56. Blumenkranz MS. LASIK and retinal detachment: should we be concerned? *Retina*. 2000;5:578-581.

57. Seiler T, McDonnell PJ. Excimer laser photorefractive keratectomy. *Surv Ophthalmol*. 1995;40:89-118.

58. Seiler T, Schmidt-Petersen J, Wollensak J. Complications after myopic photorefractive keratectomy, primarily with the Summit excimer laser. In: Salz JJ, ed. *Corneal Laser Surgery*. St. Louis, MO: Mosby-Year Book; 1995:131-142.

59. Gobbi PG, Carones F, Brancato R, et al. Acoustic transients following excimer laser ablation of the cornea. *Eur J Ophthalmol*. 1995;5:275-276.

60. Kermani O, Lubatschowski H. Structure and dynamics of photo-acoustic shock-waves in 193 nm excimer laser photoablation of the cornea. *Fortschr Ophthalmol*. 1991;88:748-753.

61. Krueger RR, Krasinski JS, Radzewicz C, et al. Photography of shock waves during excimer laser ablation of the cornea. Effect of helium gas on propagation velocity. *Cornea*. 1993;12:330-334.

62. Krueger RR, Seiler T, Gruchman T, et al. Stress wave amplitudes during laser surgery of the cornea. *Ophthalmology*. 2001;108:1070-1074.

63. Alió JL, Ruiz-Moreno JM, Artola A. Retinal detachment as a potential hazard in surgical correction of severe myopia with phakic anterior chamber lenses. *Am J Ophthalmol*. 1993;115:145-148.

64. Luna JD, Artal MN, Reviglio VE, et al. Vitreoretinal alterations following laser in situ keratomileusis: clinical and experimental studies. *Graefes Arch Clin Exp Ophthalmol*. 2001;239:416-423.

65. Smith IR, Yadarola MB, Pelizzari MF, et al. Complete bilateral vitreous detachment after LASIK retreatment. *J Cataract Refract Surg*. 2004;30:1382-1384.

66. Flaxel CJ, Choi YH, Sheety M, et al. Proposed mechanism for retinal tears after LASIK: an experimental model. *Ophthalmology*. 2004;111:24-27.

67. Mirshahi A, Schöpfer D, Gerhardt D. et al. Incidence of posterior vitreous detachment after laser in situ keratomileusis. *Graefe Arch Clin Exper Ophthalmol*. 2006;244:149-153.

68. Ruiz-Moreno JM, Alió JL, Incidence of retinal disease following refractive surgery in 9239 eyes. *J Refract Surg.* 2003;19:534-547.

69. Pollack A, Marcovich A, Bukelman A, Oliver M. Age-related macular degeneration after extracapsular cataract extraction with intraocular lens implantation. *Ophthalmology.* 1996;103:1546-1554.

70. Blair CJ, Ferguson J Jr. Exacerbation of senile degeneration following cataract extraction. *Am J Ophthalmol.* 1979;87:77-83.

71. Werb Z. How the macrophage regulates the extracellular environment. *Am J Anat.* 1983;166:237-256.

72. Lin SC, Tseng SH. Prophylactic laser photocoagulation for retinal breaks before laser in situ keratomileusis. *J Refract Surg.* 2003;19:661-665.

73. Chan CK, Tarasewicz DG, Lin SG. Relation of pre-LASIK and post-LASIK retinal lesions and retinal examination for LASIK eyes. *Br J Ophthalmol.* 2005;89:209-301.

74. Panozzo G, Parolini B. Relationships between vitreoretinal and refractive surgery. *Ophthalmology.* 2001;108:1663-1670.

75. Ruiz-Moreno JM, Alió, Pérez-Santonja JJ, de la Hoz F. Retinal detachment in phakic eyes with anterior chamber intraocular lenses to correct severe myopia. *Am J Ophthalmol.* 1999:127:270-275.

76. Michels RG, Wilkinson CD, Rice TA. *Retinal Detachment.* St Louis, Mo: Mosby; 1990;83-84.

77. Chan CK, Lawrence FC. Macular hole after laser in situ keratomileusis and photorefractive keratectomy. *Am J Ophthalmol.* 2001;131:666-667.

78. Ruiz-Moreno JM, Artola A, Pérez-Santonja JJ, Alió JL. Macular hole in a myopic eye after laser in situ keratomileusis. *J Refract Surg.* 2002;18:746-749.

79. Arevalo JF, Mendoza AJ, Velez-Vazquez W, et al. Macular hole after LASIK [letter]. *J Refract Surg.* 2004; 20:85.

80. Arevalo JF, Rodriguez FJ, Rosales-Meneses JL, et al. Vitreoretinal surgery for macular hole after laser assisted in situ keratomileusis for the correction of myopia. *Br J Ophthalmol.* 2005;89:1423-1426.

81. Arevalo JF, Mendoza AJ, Velez-Vazquez W, et al. Full-thickness macular hole after LASIK for the correction of myopia. *Ophthalmology.* 2005;112:1207-1212.

82. Arevalo JF, Rodriguez FJ, Rodriguez A. Full-thickness macular hole after laser-assisted in situ keratomileusis (LASIK) for the correction of hyperopia. In press.

83. Mansour AM, Ojeimi GK. Premacular subhyaloid hemorrhage following laser in situ keratomileusis. *J Refract Surg.* 2000;16:371-372.

84. Brancato R, Tavola A, Carones F, et al. Excimer laser photorefractive keratectomy for myopia: results in 1165 eyes. Italian Study Group. *Refract Corneal Surg.* 1993;9:95-104.

85. Kim JH, Sah WJ, Hahn TW, Lee YC. Some problems after photorefractive keratectomy. *J Refract Corneal Surg.* 1994;10(Suppl):S226-230.

86. Toda I, Yagi Y, Hara S, et al. Excimer laser photorefractive keratectomy for patients with contact lens intolerance caused by dry eyes. *Br J Ophthalmol.* 1996;80:604-609.

87. Loewenstein A, Lipshitz I, Varssano D, Lazar M. Macular hemorrhage after excimer laser photorefractive keratectomy. *J Cataract Refract Surg.* 1997;23:808-810.

88. Loewenstein A, Goldstein M, Lazar M. Retinal pathology occurring after excimer laser surgery or phakic intraocular lens implantation: Evaluation of possible relationship. *Surv Ophthalmol.* 2002;47:125-135.

89. Ruiz-Moreno JM, Artola A, Ayala MJ, et al. Choroidal neovascularization in myopic eyes after photorefractive keratectomy. *J Cataract Refract Surg.* 2000;26:1492-1495.

90. Luna JD, Reviglio VE, Juarez CP. Bilateral macular hemorrhage after laser in situ keratomileusis. *Graefes Arch Clin Exp Ophthalmol.* 1999;237:611-613.

91. Ellies P, Pietrini D, Lumbroso L, Lebuisson DA. Macular hemorrhage after laser in situ keratomileusis for high myopia. *J Cataract Refract Surg.* 2000;26:922-924.

92. Ellies P, Le Rouic JF, Dichiro P, Renard Gilles. Macular hemorrhage after LASIK for high myopia: a Causal Association? *J Cataract Refract Surg.* 2001;27:966-967.

93. Ruiz-Moreno JM, Pérez-Santonja JJ, Alió JL. Choroidal neovascularization in myopic eyes after laser-assisted in situ keratomileusis. *Retina.* 2001;21:115-120.

94. Chen YC, Ma D, Yang KJ, et al. Bilateral choroidal neovascularization after laser-assisted in situ keratomi-leusis. *Retina*. 2001;21:174-175.

95. Ruiz-Moreno JM, Montero JA. Lacquer crack formation after LASIK. *Ophthalmology*. 2003;110:1669-1671.

96. Maturi RK, Kitchens J, Spitzberg DH, Yu M. Choroidal neovascularization after LASIK. *J Refract Surg*. 2003;19:463-464.

97. Spraul CW, Müller A, Lang G.K. Visusverlust nach LASIK. *Ophthalmologe*. 2004;101:726-728.

98. Principe AH, Lin DY, Small KW, Aldave AJ. Macular hemorrhage after laser in situ keratomileusis (LASIK) with femtosecond laser flap creation. *Am J Ophthalmol*. 2004;138:657-659.

99. Pallikaris I, Siganos D LASIK complications management. In: Talamo JH, Krueger RR, eds. *The Excimer Manual. A Clinician's Guide to Excimer Laser Surgery*. Boston, MA: Little, Brown & Co; 1997:227-242.

100. Janknecht P, Soriano JM, Hansen LI. Cystoid macular oedema after excimer laser photorefractive kera-tectomy. *Br J Ophthalmol*. 1993;77:681.

Chapter 28

NIGHTMARES WITH
PRESBYOPIC CORRECTING IMPLANTS

Robert Jay Weinstock, MD

INTRODUCTION

A comprehensive study of complications in refractive surgery would be incomplete without a discussion regarding crystalline lens removal with intraocular lens implantation. More specifically, accommodating and multifocal lenses, also known together as presbyopic correcting implants, carry their own set of complications above and beyond those that are inherent to cataract and lens removal surgery with traditional monofocal lens implantation.

Today, an ophthalmologist hearing the words *refractive surgery* immediately envisions a corneal-based procedure such as laser in situ keratomileusis (LASIK). However, long before the advent of the excimer laser, refractive surgery was being performed in its primordial form with the removal of a cataract and the implantation of an intraocular lens. Albeit crude and inaccurate in its early stages, over the past 40 years the procedure has become exceedingly safe, reliable, and precise in its ability to deliver excellent uncorrected visual acuity in healthy eyes. Modern lens removal techniques and implant technologies[1-12] have become so dependable over the past decade that performing the procedure on a noncataractous eye for purely refractive reasons has become not only common but is approaching the standard of care in some situations.

PRESBYOPIC CORRECTING IMPLANTS

Until recent years, the Achilles' heel of refractive surgery, whether corneal based or with crystalline lens replacement, has been the inability to adequately address the disease of presbyopia. Planned anisometropia (ie, monovision) is a successful way to provide spectacle independence but is not well tolerated by a significant number of patients. However, with the introduction of the 3M diffractive multifocal intraocular lens (IOL) (St. Paul, Minn) implant and Array multifocal implant (AMO, Santa Ana, Calif) in the 1990s, a new option allowing simultaneous clear uncorrected vision at distance and at near in the same eye became available. These early lens designs met with limited success although some surgeons experienced excellent results and have used the Array IOL consistently since its inception. In 2005, several more presbyopic correcting lenses were approved by the US Food and Drug

Administration and CE approved and have been well received and used successfully in the ophthalmic community. Many more designs and new technologies are under development and will be introduced over the next decade. With the rapid advancement of these new technologies and the ability to correct presbyopia, it is quite possible that lens replacement surgery will surpass LASIK and other corneal-based surgery as the predominant refractive procedure in patients over 45 years of age.

These recently introduced lenses for the correction of presbyopia are Crystalens (Eyeonics, Mission Viejo, Calif), ReZoom (AMO), and ReStor (Alcon, Fort Worth, Tex). Each of the lenses differ in their design and ability. Each also carries its own set of contraindications and complications. The remainder of this chapter will focus on management, considerations, and potential complications of these 3 lens designs. There are other presbyopic correcting lenses such as the Tecnis Multifocal implant (AMO) and the Synchrony lens (Visiogen, Irvine, Calif).

CONSIDERATIONS AND COMPLICATIONS COMMON TO ALL PRESBYOPIC CORRECTING INTRAOCULAR LENSES

Some of the most important complications experienced with the use of all presbyopic correcting implants are the same as with monofocal implants: those related to the surgical removal of the crystalline lens and the postoperative course. Regardless of which lens is placed inside the eye, there is significant risk from the lensectomy procedure itself, whether cataractous or not, which should be considered and discussed at length with the patient. These complications include events such as suprachoroidal hemorrhage, aqueous misdirection, corneal wound burn, vitreous loss, IOL malpositioning, wrong lens implantation, implant damage upon insertion with need for removal, iris damage and bleeding, and nuclear or cortical material subluxation into the vitreous cavity with need for additional surgery. Postoperative complications include endophthalmitis, cystoid macular edema, retinal detachment, persistent corneal edema, and induced astigmatism, just to name a few.

In addition to these complications, the choice to implant one of the presbyopic correcting lenses adds a new dimension to the procedure that warrants additional considerations. One of the most common, disturbing, and often preventable complications associated with all the presbyopic correcting IOLs is poor patient satisfaction postoperatively. This can occur despite a normal lens removal procedure, proper placement of the intraocular lens and desired refractive results objectively. The most common reason for patient dissatisfaction with the presbyopic correcting implants is inadequate preoperative counseling resulting in the patient having falsely high expectations. Although the presbyopic correcting IOLs are a significant improvement over traditional monofocal implants with regard to providing a more spectacle-free and independent lifestyle, all of the lenses do have their short comings and are not a panacea for youthful emmetropic vision.

Each of the lenses that are used today employ different technologies to accomplish the similar goal of providing reasonably good uncorrected vision at distance, intermediate, and even near targets. Depending on the lens, there are different visual zones where the lens will not perform as well as it does in others. Preoperative and postoperative patient counseling to insure appropriate expectations is the surgeon's responsibility and is directly proportional to success with these implants. Patients' life styles, needs, and desires should be discussed at length with the surgeon so he or she can make an educated decision regarding which technology and which lens will be best suited for each individual patient. Some surgeons employ the help of a patient questionnaire to guide in this decision making. Again, the information given by the patient allows the surgeon to accurately determine which lens type to use. Therefore, careful patient selection, education, and preoperative testing are crucial to success. It is paramount to understand how each lens design works, its strengths, and its shortcomings in order to match the appropriate technology to the patient.

Of course, postoperative success is totally dependent on the right lens power calculation and this makes accurate biometry a must. Many surgeons who experience success with these lenses rely on immersion biometry as well as the IOLMaster (Zeiss, Dublin, Calif). Corneal topography is also very helpful in determining preoperative astigmatism when planning for limbal relaxing incisions or astigmatic keratotomies at the time of surgery. If more preoperative astigmatism is present than corneal relaxing incisions can correct, the patient will no doubt have postoperative astigmatism that will affect the results and performance of the presbyopic correcting intraocular lens. This can lead to significant patient dissatisfaction. Preoperative discussions are essential with these particular patients to set their expectations properly. If significant postoperative astigmatism is likely to be present, disclose this to the patient and discuss the possible need for additional corneal excimer laser treatment.

Patients who have undergone previous refractive surgery can pose a particular challenge to the surgeon in selecting the proper lens power. Differences between the changes in the anterior and posterior corneal surfaces made by the refractive procedures create inaccurate power calculations. Several formulas and technologies can help overcome this obstacle: corneal topography, IOLMaster, historical data, and contact lens over refractions. It is important to discuss with these patients that additional surgery may be needed to fine tune their vision.

In patients who have undergone RK, it may be advisable to avoid multifocal implants. After RK, there can be a multifocal effect to the cornea caused by the procedure. Adding a multifocal implant to this optical system can cause a decrease in the performance of the implant.

Dry eyes can cause significant postoperative problems regardless of the implant that is used. Since the cornea is two-thirds of refracting power of the eye, an irregular surface or tear film can cause significant degradation in the vision. Many patients who complain of unwanted visual disturbances with presbyopic correcting lenses can often be helped with correction of the dry eye and irregular tear film.

Deciding which lens technology is best suited for each patient can be challenging and is possibly the single most important step in the entire process. Consideration of each patient's primary visual need and activities is paramount. It must be understood that none of the current lens designs offers guaranteed spectacle independence and that each excels in a different visual range.

THE CRYSTALENS

The Crystalens has a monofocal optic and hinged haptics with the ability to move inside the capsular bag that allows accommodation (Figure 28-1). This can be an excellent choice for people who are more distance vision-oriented, but who would like the ability to do some intermediate work without spectacle dependence. However, the uncorrected near functioning of the Crystalens is not as good as its distance functioning and should be used cautiously in people who desire the ability to perform very close or near work for extended periods of time and who would like to be spectacle independent for these tasks.

The Crystalens is the first CE- and FDA-approved IOL to truly be considered an accommodative IOL. Work on the lens design began in the 1980s with the discovery of axial movement inside the eye with a single-piece silicone plate lens. Stuart Cumming and colleagues investigated 7 intraocular lens designs in the 1980s and 1990s to try to mimic the natural ability of a lens to move axially inside the eye. Some of the early designs were too flexible

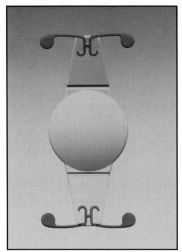

Figure 28-1. Crystalens.

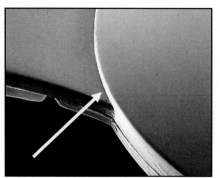

Figure 28-2. A square edge designed optic to help prevent posterior capsule opacification.

and would prolapse and dislocate anteriorly. All of the lens designs exhibited some degree of axial movement in the eye with resultant accommodative amplitude. Their final product is what is now called the Crystalens AT-45.

The Crystalens has a 4.5-mm silicone optic with attached plate style but hinged haptics. It has an overall length of 12.5 mm and has polyimide loops at the ends of the hinged haptics. These loops are designed to adhere to the capsule and prevent rotation or dislocation. The Crystalens SE is an improved model released in early 2006 that has asymmetrically shaped loops that help identify the front and back surfaces of the lens. It also incorporates a square edge designed optic to help prevent posterior capsule opacification and fibrosis (Figure 28-2). The Crystalens is made from a third-generation ultraviolet (UV)-blocking silicone. The hinged haptics theoretically allow the lens to move forward in the eye in response to the normal physiologic accommodative reflex.

A US clinical study has demonstrated the safety, efficacy, and predictability of the Crystalens with 1 year bilateral data demonstrating 98% of patients seeing 20/32 or better at distance, over 98% seeing J1 or better intermediate, and 94% seeing J2 or better at near. Why a small number of patients do not have significant accommodative effects after implantation remains a mystery and requires further study. Accommodation with the Crystalens will only work if the lens is placed inside the capsular bag and is able to move freely anteriorly and posteriorly in response to the contraction and expansion of the cilliary muscle. Contrast sensitivity testing, as reported to the FDA, exhibited similar results to a standard monofocal lens.

Considerations and Complications With the Crystalens

In addition to the complications normally associated with crystalline lens removal and posterior chamber intraocular lens placement, the Crystalens has its own set of unique complications. Most of these are due to its flexible nature and its hinged optic design.

Some major intraoperative considerations unique to the Crystalens have to do with the difficulty placing the Crystalens inside an intact capsular bag in the proper anterior/posterior orientation and the small optic size necessitates good centration. Creating a perfect capsulorrhexis is important to avoiding complications with this lens. If there is a rent in the anterior capsule the lens will likely not sit in the bag properly and may be prone to postoperative

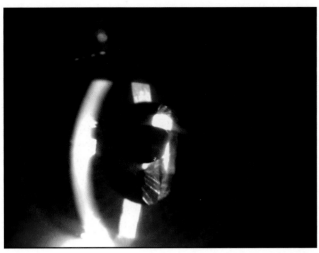

Figure 28-3. Capsular phimosis.

anterior prolapse or poor accommodative function. The capsulorrhexis should be well-centered, smooth, round, and 5.5 to 6.0 mm in diameter. A too small capsulorrhexis can cause intraoperative difficulty with removal of nuclear and cortical material removal leading to a compromise in the integrity of the capsule or zonulolyis. Postoperatively it can lead to late capsular phimosis (Figure 28-3) or anterior capsular contraction. Any tensile forces such as these can cause abnormal movement or position of the lens in the eye. On the other hand, too large of a capsulorrhexis may not provide adequate support for the lens edge and haptics that will predispose to lens anterior prolapse. If the capsulorrhexis is not the proper size, if the capsular bag is not perfectly intact, or if the zonules are compromised, it is best not to place a Crystalens inside the eye. It is not designed to be placed in the ciliary sulcus.

A slightly enlarged incision of approximately 3.8 mm is required to place the Crystalens inside the eye unfolded. An injector system is available for the Crystalens that will reduce the incision size to the same as needed for a monofocal implant. Wound construction is very important because good visual results with the Crystalens are dependent on minimal astigmatism postoperatively. With the enlarged incision, there needs to be special attention on constructing an astigmatically neutral incision. It is also advisable to place a suture through the enlarged wound to ensure no chance of a postoperative wound leak, shallowing of the anterior chamber, and bowing forward of the optic causing a myopic shift. If this should occur, surgical intervention to reposition the lens to an optic posterior configuration may be required. In some cases of mild myopic shift without a wound leak, atropinization can allow the Crystalens to take a more posterior position

Due to the flexible nature of the haptics, inserting the lens can be slightly difficult. It is very important that the haptics be placed inside the capsular bag with the optic being well centered in the middle of the eye. All viscoelastic material must be removed from the capsular bag, especially behind the lens, so there is no anterior vaulting of the lens post operatively. One must be sure not to place the implant in the eye upside down or it will be vaulted enough to cause a myopic shift and not function as intended. The hinged haptics have a groove on the posterior side of the lens at the junction of the optic. This groove can be seen under high magnification on the posterior side of the lens in vitro. Also, the asymmetric polyimide loops at the end of the haptics help in identifying the proper anterior posterior orientation. The distal haptic should have the round loop on the right side and the oval loop on the left if the lens is properly placed. Once the lens is in the capsular bag and the viscoelastic is removed, it should take a well-centered position with the optic flush against the posterior capsule centrally and the haptics tilted slightly (15 to 30 degrees) anteriorly. No posterior capsule striae should be present at the end of the case. Striae signify the optic is not positioned posterior enough or the eye is not sealed. If striae are still present despite attempts to reposition the lens and the eye is well sealed without a leak, it may signify poor capsular integrity and may be advisable to replace the Crystalens with a monofocal implant. The same holds true if it is not possible to center the Crystalens in the eye.

As with any implant, choosing the wrong power is always a significant complication. Poor biometry will often lead to ammetropic results and suboptimal patient satisfaction. Immersion ultrasound, IOLMaster biometry, and corneal topography have all been used in conjunction to successfully ensure proper lens selection. Plano to -0.50 is the desired target for the Crystalens.

Lens vaulting creates refractive problems for the patient and can either occur early or late in the postoperative period. Early posterior vaulting can either be anterior or posterior. Posterior lens vaulting early in the postoperative period is usually due to a hyperinflation syndrome at the time of surgery because the eye is overpressurized at the end of the case. This forces the flexible lens posteriorly and causes a hyperopic shift. This condition may require surgical intervention to resolve.

Early in the postoperative period, there can also be symmetrical or asymmetrical anterior vaulting of the lens. This is usually due to a wound leak, allowing the flexible optic to prolapse anteriorly. Usually in this situation, there is a myopic shift of 1.00 to 2.00 D. Often in these cases, striae in the posterior capsule can be seen and the lens may be observed in a slightly anterior position at the slit lamp. Surgical intervention is often required to remedy the situation by inflating the capsular bag with a viscoelastic material and pushing the Crystalens posteriorly into the capsular bag, making sure the wound is well sealed at the end of the case. Cycloplegia may reduce the anterior vaulting without surgical intervention and should always be tried first.

Another cause for early anterior vaulting postoperatively can be due to slow encapsulation of the loop haptics. The loops usually fibrose quickly to the equatorial capsule but if they do not contact it well or are blocked by residual cortex, the haptics may dislocate from the sulcus with accommodation and the lens will move anteriorly.

Late postoperative vaulting of the Crystalens also can occur. It can be either posterior or anterior vaulting of the lens due to late anterior capsular fibrosis or capsular contraction syndromes leading to an abnormal position of the lens inside the capsular bag. Anterior capsular fibrosis is typically ovoid in shape, causing irregular astigmatism and an abnormal orientation of the Crystalens inside the capsular bag. It can cause the lens to either symmetrically vault anterior or posterior, or develop an asymmetric vault in which one haptic is positioned more posteriorly than the other haptic. This will induce a tilt in the lens and result in refractive astigmatism.

On slit-lamp examination, the capsular contraction syndrome is usually obvious with a whitening of the capsule and a contracture in either the horizontal or longitudinal axis. In addition to capsular contraction syndrome, residual cortex left in the capsular bag can also result in asymmetrical vault, either anteriorly or posteriorly. The residual cortex can cause fibrosis locally of the capsule that will cause striae to be seen in a localized area in the posterior capsule. This can cause a shift of the lens position and a possible vaulting either anteriorly or posteriorly of the haptic and lens near the residual cortex.

Treatment of both residual cortex with capsular contraction as well as anterior capsular fibrosis is primarily done using the YAG laser. The YAG laser reduces the tensile forces on the capsular bag that are causing the distortion and abnormal position of the lens. With capsular contraction syndrome, YAG laser is used to treat the anterior capsule. Usually with anterior capsular fibrosis, a hyperopic shift is seen and after the YAG treatment to the anterior capsule

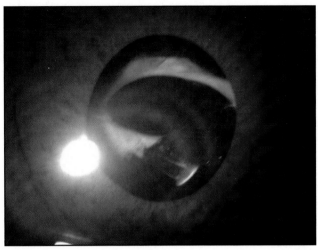

Figure 28-4. YAG laser done to treat the capsular phimosis.

there is resolution of the anterior vaulting (Figure 28-4). YAG treatment is best done by applying laser treatment to the fibrotic areas of the anterior capsule to release the forces enacting on the Crystalens. One or 2 applications along the long axis of the capsular opening should be enough to resolve the contraction. Sometimes several days are needed to see the posterior movement of the lens take effect.

Early Crystalens use was performed with a very small capsulorrhexis opening of approximately 4 to 5 mm. In these early cases, there was a higher rate of capsular contraction syndrome and since then surgeons have moved to a more enlarged capsulorrhexis of 5 to 6 mm that has decreased the rate of capsular phimosis.

YAG laser treatments in cases of residual cortex and capsular contraction are best applied to the posterior capsule. Once the residual cortex is located, and the striae adjacent to the residual cortex are identified, YAG laser capsulotomy can be performed locally in that area to reduce the tensile forces on the capsular bag and allow the Crystalens to be positioned centrally in the eye. Frequent postoperative visits and vision checks as well as refraction post-YAG are paramount to success with the Crystalens in these situations.

Although the vast majority of Crystalens patients are successful in gaining excellent distance visual acuity and excellent intermediate visual acuity with moderate near function, there is a subset of patients who will have difficulty with reading either immediately postoperatively or who will lose their ability in the distant postoperative period. It is difficult to predict which patients will have this phenomenon, therefore, preoperative counseling is important due to the possible loss of accommodative ability of the lens with time. It has been noted that the accommodative effects improve with time and with proper training in some cases.

THE REZOOM IMPLANT

The ReZoom (AMO) multifocal refractive intraocular lens may be better than the ReStor (Alcon) in that it provides good visual acuity at all ranges of vision, including intermediate vision. However, there are significant night visual disturbances and dysphotopsias with this lens, and like the Array lens, it is almost impossible to predict why a particular patient will be incapacitated by these symptoms. The near vision does not supply as much add at the spectacle plane and may be better suited than the ReStor for someone who needs excellent vision in the intermediate range (such as heavy computer users).

The ReZoom lens is a second-generation acrylic refractive multifocal IOL. It features 5 refractive optical zones that distribute light to provide good, near, intermediate, and distance vision. The central zone is distant dominant and the second zone is near dominant. Aspheric transition provides intermediate vision in all light conditions. It is a 3-piece acrylic IOL with PMMA haptics. The optic size is 6 mm with a 13-mm overall length. It can be injected into the eye with an unfolder implantation system through a sub-3-mm incision intended for placement inside the capsular bag.

In clinical studies, 93.4% of patients studied function without glasses for distance vision, 92.6% function for intermediate vision without glasses, and 81.4% function at near without glasses. The optic is designed with a rounded anterior edge to reduce internal reflections, a sloping side edge to minimize edge glare, and a square posterior edge to facilitate capsular contact and possibly avoid posterior capsular opacification.

The ReZoom lens is the second iteration based on the initial AMO multifocal IOL called the Array lens. As compared to the Array lens, zone 1 is unchanged, zone 2 is 5% larger, zone 3 is 80% larger, zone 4 is 55% smaller, and zone 5 is the same. These changes were made in order to reduce the night-time visual disturbances and dysphotopsias that were noted in some patients who were implanted with the Array lens. The reduction in the zone 4 (near dominant portion) of the lens was made to improve quality of vision in mesopic pupillary conditions such as night driving.

With the ReZoom design, in bright light conditions and a 2-mm pupil approximately 84% of light is distributed to the distance dominant central zone. In low light conditions and a 5-mm pupil, approximately 60% of light is distributed to the distance dominant zone and 40% to intermediate and near zones. Very small pupils, whether physiologic or secondary to extreme bright light conditions, may impair near vision performance.

Considerations and Complications With the ReZoom Implant

As mentioned previously, correct patient selection is paramount in success with the ReZoom multifocal IOL. Many of the complications seen with this lens are related to poor patient satisfaction postoperatively if the patient engages in a significant amount of night driving activities or other distant vision activities performed under mesopic conditions. Many of these complications can be avoided with proper patient screening as well as careful preoperative patient counseling. The options for different lens technologies need to be discussed at length with the patient so that they understand the strengths and limitations of the different technologies available. Patients should be aware that there may be halos or glare around point sources of light at night, that a longer adaptation period may be required, that they may experience fuzzy near vision at times, and that reading glasses may still be needed, especially for very fine print.

Additionally, experience with the Array and the ReZoom lenses has shown that there is an adaptation process that transpires over a 3-week to 6-month period of time where a person learns to adjust to the pseudoaccommodative effects of the multifocal optics. This process has been termed *neuroadaptation*. It is not uncommon for patients to notice significant halos, glare, and night-time visual disturbances early on in the postop period that tend to diminish with time. With appropriate preoperative and postoperative education, patients will be prepared for the halos seen at night initially and have the confidence that they will adapt with time.

Halos are a visual disturbance well known to hyperopes and cataract patients. Therefore, the ReZoom lens may be better tolerated in hyperopic individuals who are accustomed to seeing a halo around a point source of light. In contrast, a low to moderate myope typically sees star bursts of light and is more used to this type of dysphotopsia. When previously myopic patients notice postoperative halos that are possible with the ReZoom lens, they may be more concerned by them because it is unfamiliar. The hyperope, who is accustomed to seeing such visual disturbances, may not even notice the postoperative halos around a point source of light. In addition to a more noticeable appearance of halos around point sources of light as seen by previously myopic patients, they may also be more dissatisfied with the quality of the near visual acuity afforded by the ReZoom IOL. Moderate myopes are accustomed to having excellent sharp vision up close due to their natural myopia and the pseudoaccommodative effect of the ReZoom lens may not duplicate this crisp near vision.

Additional predictors of unhappy ReZoom multifocal IOL patients are character traits. Persons who are not motivated to be less dependent on glasses, who are unwilling to adapt to a new visual system, or who are demanding and expecting perfect vision will certainly be poor candidates for this lens. Other factors that identify poor candidates (and therefore greater opportunity for postoperative patient dissatisfaction) include patients with unstable capsular support, those with significant dry eyes, corneal scarring, mild to moderate myopia, pupil size less than 2.5 mm, a monofocal implant in their first eye, or uncorrected postoperative astigmatism greater than a half of a diopter.

Postoperative emmetropia, whether achieved with the primary implantation of the lens, with or without limbal relaxing incisions, or postoperatively with the use of excimer laser is the goal with the ReZoom IOL as well as any PCLS. Significant postoperative astigmatism, although not a true complication, can be classified as such with the multifocal lenses. Residual astigmatism is more likely to cause visual disturbances and possibly further worsen the night time halos. Preoperatively, astigmatism should certainly be assessed with manual keratotomy as well as corneal topography or wavefront analysis and can be addressed intraoperatively with astigmatic keratectomies, limbal relaxing incisions, or a combination of both. Postoperatively, the astigmatism can also be managed with the excimer laser.

Postoperative complaints heard from patients include distance blur, which is usually due to ammetropic results; monocular diplopia, which can be due to poor ocular surface or poor IOL centration; object glow, which is likely related to dry eye syndrome or a posterior capsular opacification; or ghosting, which can be due to uncorrected astigmatism. Halos at night in the early postoperative period can be addressed by asking the patient to wait 3 months for neuroadaptation to occur. Additionally, turning on the dome light in the car can shrink the pupils and reduce the unwanted visual disturbances. However, when severe and disabling symptoms persist longer than 3 months, lens removal may be indicated. Inducing pharmacological miosis with brimonidine tartrate 0.2% or Pilocarpine 0.5% is also helpful in reducing these unwanted night time visual disturbances. However, if the pupil is too small either naturally or pharmacologically, as in bright light conditions, the reading vision may suffer because the iris covers the second zone (near), eliminating its image.

Another known complication of any PCL, and especially the ReZoom, is postoperative lens decentration. The zonal progressive nature of the ReZoom is fairly sensitive to decentration due to the small central distance portion of the lens. Usually up to 1 mm of decentration is tolerated whereas 3 to 4 mm may be tolerable with a monofocal implant. Eyes with irregular pupils may require pupilloplasty to remedy visual disturbances. If the lens is found to be truly decentered and causing dysphtopsias, it is best to treat by first determining the cause of decentration. It can be due either to the lens or to the capsule. If one of the haptics is bent or kinked during loading or during the injection process, the lens may initially take an eccentric position. If it does not centralize within 1 or 2 minutes, there are two options. One is to tease the bent haptic out of the capsular bag and out of the wound and attempt to straighten or unkink the irregularity. If when it is dialed back into the capsule it again does not center, it is advised to remove the damaged lens from the eye and replace it. Decentration in the early postoperative period is likely due to movement of the lens inside the bag. This is sometimes

Figure 28-5. ReStor implant.

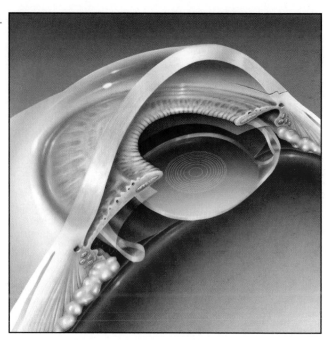

seen if residual cortex is inadvertently left behind which can hydrate, pushing on the haptic or optic. It may be necessary to reposition the lens surgically. In the late postoperative period, asymmetric posterior or anterior capsular contraction can also cause a shift in the lens position. This situation can be remedied with strategically placed YAG laser capsulotomies.

ReStor Implant

In contrast to the Crystalens, the ReStor, a multifocal apodized diffractive IOL (Figure 28-5), does achieve excellent near vision with a +4 add at the lens plane translating into approximately +3 add at the spectacle plane. With this, most patients are able to achieve spectacle independence for typical near work and reading at 14 inches, although the intermediate vision may not be as sharp. The multifocal technology employed in this lens has rendered it susceptible to night vision dysphotopsias and distance vision disturbances as reported by some patients. For most patients, however, distance vision with the ReStor has achieved excellent results and the glare or halos around point sources of light are well tolerated. The loss of low light contrast sensitivity can be disturbing to people who do a lot of night driving or are extremely distance vision oriented. With this said, the ReStor may not be the best selection of lens for someone who enjoys night time activities, drives a lot at night, or performs a lot of long distance vision activities at dusk or early in the morning.

The Acrysof ReStor multifocal intraocular lens is a biconvex apodized diffractive optic posterior chamber implant. It is available in a single piece or 3-piece model. The optic size is 6 mm and the overall haptic length is 13 mm in both models. It can be injected into the eye with an unfolder implantation system through a sub-3-mm incision intended for placement inside the capsular bag.

The biconvex optic with the apodized diffractive structure provides an increased depth of focus. The lens has 12 concentric steps of gradually decreasing step heights. In the lenticular plane, it creates +4.00 D of additional power resulting in 3.20 D at the spectacle plane. This is all contained within a central apodized diffractive region of 3.6 mm. The peripheral refractive region contributes to distance vision for large pupil diameters. This peripheral portion is dedicated to distance vision only. Therefore, the reading portion of this lens is designed to work in a small pupil situation in bright light, which is in contrast to the ReZoom lens, which is better suited for a medium to larger size pupil in less illumination. The apodized diffractive steps spilt light energy between the near and distance focal points regardless of the light situation.

Considerations and Complications With the ReStor Implant

Some unwanted visual effects may be expected due to the superposition of focused and unfocused multiple images. These may include halos or radial lines around a point source of light under night time conditions. A reduction in contrast sensitivity as compared to a monofocal IOL may be experienced by some patients and may be more prevalent in low light conditions. In order to achieve success with the ReStor IOL, the surgeon must target emmetropia. Patients with significant preoperative or predicted postoperative astigmatism of greater than 1.00 D are less likely to be happy with their visual outcomes with the ReStor lens.

IOL centration is as important as with the ReZoom lens since lens decentration may result in a patient experiencing visual disturbances under certain lighting conditions. Most patients will only tolerate decentration of approximately 1 mm. This is quite common in the elderly population where there is a somewhat more nasal orientation of the center of the pupil in regards to the capsular bag.

Postoperatively, posterior capsular opacification may cause earlier clinical symptoms with the ReStor lens as compared to monofocal lenses. Therefore, earlier YAG laser capsulotomy may be necessary to restore adequate visual function with the ReStor lens.

Common judgment should be used by the surgeon prior to implanting the ReStor as well as other multifocal lenses. The cornea should be assessed for any significant irregular astigmatism or aberrations. Pre-existing retinal conditions, such as diabetic retinopathy or macular degeneration, should be monitored and considered prior to lens insertion. Additionally, any unexpected intraoperative complications should preclude the surgeon from implanting the ReStor implant. For example, significant deformation or mechanical manipulation of the pupil during the surgery, significant vitreous loss, significant anterior chamber bleeding, and compromise of the stability of the capsular bag should be relative contraindications to placement of the ReStor IOL. In these situations, it is best to choose a standard monofocal implant. Controlled clinical studies revealed that a maximum visual performance with the ReStor lens was achieved when implanted bilaterally. When implanted monocularly, a statistically significant decrease in mean uncorrected visual acuity (UCVA) and best corrected distance vision was observed in subjects with ReStor as compared with monofocal controls. Older subjects implanted with the ReStor lens (greater than 80 years old) demonstrated a trend for poorer UCVA than the monofocal control patients.

A binocular refraction defocused curve from the United States intermediate vision study displays 2 peaks, one at the zero base line corresponding to the distance focal point of the lens and one near -3.00 which corresponds to the near focal point of the lens. This curve demonstrates that ReStor IOL patients can achieve 20/20 or better vision at distance with an additional increase of the focus of approximately 3.00 D for 20/20 near vision as compared to monofocal control patients. There is a slight dip in the defocus curve of intermediate vision to the visual acuity level of 20/40 or better. In clinical practice, this translates into a patient experiencing theoretical excellent distant visual acuity uncorrected as well as excellent uncorrected near visual acuity. However, there does seem to be a relative loss in intermediate vision. Therefore, patients with these lenses tend to have more difficulty with intermediate tasks such as computer vision. This fact should be a strong consideration when discussing lens options with patients.

Clinical studies have also shown a tendency for slightly reduced contrast sensitivity and low contrast acuity in ReStor IOL patients under low lighting (mesopic) conditions when exposed to a glare source. A study using a night driving simulator was performed using the ReStor IOL. The test simulated driving scenes, including a city street at night with streetlights and a rural highway with low beam headlights. Testing of both driving scenes was conducted under clear and foggy driving conditions as well as with glare conditions. This study revealed that the ability of the ReStor IOL patients to detect and identify road signs and hazards was similar to the monofocal controls under normal visibility conditions. However, the ReStor lens did not perform as well as the monofocal lens when both fog and glare were present.

Under glare conditions, the ability of the ReStor lens subjects to identify the text sign was reduced on average by 28%, although there was only a small difference under these conditions for the warning signs. In the FDA studies for the ReStor, mean visual disturbance ratings with the ReStor PCL compared to a monofocal IOL showed that 13% of patients had moderate or severe night vision disturbances in the ReStor group compared to 6% in the monofocal group. With regard to glare, 26% experienced moderate or severe glare in the ReStor group compared to 9% in the monofocal group.

Additionally, in the ReStor group, 24% experienced moderate or severe halos with the ReStor lens compared to 3% with the monofocal lens. These results were gathered between 120 and 180 days postoperatively. These data indicate that there is a significantly higher proportion of ReStor patients who will experience night time visual disturbances, glare, and halos compared with patients who have monofocal implants. As with the ReZoom lens, clinical experience suggests that a neuroadaptation period of several months may improve patients' symptoms with these disturbances. However, it is still advisable to counsel patients appropriately as to the potential problems with night vision and to screen patients properly to avoid dissatisfaction postoperatively.

CONCLUSION

Presbyopic correcting implants have opened the door to a new level of sophistication in lenticular-based surgery. If used properly, patients can experience a level of spectacle independence previously unavailable with conventional monfocal implants. However, these lenses are not applicable to all patients and each has its own strengths and weaknesses. With a complete understanding of each implant and the knowledge of how to avoid and manage complications, a surgeon is likely to experience good outcomes and have happy and satisfied patients.

KEY POINTS

1. Accommodating and multifocal lenses, also known together as presbyopic correcting implants, carry their own set of complications above and beyond those that are inherent to cataract and lens removal surgery with traditional monofocal lens implantation.

2. The most common reason for patient dissatisfaction with the presbyopic correcting implants is inadequate preoperative counseling resulting in the patient having falsely high expectations.

3. Some major intraoperative considerations unique to the Crystalens have to do with the difficulty placing the Crystalens inside an intact capsular bag in the proper anterior/posterior orientation and the small optic size necessitates good centration.

4. Many of the complications seen with the ReZoom lens are related to poor patient satisfaction postoperatively if the patient engages in a significant amount of night driving activities or other distant vision activities performed under mesopic conditions.

5. In order to achieve success with the ReStor IOL, the surgeon must target emmetropia. Patients with significant preoperative or predicted postoperative astigmatism of greater than one diopter are less likely to be happy with their visual outcomes with the ReStor lens.

REFERENCES

1. Arens B, Freudenthaler N, Quentin CD. Binocular function after bilateral implantation of monofocal and refractive multifocal intraocular lenses. *J Cataract Refract Surg.* 1999;25:399-404.

2. Brydon KW, Tokarewicz AC, Nichols BD. AMO Array multifocal lens versus monofocal correction in cataract surgery. *J Cataract Refract Surg.* 2000;26:96-100.

3. Dell S, Doane J, Slade S. *Lens Vaulting With the Crystalens Accommodating Intraocular Lens* [In press]; 2006.

4. Haring G, Dick HB, Krummenauer F, et al. Subjective photic phenomena with refractive multifocal and monofocal intraocular lenses. Results of a multicenter questionnaire. *J Cataract Refract Surg.* 2001; 27:245-249.

5. Haring G, Gronemeyer A, Hedderich J, et al. Stereoacuity and aniseikonia after unilateral and bilateral implantation of the Array refractive multifocal intraocular lens. *J Cataract Refract Surg.* 1999;25:1151-1156.

6. McDonald JE, El-Moatassem Kotb AM, Decker BB. Effect of brimonidine tartrate ophthalmic solution 0.2% on pupil size in normal eyes under different luminance conditions. *J Cataract Refract Surg.* 2001;27:560-564.

7. Montes-Mico R, Alio JL. Distance and near contrast sensitivity function after multifocal intraocular lens implantation. *J Cataract Refract Surg.* 2003;29(4):7032-7011.

8. Packer M., Hoffman RS, Dick B, Fine IH. *Refractive Lens Exchange: Outcomes, Complications and Management* [In press]; 2006.

9. Pieh S, Weghaupt H, Skorpik C. Contrast sensitivity and glare disability with diffractive and refractive multifocal intraocular lenses. *J Cataract Refract Surg.* 1998;24:659-662.

10. Richter-Mueksch S, Weghaupt H, Skorpik C, Velikay-Parel M, Radner W. Reading performance with a refractive multifocal and a diffractive bifocal intraocular lens. *J Cataract Refract Surg.* 2002;28(11):1957-1963.

11. Steinert RF, Aker BL, Trentacost DJ, Smith PJ, Tarantino N. A prospective comparative study of the AMO Array zonal progressive multifocal silicone intraocular lens and a monofocal intraocular lens. *Ophthalmology.* 1999;106:1243-1255.

12. Steinert RF, Post CT, Brint SF, et al. A progressive, randomized, double-masked comparison of a zonal-progressive multifocal intraocular lens and a monofocal intraocular lens. *Ophthalmology*. 1992;99:853-861.

Please see Hyperopic Shift After Phacoemulsification in Eyes With Previous Radial Keratotomy video on enclosed CD-ROM.

Chapter 29

Toxic Anterior Segment Syndrome

Simon P. Holland, MB, FRCSC; Douglas W. Morck, DVM, PhD; Gina Chavez, BSc; Yumi G. Ohashi, BSc; and Tracy L. Lee, BSc

Introduction

Toxic anterior segment syndrome (TASS) is more widely reported after first being recognized as a specific entity in 1992.[1] The classic features of TASS[1-11] are early and intense postoperative inflammation after anterior segment surgery without vitreal involvement. Presently, we do not know whether the increased awareness of the condition is the cause for the increase in reporting or if there is a real rise in incidence after cataract surgery. Previously, postoperative inflammation that appeared to be non-infectious was sometimes described as sterile endophthalmitis or postoperative uveitis of unknown origin. We suggest that the pathogenesis of TASS may be related to the bacterial biofilm contamination of sterilizer reservoirs and may present some critical parallel concepts to that of diffuse lamellar keratitis (DLK).

Definition

TASS is described as a group of signs and symptoms but lack of a precise definition due to the overlap with early infectious endophthalmitis, uveitis from retained cortex, and prior history of iritis. The expected characteristics are early onset (24 to 72 hours); intense anterior segment inflammation, including fibrin deposition and corneal edema; minimal or no pain; and the absence of vitritis. Infectious endophthalmitis can be differentiated by later presentation (peaks between day 3 and day 7), pain, and vitritis. However, early cases of endophthalmitis may present as TASS and wherever there is doubt regarding the diagnosis, the case should be treated as infectious endophthalmitis. The case illustrated (Figure 29-1) shows the appearance 8 hours after cataract surgery and was initially thought to be TASS. The patient was subsequently diagnosed as having endophthalmitis, culture positive for *Staphylococcus aureus*. The second case shows a more classical presentation on day 1 (Figure 29-2). Table 29-1 summarizes the differentiating features between infectious endophthalmitis and TASS.

Figure 29-1. Early endophthalmitis presenting on the day of surgery.

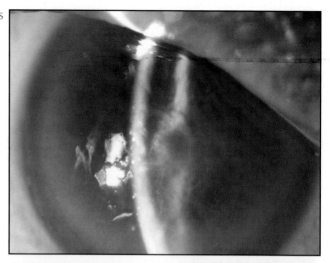

Figure 29-2. TASS on the first post-operative day.

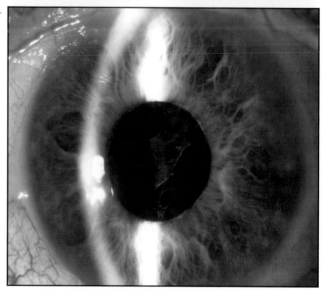

CLINICAL FEATURES

Acute onset of anterior segment inflammation is the hallmark of TASS.

Symptoms

Although severe pain is uncommon, patients will admit to some discomfort but their main concern is blurred vision. Ciliary injection is less common.

Cornea

Corneal edema, extending limbus to limbus, has been frequently described.[2] In cases in which this is the predominant feature, the condition has been termed toxic endothelial cell destruction syndrome (TECDS).[3-5]

	Table 29-1	
Differential Diagnosis: Toxic Anterior Segment Syndrome Versus Infectious Endophthalmitis		
Characteristics	*TASS*	*Infectious Endophthalmitis*
Onset	1 to 3 days	3 to 7 days
Symptoms	Blurred vision	Pain and blurred vision
Cornea	Edema 1+	Edema 2+
Anterior chamber	Cells 1 to 3+	Cells 3+
	Fibrin 1 to 3+	Fibrin variable
	Hypopyon 1+	Hypopyon 3+
Vitreous	Clear	Vitritis

Anterior Chamber Reaction

An intense cellular and fibrinous reaction is common and may progress to hypopyon formation if treatment is delayed. Fibrin membranes can develop and this may lead to glaucoma and visual loss as was seen in 2 of our cases.

Prognosis

Most cases obtain full recovery with early treatment using topical steroids. Delayed treatment or severe cases may develop posterior synechiae, distorted irregular pupils, and glaucoma.

Vitritis

Vitritis is almost never associated with TASS and indicates infectious endophthalmitis. However, it is possible that some cases of culture-negative endophthalmitis may also be caused by toxins and contaminating agents that cause TASS and be a "spill over" of the anterior segment inflammation. Better differentiation between infectious endophthalmitis, culture-negative or sterile endophthalmitis, and TASS may occur with newer techniques such as polymerase chain reaction (PCR) analysis of aqueous and vitreal aspirates.

Response to Steroids

TASS cases usually respond rapidly to frequent topical steroids without need for surgical intervention and thus this feature has been used as a confirmation of the diagnosis of TASS.

TOXIC ANTERIOR SEGMENT SYNDROME ETIOLOGY

TASS is multifactorial and determining the cause can be difficult. Surgeons in centers experiencing a TASS outbreak are likely to make multiple, simultaneous changes and thus retrospectively determining the causative agent is frequently impossible. Multiple possible factors have been demonstrated to be associated with TASS (Table 29-2).

TASS is rarely described as sporadic. It is possible that apparent sporadic cases are more attributable to other factors such as surgical complications (eg, retained cortex, prolonged surgery, and increased inflammation due to iris stretching).

> ## Table 29-2
> ### Conditions Implicated in Toxic Anterior Segment Syndrome
>
> *Intraocular Causes*
>
> Incomplete cortex removal, pupil stretching, and possible immunological differences (as with DLK in atopic patients).
>
> *Intraocular Medication*
>
> Dosing errors with antibiotics, preservatives, ointments,[6] and pH imbalance.
>
> *Instrument Contamination*
>
> Bacterial endotoxins, dried debris (eg, inadequate cleaning of cannulas, persistence of detergents, irrigating solutions, endotoxins in irrigating fluids [Endosol],[7] incorrect pH or composition of irrigating fluids).

Irrigating Solutions

Multiple TASS outbreaks have been attributed to irrigating solution contaminants, endotoxins, incorrect compositions, and pH imbalance. Presence of preservatives in intraocular saline has also been associated with TASS outbreaks. Lui et al[4] attributed an outbreak to the use of an external eye rinse, Eye Stream (Alcon, Ft Worth, Tex) that is preserved with benzalkonium chloride (BAK) 0.01% as an intraocular solution. Features described were more characteristic of endothelial toxicity than the inflammatory response seen with TASS. However, inadvertent use of preservatives in the anterior chamber can be a significant cause of corneal decomposition and anterior segment inflammation. It may be useful to consider endothelial toxicity from preservatives and inappropriate drug dosages separately from the more classic TASS.

Balanced Salt Solution and Endotoxin

Multiple TASS outbreaks reported in 2004 and 2005 were associated with a balanced salt solution (BSS) manufactured by Cytosol Laboratories (Lenoir, NC) (also marketed under AMO Endosol [Santa Ana, Calif] and Acorn BSS). Endotoxin was identified in Cytosol BSS and 6 clinics reported TASS outbreaks with this association to the FDA by January 2006. Cytosol BSS was issued a withdrawal notice by FDA on February 13, 2006.

Sterilization

All aspects of the sterilization process have been associated with TASS.

Detergent and Ultrasonic Bath Endotoxin

One of the earlier studies on TASS identified *Klebsiella pneumonia* and bacterial endotoxin in the ultrasonic cleaning bath and liquid instrument detergent. The authors postulated that the endotoxins remaining on the instruments after cleaning and sterilization were responsible for an outbreak of TASS affecting five of 16 patients.[8]

Endotoxin Instrument Contamination and Short Cycle Sterilization

Our previous work with DLK outbreaks linked reservoir contamination with endotoxin-forming bacteria and biofilm in Statim sterilizers (SciCan, Toronto, Canada). Short cycle sterilization is bactericidal but does not fully inactivate bacterial endotoxins.[9] It has also been shown that endotoxins can be present in the autoclave steam of the STATIM sterilizer although possibly not in concentrations needed to cause DLK.[10] In the investigation of our own TASS epidemic, Outbreak A, we demonstrated an association between TASS and short cycle steam sterilization. In addition, we have had anecdotal reports of an increase in incidence of TASS associated with DLK outbreaks in ambulatory surgical centres performing both cataract surgery and LASIK using the same.[9]

Impurities in Sterilizer Steam

Inadequate maintenance of sterilizers has been linked to TASS.[11] In one investigated TASS outbreak, involving 8 of 21 surgeries, the condition was associated with impurities such as sulfates, copper, zinc and silica in autoclave steam moisture and a change in cleaning personal. Resolution was achieved with elimination of the autoclave steam moisture impurities.

Inadequate Cleaning of Surgical Instruments and Reusable Cannulas

Detergent residues on instruments may lead to endothelial toxicity.[3] We experienced an unreported TASS outbreak associated with dried residue from reusable cannulas; this affected eight patients undergoing penetrating keratoplasty who were injected with methyl choline at the completion of the surgery using the reusable cannulas. An immediate fibrin response occurred and was initially attributed to the use of generic methyl choline but on reintroduction of Carbachol (Alcon), the reaction still occurred. This was resolved by using only disposable cannulas. It was subsequently found that inadequate cleaning of the reusable cannulas was likely responsible for the outbreak. A similar situation may occur when phacoemulsification tips are reused and not cleaned sufficiently to remove any dried material that may be caught in the lumen.

Intraocular Ointment

A recent Canadian study has linked the presence of anterior chamber oily droplets and TASS. It was due to ointments applied postoperatively and tight patching of the eye.[6]

OUTBREAK INVESTIGATION

After recognition of an outbreak, specific cause or causes need to be rapidly identified and corrective action taken. Investigation is usually challenging and the etiology difficult to determine due to the often multiple and simultaneous changes made in the affected surgical center. The following steps may prove useful.

Case Definition

TASS can be defined by intense anterior segment inflammation occurring within 72 hours of surgery with clear vitreous.

Data Collection

Case details should be collected on each patient presenting with TASS like signs and symptoms. Any changes made in the surgical centre over the period of the outbreak should also be carefully noted.

One of the most difficult aspects of outbreak investigation is obtaining sufficient data retrospectively and determining when and which changes were made that may have controlled the outbreak. Retrieval of all cases is necessary and can prove difficult in an outpatient-based surgical center especially when diagnostic criteria vary between surgeons and office locations, making standardization challenging. Creation of an epidemic curve documenting any changes before and after the onset of the epidemic is optimal if data is available.

Microbial Investigations

Specific investigations may prove helpful in determining the causal agents involved in the TASS outbreak. Common sampling sites include the sterilizer reservoir, internal tubing, ultrasound baths, cannulas, and the air and water supplies.

Management Issues

Managing an outbreak involves issues that may require strict confidentiality, thus, it is advised to designate one staff member to be responsible for data collection and documentation of all changes, ensuring that the case log is accurate. In addition, allocate a senior manager and/or physician as a spokesperson for media enquires and communication with regulatory authorities (eg, FDA). Appropriate internal communication is needed to ensure staff members are well informed of all protocol changes required to resolve the outbreak.

TREATMENT

Frequent topical steroids every 30 to 60 minutes are usually effective with improvement within the first 24 to 48 hours. Three patients in Outbreak A underwent anterior chamber washout after diagnosis on the day of surgery but the value of this is uncertain. In cases where corneal and endothelial toxicity occurs, a corneal transplantation may be necessary.

OUTCOMES

Early diagnosis and treatment invariably lead to excellent outcomes with the majority of patients achieving a BSCVA of 20/40 or better. Patients can develop glaucoma from initial trabeculitis and long-term as a result of fibrin membranes.

CONCLUSION

Investigation of a TASS outbreak is usually prolonged and challenging but the underlying cause or causes can usually be found. All aspects of the surgical process need to be reviewed and outside assistance and opinions are useful. The recent upsurge in TASS outbreaks is of concern and probably represents a true increase in incidence rather than improved reporting of a previously present problem. This may be related to the increase in high volume surgery with rapid turn over times requiring short cycle sterilization. The prognosis is excellent for TASS if recognized early and treated aggressively with topical steroids. Differentiation from infectious endophthalmitis is critical and continued surveillance and monitoring of operating room protocols is essential to prevent reoccurrences.

KEY POINTS

1. The classic feature of TASS is early and intense postoperative inflammation after anterior segment surgery without vitreal involvement.
2. Vitritis is almost never associated with TASS and indicates infectious endophthalmitis.
3. Infectious endophthalmitis can be differentiated by later presentation (peaks between day 3 and day 7), pain, and vitritis.
4. Early cases of endophthalmitis may present as TASS and wherever there is doubt regarding the diagnosis, the case should be treated as infectious endophthalmitis.
5. Most cases obtain full recovery with early treatment using topical steroids. Delayed treatment or severe cases may develop posterior synechiae, distorted irregular pupils, and glaucoma.

REFERENCES

1. Monson MC, Mamalis N, Olson RJ. Toxic anterior segment inflammation following cataract surgery. *J Cataract Refract Surg.* 1992;18:184-189.
2. Mamalis N, Edelhauser HF, Dawson DG, et al. Toxic anterior segment syndrome. Review/update. *J Cataract Refract Surg.* 2006;32:324-333.
3. Breebaart AC, Nuyts RMMA, Pels E, et al. Toxic endothelial destruction of the cornea after routine extracapsular cataract surgery. *Arch Ophthalmol.* 1990;108:1121-1125.
4. Liu H, Routley I, Teichmann KD. Toxic endothelial cell destruction from intraocular benzalkonium chloride. *J Cataract Refract Surg.* 2001;27:1746-1750.
5. Eleftheriadis H, Cheong M, Saneman S, et al. Corneal toxicity secondary to inadvertent use of benzalkonium chloride preserved viscoelastic material in cataract surgery. *Br J Ophthalmol.* 2002;86:299-305.
6. Werner L, Sher JH, Taylor JR, et al. Toxic anterior segment syndrome and possible association with ointment in the anterior chamber following cataract surgery. *J Cataract Refract Surg.* 2006;32:277-235.
7. Holland SP, Chavez G, Morck D, Mathias R. 2006. Toxic Anterior Segment Syndrome (TASS) associated with short cycle sterilization and BSS. Presented at American Society of Cataract and Refractive Surgeons (ASCRS) Annual meeting; March 17-22, 2006; San Francisco, Calif.
8. Kreisler KR, Martin SS, Young CW, et al. Postoperative inflammation following cataract extraction caused by bacterial contamination of the cleaning bath detergent. *J Cataract Refract Surg.* 1992;18:106-110.
9. Holland SP, Mathias RG, Morck DW, et al. Diffuse lamellar keratitis related to endotoxins released from sterilizer reservoir biofilms. *Ophthalmology.* 2000;107:1227-1233.
10. Whitby JL, Hitchins VM. Endotoxin levels in steam and reservoirs of table-top steam sterilizers. *J Cataract Refract Surg.* 2002;18:51-52.
11. Hellinger WC, Hasan SA, Bacalis LP et al. Outbreak of toxic anterior chamber syndrome following cataract surgery associated with impurities of autoclave steam moisture. *Infect Control Hosp Epidemiol.* 2006;27(13):294-298.

Chapter 30

PHAKIC INTRAOCULAR LENS COMPLICATIONS

Benjamin F. Boyd, MD, FACS; Samuel Boyd, MD;
Soosan Jacob, MS, FRCS, FERC, Dip NB; and
Amar Agarwal, MS, FRCS, FRCOphth

INTRODUCTION

Phakic intraocular lenses (IOLs) have recently gained popularity for the management of high refractive errors. This has been partly due to the inability of corneal refractive procedures to satisfactorily correct higher refractive errors due to the problems associated with regression,[1] ectasia, and poor quality of the corneal refractive surface[2,3] after ablation for higher powers.

The increasing use of phakic IOLs has also been due to tremendous improvements in the designs and materials used for these IOLs and also due to better microsurgical techniques and vastly improved surgical skills as also due to better viscoelastic devices. Major advantages associated with the use of phakic IOLs include ability to correct higher amounts of ametropia, fast visual recovery, better quality of vision with lesser induction of higher-order aberrations, and preservation of accommodation. All these factors combined with the ease for the regular cataract surgeon to also enter the field of refractive surgery have contributed to the rapidly gaining popularity of phakic IOLs.

Phakic IOLs can be classified into anterior chamber phakic IOLs (ACPIOLs) and posterior chamber phakic IOLs (PCPIOLs). ACPIOLs can be subclassified as angle supported or iris supported. These can be implanted for both myopia and hypermetropia as well as for astigmatism and presbyopia. Despite the popularity and success that they are enjoying, phakic IOLs may still be associated with complications, and these patients need to be under constant surveillance for early detection of any possible complications.

ANGLE-SUPPORTED PHAKIC INTRAOCULAR LENSES

The haptics of an appropriately sized angle-supported phakic IOL are supposed to rest on the scleral spur. Perfect sizing of the IOL is difficult and not always possible. The haptics of an excessively large IOL may press on the corneoscleral trabeculae, Schlemms canal, and the blood vessels and nerves in the angle. This pressure may lead to the erosion of angle tissues with displacement of the haptics onto the ciliary body and iris ischemia and atrophy with progressive pupillary ovalization. An excessively small IOL may damage the corneal endothelium due to its moving around in the anterior chamber.

Figure 30-1. Insertion technique of the APC IOL. The forceps retain a grasp on the optic and the IOL is placed into the anterior chamber (arrow). The forceps (F) are repositioned to grasp the elbow (H) of the proximal haptic and the IOL is continued into the anterior chamber. This technique avoids the insertion of an instrument into a phakic eye all the way into the pupillary area. The distal footplates are directed toward the angle. The proximal haptic is then placed in the incision, but the proximal footplates remain outside the eye. (Courtesy of Benjamin F. Boyd, MD, FACS, Editor-in-Chief, *Atlas of Refractive Surgery* with permission from Highlights of Ophthalmology, English Edition, 2000.)

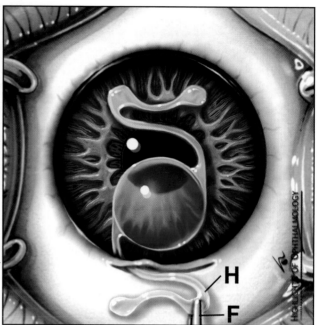

IOL size, design, and positioning are important in the prevention of complications. The patient must undergo thorough examination of the eye and its anatomy before implanting a phakic IOL. The fifth-generation ZSAL-4/Plus phakic lens (Morcher, Stuttgart, Germany) is an angle-supported lens, which has been modified to have a larger optic diameter, and a new haptic geometry. This increases haptic flexibility and disperses compression forces equally against the angle structures.[4]

The ZB5M generation of the Baïkoff angle-supported lenses (Chiron-Domilens, France) also have better efficacy and predictability and the potential risk for damage to the corneal endothelium has been greatly reduced.[5,6] Problems like night halos with pupillary dilation exceeding the optic size and pupillary ovalization in the meridian of the haptics are still present. The designs are being continuously modified and upgraded to avoid these problems.

The NuVita lens (Bausch & Lomb, Rochester, NY), formerly the Baïkoff AC-IOL is based on the Kelman Multiflex style (Alcon, Ft. Worth, Tex). The one style of aphakic anterior chamber lens that has survived during the last 15 years is the Kelman Multiflex style (Figure 30-1). This technology takes advantage of the fact that most surgeons can place an anterior chamber lens more easily than the other styles.

IRIS-SUPPORTED PHAKIC INTRAOCULAR LENSES

Worst introduced the iris claw lens in 1977 and implanted an opaque iris claw lens in the phakic eye of a patient who had unbearable diplopia in 1979. In 1986, Fechner and Worst introduced the iris claw phakic myopic lens. These have become popular now as the Artisan (Ophtec, Netherlands) and the Verisyse lenses (AMO, Santa Ana, Calif). These remain in place due to iris enclavation and so no angle complications are generally encountered, though they may be associated with various other complications.

The pupil should be kept moderately constricted. One or 2 stab incisions are made according to the technique to be used (Figure 30-2) and the anterior chamber filled with high molecular weight viscoelastic. A 5- to 6-mm incision is made (Figure 30-3). A periph-

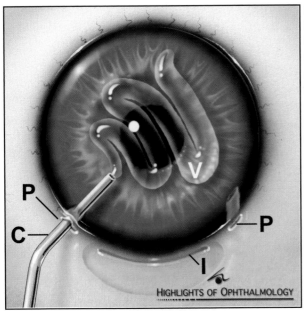

Figure 30-2. Artisan IOL surgical implantation technique—incisions. One or 2 paracentesis stab incisions (P) are made according to the technique to be used. The anterior chamber is filled with a high molecular weight viscoelastic via a cannula (C) placed through one of the paracentesis. A 5- to 6-mm incision (I) is then made. A peripheral iridotomy must be made now or at the end of the procedure. (Courtesy of Benjamin F. Boyd, MD, FACS, Editor-in-Chief, *Atlas of Refractive Surgery* with permission from Highlights of Ophthalmology, English Edition, 2000.)

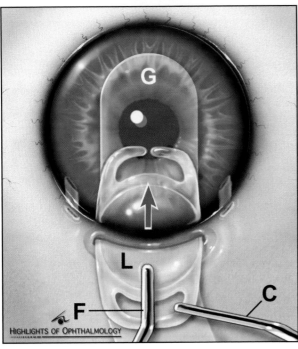

Figure 30-3. Artisan IOL Surgical Implantation Technique—insertion. A lens glide (G) is placed through the incision and across the anterior chamber. With viscoelastic filling the anterior chamber, the Artisan lens (L) is grasped with a special forceps (F) and inserted into the wound on the lens glide. A second instrument, an irrigating cannula (C), is placed inside the haptic loop and pushes the lens (arrow) inside the anterior chamber. (Courtesy of Benjamin F. Boyd, MD, FACS, Editor-in-Chief, *Atlas of Refractive Surgery* with permission from Highlights of Ophthalmology, English Edition, 2000.)

eral iridotomy must be made, now or at the end of the procedure, and the iris reposited completely. The lens is gently and slowly nudged into the eye (Figure 30-4), rotated into the 3- to 9-o'clock axis, and centered over the pupil. The wound is partially sutured, leaving an opening sufficient to introduce a forceps.

The lens is centered over the pupil and gently pressed onto the iris with an Artisan forceps. The longer inferior blade of this forceps is an important feature, ensuring stability of the lens while it is attached to the iris. An Operaid enclavation instrument (Ophtec) is introduced

Figure 30-4. Artisan IOL surgical implantation technique—enclavation. The special Operaid irrigating enclavation instrument (E) is introduced through the stab incision (P) or through the main incision under the Artisan loop tip. Using the instrument, a fold of iris is lifted (arrow) through the slot in the tip of the lens haptic. The instrument is withdrawn slowly, being careful that it does not catch the iris. The Artisan forceps (F) stabilize the lens during this maneuver. (Courtesy of Benjamin F. Boyd, MD, FACS, Editor-in-Chief, *Atlas of Refractive Surgery* with permission from Highlights of Ophthalmology, English Edition, 2000.)

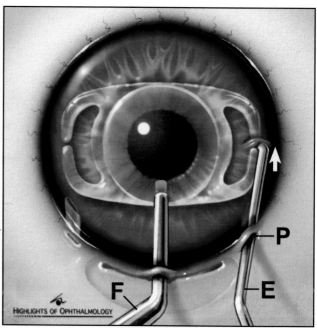

Figure 30-5. Artisan IOL surgical implantation technique—enclavation detail. This magnified portion of the lens haptics shows how the enclavation instrument (E) engages a small fold of the iris (I) beneath the distal haptic (H). The iris fold is "snow-plowed" forward (white arrow) and gently captured in the slot (S) of the haptics. The IOL and its haptics are pushed posteriorly (black arrows) to assist this enclavation of the iris. (Courtesy of Benjamin F. Boyd, MD, FACS, Editor-in-Chief, *Atlas of Refractive Surgery* with permission from Highlights of Ophthalmology, English Edition, 2000.)

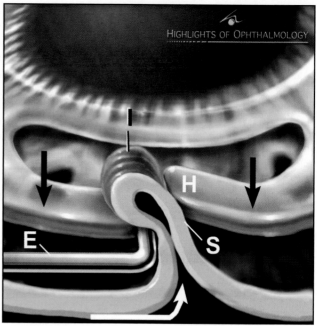

through the stab incision superior to the Artisan loop tip. This instrument comes double armed, in right and left hand configurations, depending which loop of the IOL the iris is being attached.

Using the enclavation instrument, a fold of iris is lifted through the slot in the tip of the lens haptic (see Figure 30-4 and detail in Figure 30-5). The instrument is withdrawn slowly, being careful that it does not catch the iris. The maneuver is repeated for the other tip of the lens. If a peripheral iridotomy has not already been made, it must be made now. The

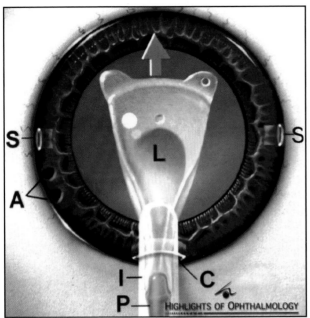

Figure 30-6. Foldable posterior chamber phakic lens (ICL)—insertion technique, step 1. A double YAG laser peripheral iridotomy (A) to avoid iris blockage is performed the week prior to lens implantation in order to avoid iris pigment deposition on the lens. Iridotomies would be very difficult to do intraoperatively because of the widely dilated pupil. First, a 3.0-mm temporal clear corneal incision (C) is performed, as well as 2 side port incisions (S) 90 degrees away from the main incision and 180 degrees away from each other. The chamber is filled with viscoelastic material (not shown). The foldable posterior chamber lens will be placed between the iris and natural lens. The folded lens (L) is inserted into the eye via the special inserter (I), which has been placed through the corneal incision. A plunger (P) inside the inserter pushes the distal haptics of the ICL into the anterior chamber (arrow) while unfolding as shown. The lens haptics will be placed in the posterior chamber later. This illustration is shown from the surgeon's point of view as he or she is operating. The lens is implanted from the temporal side of the eye. (Courtesy of Benjamin F. Boyd, MD, FACS, Editor-in-Chief, *Atlas of Refractive Surgery* with permission from Highlights of Ophthalmology, English Edition, 2000.)

iridotomy is a vital part of the procedure and must not be omitted. Lens position and fixation are inspected. When perfect, the wound is closed carefully. All viscoelastic is patiently removed while maintaining the depth of the anterior chamber with balanced salt solution (BSS). Steroid and antibiotic drops are placed. If there might be residual viscoelastic, prophylactic Iopidine or Latanoprost may be used to control any rise in pressure.

POSTERIOR CHAMBER PHAKIC INTRAOCULAR LENSES

The initial PCPIOL were made of silicone,[7,8] but they lead to complications such as development of cataract, endothelial loss, and chronic uveitis. The new generation of PCPIOLs are made of Collamer,[9] a copolymer of hydroxyethylmethacrylate and porcine collagen (ICL-STAAR, Switzerland) (Figures 30-6 to 30-8).

IOL–iris touch, IOL–crystalline lens touch, and anterior chamber shallowing[10] may cause pigmentary dispersion,[11,12] cataract formation,[13-15] and shallowing of the iridocorneal angle.[16] IOL decentration[14] has also frequently been described. The ideal position of the PCPIOL is for the haptics to rest on the zonules with an appropriate vault over the anterior lens capsule. Positioning in the sulcus can lead to pigment dispersion[17] and inflammation and is, therefore, not desirable. The PCPIOL produces resistance to the flow of aqueous across the pupil and this situation is worsened with the increase in size of the crystalline lens with age. Proper sizing of the IOL is of great importance. A small size IOL applies pressure against the natural lens, the ciliary body, and the posterior surface of the iris, causing cataract, uveitis, and pigment dispersion respectively.

Figure 30-7. Foldable posterior chamber phakic lens (ICL)—Insertion technique of the haptics. The distal haptics of the ICL are placed in behind the iris before the proximal haptics. With a spatula (S), inserted through one of the side ports, the distal extremity of the ICL is gently pushed (arrow) into the posterior chamber, to the ciliary sulcus. The same movement is used to place the proximal haptics into the posterior chamber. This illustration is shown from the surgeon's point of view as he/she is operating. (Courtesy of Benjamin F. Boyd, MD, FACS, Editor-in-Chief, *Atlas of Refractive Surgery* with permission from Highlights of Ophthalmology, English Edition, 2000.)

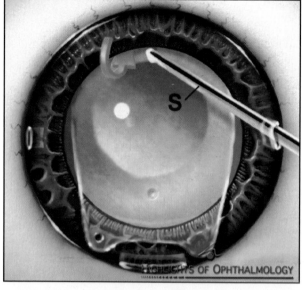

Figure 30-8. Conceptual cross section of all stages for implantation of a foldable posterior chamber phakic lens (ICL). This conceptual cross section shows the insertion and unfolding of the (ICL) compared to the final configuration of the ICL in position behind the iris and in front of the crystalline lens. (1) The plunger (P) inside the inserter pushes the distal haptics of the ICL into the anterior chamber (blue arrows) while unfolding as shown. (2) In separate maneuvers, the haptics are then placed (red arrows) into the posterior chamber behind the iris and into the ciliary sulcus. The iris will then be constricted. The inset shows a surgeon's view of this final configuration. This illustration is a section of the eye taken from 3 to 9 o'clock, as the ICL is inserted through

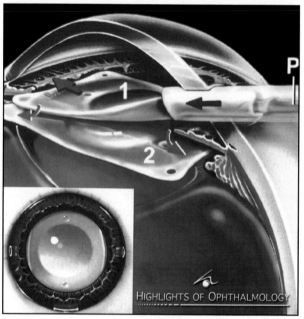

the temporal approach. (Courtesy of Benjamin F. Boyd, MD, FACS, Editor-in-Chief, *Atlas of Refractive Surgery* with permission from Highlights of Ophthalmology, English Edition, 2000.)

COMPLICATIONS ASSOCIATED WITH THE USE OF PHAKIC INTRAOCULAR LENSES

Proper preoperative selection of the patient goes a long way in preventing problems. It is advisable to include patients with a deep anterior chamber (more than 3.2 mm) and with a healthy endothelium. Patients with preoperative ocular pathology such as inflammation of the eye, pigment dispersion, glaucoma, or with other conditions such as diabetes should be excluded. Hyperopes should also fulfill all the inclusion criteria before being considered for phakic IOLs.

In all phakic IOLs, increased crystalline lens size with increasing age and cataract formation leading to a decrease in the depth of the anterior chamber and crowding in the posterior chamber tend to exaggerate the pathologic processes. While the results of phakic IOLs are highly predictable, long-term data are limited. Normal blinking of the eyes does not generally cause problems, though forcible rubbing of the eyes may cause a variety of complications, including damage to the endothelium, crystalline lens, pigment dispersion, etc.

Residual Refractive Error

This can be avoided with careful preoperative planning. Any pre-existing astigmatism can be taken care of by positioning the incision in the meridian of the steeper axis. It can also be combined with arcuate keratotomy for pre-existing astigmatism. One can also combine this procedure with surface ablation procedures to take care of very high refractive errors or any coexisting astigmatism. Here, the flap is first made on the cornea, followed by introducing the phakic IOL. The patients refractive status is again evaluated and either the residual spherocylindrical error alone can be treated or a custom treatment may be done based on the topography and aberrometry.

Corneal Endothelial Damage

Corneal endothelial damage was one of the main problems associated with phakic anterior chamber IOLs. The cause for this seemed to be due to intermittent contact between the optic edge and the peripheral endothelium[18,19] especially due to eye rubbing. Other contributing causes are trauma due to the surgery, low grade or frank inflammation,[20-22] and endothelial damage due to the angle fixation or iris fixation of the IOL.

Endothelial cell loss with the Baïkoff ZB angle-supported IOL ranged from 16.0% to 18.8% at 1 year and from 20.0% to 28.0% at 2 years.[18,23-26] This lens had a 4.5-mm diameter biconcave optic and 25-degree angulated haptics, and intermittent contact between the optic edge and the endothelium was responsible for the high endothelial cell loss.[19,23] Lesser distance between the optic edge and the endothelium contributes to corneal endothelial damage in eyes with angle-supported phakic lenses.[18,19,25] The new design of the ZB5M lens has a thinner optic edge with a smaller optic diameter of 4.0 mm (total optical diameter of 5.00 mm) and lesser haptic angulation of 20 degrees.[5] This resulted in an increase in the lenticulo-corneal distance and therefore lesser chances of endothelial damage.[5,6,27] Baïkoff et al[5] attributed most of the endothelial loss (3.8%) with the ZB5M lens to be secondary to the surgery. The progressive cell loss was calculated to be 0.7% per year. Alió et al[6] had similar results with continuing cell loss, similar to that after posterior chamber IOL implantation in cataract surgery.[28]

The distance of the ZSAL-4 angle-supported phakic IOL from the endothelium by high-frequency ultrasound biomicroscopy (UBM)[29] also appeared sufficient to prevent corneal endothelial damage due to contact between the optic edge and the endothelium from eye rubbing.

The Worst-Fechner iris-fixated lenses (Ophtec) have also been modified due to reports of continuous endothelial cell loss.[30-32]

Endothelial contact of the IOL during surgery by inexperienced surgeons may be more common with the Verisyse lens, especially during enclavation. Jiménez-Alfaro et al[33] attribute most of the endothelial cell loss (4.41%) present at 6 months after surgery to the traumatic effect of surgery and consider progressive cell loss due to PCPIOL to be similar with those of the recent reports on angle-supported lenses and therefore within safety limits.

Cataract

Cataract formation was the most significant complication seen with the early prototypes of the collamer posterior chamber ICL. Cataract formation[15,34,35] is mainly due to mechanical irritation of the anterior capsule by contact between the PCPIOL and the crystalline lens. Accidental surgical trauma and damage during nd:YAG laser iridotomy is also possible.[15] Obstruction of the aqueous humor circulation toward the anterior surface of the crystalline lens, subclinical ocular inflammation, and IOL biocompatibility are also implicated.[34-36]

Uveitis

Among other problems, the Worst-Fechner iris-fixated lenses were also associated with chronic subclinical inflammation and an altered blood–aqueous barrier[37-39] and are no longer used. Its design has now been modified to reduce the incidence of these complications. Iris chafing may occur due to the lenses. There may be chronic iritis due to continued compression of the enclaved iris tissue. Enclavation of excess iris in the claws pushes the ACPIOL against the iris and the crystalline lens. This may interfere with aqueous circulation through the pupil, leading to increased intraocular pressure (IOP), uveitis, neovascularization, and other sequelae.

Subclinical inflammation also exists after implantation of a phakic IOL in the anterior chamber.[38-41] PCPIOLs should ideally rest on the zonules and if placed in the sulcus, they induce pain and inflammation.[42,43] This chronic inflammation may be responsible for endothelial loss and decrease in the lens transmittance.[38,40,41]

Pérez-Santonja et al found evidence of chronic inflammation even 2 years after surgery with iris-fixated or angle-supported phakic lenses.[38] The Worst-Fechner lens incarcerates the iris in the claw, leading to insidious trauma. Angle-supported lenses also cause prolonged compression on the iris and ciliary body band by the haptics,[42] leading to chronic inflammation and uveitis-glaucoma-hyphema (UGH) syndrome, though lesser than with Worst-Fechner lenses.[41]

Jiménez-Alfaro et al attribute the constantly elevated flare values in their series of patients to the presence of the PCPIOL. Because Collamer is highly biocompatible,[44] they postulate the constant friction between the posterior iris surface and the PCPIOL or by the haptic on the ciliary sulcus to lead to the inflammation, the contact between the iris and the PCPIOL being more significant.

Pigmentary Dispersion Syndromes

One case of pigmentary dispersion, without transilluminating defects, in which the PCPIOL was decentered, has been reported.[8] The vaulting of the PCPIOL, though it prevents contact with the anterior capsule of the lens, pushes the iris forward, resulting in continuous contact pressure and friction and hence shedding of the posterior pigment epithelium. This may be exacerbated by blinking, squeezing, and rubbing of the eyes. Similarity between the PCPIOL material and the anterior capsule prevents this.[9] In a series of cases by Jiménez-Alfaro et al,[33] none of the patients had pigmentary dispersion.

Increased Intraocular Pressure

There have been reports of pupillary block after phakic PC IOL implantation.[8,9,45-47] This condition presents within the first 1 or 2 days postoperatively with an elevated IOP associated with a high phakic PCPIOL vault and impermeable or insufficient iridotomies. The aqueous humor trapped in the posterior chamber increases the forward vaulting of the PCPIOL and creates peripheral anterior chamber shallowing with angle closure. The entire iris is pushed forwards by the PCPIOL and there is, therefore, no typical iris bombe pattern seen. This generally responds to pupillary dilatation but requires a new, functional peripheral iridotomy as definitive treatment.[48]

Other causes for increased IOP after phakic IOL implantation include retained viscoelastics, aqueous misdirection syndrome, crowding of the angle of the anterior chamber by a PCPIOL, pigment dispersion leading to pigmentary glaucoma, postinflammatory glaucoma, steroid-induced rise in IOP, etc. The ACPIOL may also cause a pupillary block type of glaucoma.

Pupillary Ovalization

Progressive pupillary ovalization is a problem present with all ACPIOLs. It can occur despite an initially successful surgery and happy patient. Other than being cosmetically noticeable in light colored eyes, it can also lead to optical problems, low-grade uveitis, and decentration or dislocation of the IOL. It occurs due to fibrous tissue formation and contraction near the footplates of the IOL. It may also be due to sectorial iris hypoperfusion and the resultant secondary ischemia.[49] Such patients should have regular follow-up and may even require lens explantation. Sometimes, the pupil becomes partially dilated and does not respond to the usual miotics.

Secondary Visual Alterations

Patients with phakic IOLs can complain of reduced vision, prism effect, glare, halos, difficulty in night time driving, and diplopia. These secondary visual alterations may occur due to decentered phakic IOLs or due to small-sized optic zones. It may also occur due to pupillary ovalization and early cataract formation or early corneal decompensation. Night halos may be less frequent with PCPIOLs than what is to be expected because the effective optic zone of the lens is increased due to the retropupillary position of the IOL.[33]

Decentration

Decentration occur with inappropriately sized or damaged phakic IOLs. It may also occur secondary to inappropriate positioning and inadequate fixation. Iris atrophy and pupillary ovalization with ACPIOLs can lead to a well-centered IOL becoming decentered. It can generally be avoided by careful measurement of white-to-white distance for proper sizing of the IOL and appropriate care during surgery. Late dislocation of the IOL may be caused by trauma. In case of iris-fixated ACPIOLs, the iris tissue in the claw may undergo atrophy and lead to dislocation.

Lens Repositioning or Removal

This could be indicated for a variety of reasons ranging from wrong biometry, inappropriately sized IOL or for management of complications such as cataract formation, endothelial loss, pupillary ovalization, etc. Removal, repositioning, or exchange of the lens does expose the patient to the risks of another operation

Retinal Detachment

An incidence of retinal detachment (RD) from 0.61% to 4.8% and an interval between lens implantation and retinal detachment of 17.43 ± 16.4 months has been reported in patients with severe myopia corrected by ACPIOL.[6,50-53] Scleral surgery had a success rate of 87.5% with a single procedure.

Figure 30-9. (A) Color fundus photograph of cystoid macular edema.
(B) Capillary leakage in the macular
area. (C) Early flower petal appearance. (D) Late flower petal appearance. (Courtesy of Dr. Agarwal's Eye
Hospital, India.)

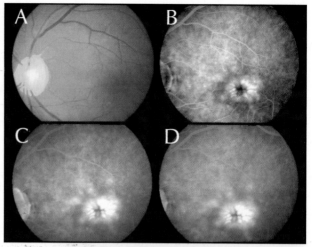

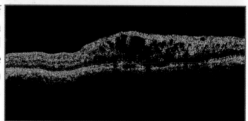

Figure 30-10. Ocular coherence tomography of
cystoid macular edema. Line scan of the macula
shows loss of foveal contour. Increased retinal
thickness in the macula with multiple large
optically clear low reflective cystic spaces with
septae seen in the inner retina. (Courtesy of Dr.
Agarwal's Eye Hospital, India.)

There are also reports of RD in patients with high-degree myopia treated with PCP
IOLs[8,54,55] with the incidence ranging from 0.8% (4) to 2.07%. These RDs could occur either
secondary to the IOL insertion, causing traction on the anterior and/or posterior margin of
the vitreous base, or as part of the natural history of retinal detachment in high-degree myopia. Martínez-Castillo et al[54] do not attribute any increased incidence of RD after PCPIOL
implantation for surgical correction of high myopia.

Controversy exists regarding the best surgical option for the management of RD in these
patients.[52,56,57] These RDs can be handled with scleral buckling (SB), which gives good
anatomic and functional results,[52] or with pars plana vitrectomy (PPV) and pneumatic retinopexy, which also avoids any change in the refractive status.[56,57] Martínez-Castillo et al[54]
did not have any increased difficulty due to the presence of the PCPIOL in identifying and
locating causative breaks when SB or PPV were performed. They also found both SB and
PPV to be effective in the management of these RDs. PPV could increase the risk of nuclear
sclerosis, which is partly age related[58,59] and partly due to the anterior movement of the lens
increasing the PCPIOL-lenticular contact after RD surgery.

Cystoid Macular Edema

This may occur secondary to any intraocular procedure or may be due to chronic uveitis
and anterior segment inflammation (Figures 30-9 and 30-10).

Endophthalmitis

As with any other intraocular procedure, the risk of endophthalmitis exists. It is especially
devastating since this procedure is often performed on a person with good BCVA who is
generally undergoing surgery only for cosmetic purposes. It is therefore not advisable to

operate on both eyes in the same sitting. The investigations, diagnosis, and management of endophthalmitis would be similar to that occurring after cataract surgery.

RECENT ADVANCES

The latest models of all types of phakic IOLs[60] including the Artisan lenses, the Baïkoff and NuVita angle-supported IOLs, the ICL, the Medenium silicone PCPIOL etc, have all improved vastly over the previous prototypes and recent data for most of them are encouraging.

KEY POINTS

1. Phakic IOLs can be classified into anterior chamber phakic IOLs (ACPIOLs) and posterior chamber phakic IOLs (PCPIOLs). ACPIOLs can be subclassified as angle supported or iris supported.

2. Proper preoperative selection of the patient goes a long way in preventing problems. It is advisable to include patients with a deep anterior chamber (more than 3.2 mm) and with a healthy endothelium. Patients with preoperative ocular pathology such as inflammation of the eye, pigment dispersion, glaucoma or with other conditions such as diabetes should be excluded. Hyperopes should also fulfill all the inclusion criteria before being considered for phakic IOLs.

3. While the results of phakic IOLs are highly predictable, long-term data are limited. Normal blinking of the eyes does not generally cause problems, though forcible rubbing of the eyes may cause a variety of complications including damage to the endothelium, crystalline lens, pigment dispersion, etc.

4. They can be associated with numerous complications such as endothelial loss, cataract, pigment dispersion, increased IOP, pupillary ovalization, IOL decentration, visual phenomena, etc.

5. Latest models of all types of phakic IOLs have encouraging post-operative data and improved safety profile.

REFERENCES

1. Pérez-Santonja JJ, Bellot JJ, Claramonte P, et al. Laser in situ keratomileusis to correct high myopia. *J Cataract Refract Surg.* 1997;23:372-385.

2. Applegate RA, Howland HC. Refractive surgery, optical aberrations, and visual performance. *J Refract Surg.* 1997;13:295-299.

3. Oliver KM, Hemenger RP, Corbett MC, et al. Corneal optical aberrations induced by photorefractive keratectomy. *J Refract Surg.* 1997;13:246-254.

4. Pérez-Santonja JJ, Alió JL, Jiménez-Alfaro I, Zato MA. Surgical correction of severe myopia with an angle-supported phakic intraocular lens. *J Cataract Refract Surg.* 2000;26:1288-1302.

5. Baïkoff G, Arne JL, Bokobza Y, et al. Angle-fixated anterior chamber phakic intraocular lens for myopia of −7 to −19 diopters. *J Refract Surg.* 1998;14:282-293.

6. Alió JL, de la Hoz F, Pérez-Santonja JJ, et al. Phakic anterior chamber lenses for the correction of myopia. A 7-year cumulative analysis of complications in 263 cases. *Ophthalmology.* 1999;106:458-466.

7. Fechner PU, Haigis W, Wichmann W. Posterior chamber myopia lenses in phakic eyes. *J Cataract Refract Surg.* 1996;22:178-182.

8. Zaldivar R, Davidorf JM, Oscherow S. Posterior chamber phakic intraocular lens for myopia of −8 to −19 diopters. *J Refract Surg.* 1998;14:294-305.

9. Assetto V, Benedetti S, Pesando P. Collamer intraocular contact lens to correct high myopia. *J Cataract Refract Surg.* 1996;22:551-556.

10. Trindade F, Pereira F, Cronemberger S. Ultrasound biomicroscopic imaging of posterior chamber phakic intraocular lens. *J Refract Surg.* 1998;14:497-503.

11. Maden A, Gunenc U, Erkin E. Gonioscopic changes in eyes with posterior chamber intraocular lenses. *Doc Ophthalmol.* 1992;82:231-238.

12. Abela-Formanek C, Kruger AJ, Dejaco-Ruhswurm I, et al. Gonioscopic changes after implantation of a posterior chamber lens in phakic myopic eyes. *J Cataract Refract Surg.* 2001;27:1919-1925.

13. Brauweiler PH, Wehler T, Busin M. High incidence of cataract formation after implantation of a silicone posterior chamber lens in phakic, highly myopic eyes. *Ophthalmology.* 1999;106:1651-1655.

14. Menezo JL, Peris-Martinez C, Cisneros A, Martínez-Costa R. Posterior chamber phakic intraocular lenses to correct high myopia: a comparative study between Staar and Adatomed models. *J Refract Surg.* 2001;17:32-42.

15. Fink AM, Gore C, Rosen E. Cataract development after implantation of the STAAR Collamer posterior chamber phakic lens. *J Cataract Refract Surg.* 1999;25:278-282.

16. Arne JL, Lesueur LC. Phakic posterior chamber lenses for high myopia: functional and anatomical outcomes. *J Cataract Refract Surg.* 2000;26:369-374.

17. Brandt JD, Mockovak ME, Chayet A. Pigmentary dispersion syndrome induced by a posterior chamber phakic refractive lens. *Am J Ophthalmol.* 2001;131:260-263.

18. Mimouni F, Colin J, Koffi V, Bonnet P. Damage to the corneal endothelium from anterior chamber intraocular lenses in phakic myopic eyes. *Refract Corneal Surg.* 1991;7:277-281.

19. Saragoussi JJ, Cotinat J, Renard G, et al. Damage to the corneal endothelium by minus power anterior chamber intraocular lenses. *Refract Corneal Surg.* 1991;7:282-285.

20. Rao GN, Stevens RE, Harris JK, Aquavella JV. Long-term changes in corneal endothelium following intraocular lens implantation. *Ophthalmology.* 1981;88:386-397.

21. Long-term corneal endothelial cell loss after cataract surgery. Results of a randomized controlled trial. Oxford Cataract Treatment and Evaluation Team (OCTET). *Arch Ophthalmol.* 1986;104:1170–1175.

22. Matsuda M, Miyake K, Inaba M. Long-term corneal endothelial changes after intraocular lens implantation. *Am J Ophthalmol.* 1988;105:248-252.

23. Baïkoff G. The refractive IOL in a phakic eye. *Ophthalmic Pract.* 1991;9:58–61,80.

24. Iradier MT, Hernandez JL, Estrella J, et al. Lente de Baïkoff: estudio de los resultados refractivos. *Arch Soc Esp Oftalmol.* 1992;62:259-265.

25. Bour T, Piquot X, Pospisil A, Montard M. Répercussions endothéliales de l'implant myopique de chambre antérieure ZB au cours de la première année. Etude prospective avec analyse statistique. *J Fr Ophtalmol.* 1991;14:633-641.

26. Alió JL, Pérez-Santonja JJ, Artola A. Surgical correction of myopia. In: Nema HV, Nema N, eds. *Recent Advances in Ophthalmology.* New Delhi, India: Jaypee Brothers; 1996:1-28.

27. Saragoussi J-J, Puech M, Assouline M, et al. Ultrasound biomicroscopy of Baïkoff anterior chamber phakic intraocular lenses. *J Refract Surg.* 1997;13:135-141.

28. Bourne WM, Nelson LR, Hodge DO. Continued endothelial cell loss ten years after lens implantation. *Ophthalmology.* 1994;101:1014-1023.

29. Jiménez-Alfaro I, García-Feijoó J, Pérez-Santonja JJ, et al. Ultrasound biomicroscopy of ZSAL-4 anterior chamber phakic intraocular lens for high myopia. *JCRS.* 2001;27(10):1567-1573.

30. Pérez-Santonja JJ, Iradier MT, Sanz-Iglesias L, et al. Endothelial changes in phakic eyes with anterior chamber intraocular lenses to correct high myopia. *J Cataract Refract Surg.* 1996;22:1017-1022.

31. Fechner PU, Haubitz I, Wichmann W, Wulff K. Worst-Fechner biconcave minus power phakic iris-claw lens. *J Refract Surg.* 1999;15:93-105.

32. Menezo JL, Cisneros AL, Rodriguez-Salvador V, et al. Endothelial study of iris-claw phakic lens: four year follow-up. *J Cataract Refract Surg.* 1998;24:1039-1049.

33. Jiménez-Alfarol, Benítez del Castillo JM, García Feijoó J, et al. Safety of posterior chamber phakic intraocular lenses for the correction of high myopia : Anterior segment changes after posterior chamber phakic intraocular lens implantation. *Ophthalmology*. 2001;108(1):90-99.

34. Zaldivar R, Davidorf JM, Oscherow S, et al. Combined posterior chamber phakic intraocular lens and laser in situ keratomileusis: bioptics for extreme myopia. *J Refract Surg*. 1999;15:299-308.

35. Apple DJ, Werner L. Complications of cataract and refractive surgery: a clinicopathological documentation. *Trans Am Ophthalmol Soc*. 2001;99:95-107, discussion 107–109.

36. Kashani AA. Phakic intraocular lens. *J Cataract Refract Surg*. 1999;25:1033-1034[letter].

37. Pérez-Santonja JJ, Bueno JL, Zato MA. Surgical correction of high myopia in phakic eyes with Worst-Fechner myopia intraocular lenses. *J Refract Surg*. 1997;13:268-284.

38. Pérez-Santonja JJ, Iradier MT, Benítez del Castillo JM, et al. Chronic subclinical inflammation in phakic eyes with intraocular lenses to correct myopia. *J Cataract Refract Surg*. 1996;22:183-187.

39. Pérez-Santonja JJ, Hernandez JL, Benítez del Castillo JM, et al. Fluorophotometry in myopic phakic eyes with anterior chamber intraocular lenses to correct severe myopia. *Am J Ophthalmol*. 1994;118:316-321.

40. Benítez del Castillo JM, Hernandez JL, Iradier MT, et al. Fluorophotometry in phakic eyes with anterior chamber intraocular lens implantation to correct myopia. *J Cataract Refract Surg*. 1993;19:607-609.

41. Alió JL, de la Hoz F, Ismail MM. Subclinical inflammatory reaction induced by phakic anterior chamber lenses for the correction of high myopia. *Ocular Inmunol Inflam*. 1993;1:219-223.

42. Miyake K, Asakura M, Kobayashi H. Effect of intraocular lens fixation on the blood-aqueous barrier. *Am J Ophthalmol*. 1984;98:451-455.

43. Othenin-Girard P, Pittet N, Herbort CP. La barriére hémato-aqueuse aprés opération de cataracte: comparaison de l'implantation dans le sac capsulaire et dans le sulcus. *Can J Ophthalmol*. 1993;28:55-57.

44. Brown DC, Grabow HB, Martin G, et al. Staar Collamer intraocular lens: clinical results from the phase I FDA core study. *J Cataract Refract Surg*. 1998;24:1032-1038.

45. Rosen E, Gore C. Staar Collamer posterior chamber phakic intraocular lens to correct myopia and hyperopia. *J Cataract Refract Surg*. 1998;24:596-606.

46. Davidorf JM, Zaldivar R, Oscherow S. Posterior chamber phakic intraocular lens for hyperopia of +4 to +11 diopters. *J Refract Surg*. 1998;14:306-311.

47. Pesando PM, Ghiringhello MP, Tagliavacche P. Posterior chamber collamer phakic intraocular lens for myopia and hyperopia. *J Refract Surg*. 1999;15:415-423.

48. Bylsma SS, Zalta AH, Foley E, et al. Phakic posterior chamber intraocular lens pupillary block. *JCRS*. 2002;28(12):2222-2228.

49. Fellner P, Vidic B, Ramkissoon Y et al. Pupil ovalization after phakic intraocular lens implantation is associated with sectorial iris hypoperfusion. *Arch Ophthalmol*. 2005;123(8):1061-1065.

50. Baïkoff G. Phakic anterior chamber intraocular lenses. *Int Ophthalmol Clin*. 1991;31:75–86.

51. Foss AJ, Rosen PH, Cooling RJ. Retinal detachment following anterior chamber lens implantation for the correction of ultra-high myopia in phakic eyes. *Br J Ophthalmol*. 1993;77:212–213.

52. Ruiz-Moreno JM, Alió JL, Pérez-Santonja JJ, de la Hoz F. Retinal detachment in phakic eyes with anterior chamber lenses to correct severe myopia. *Am J Ophthalmol*. 1999;127:270–275.

53. Alió JL, Ruiz-Moreno JM, Artola A. Retinal detachment as a potential hazard in surgical correction of severe myopia with phakic anterior chamber lenses. *Am J Ophthalmol*. 1993;115:145–148.

54. Martínez-Castillo V, Boixadera A, Verdugo A et al. Rhegmatogenous retinal detachment in phakic eyes after posterior chamber phakic intraocular lens implantation for severe myopia. *Ophthalmology*. 2005; 112(4):580-585.

55. Panozzo G, Parolini B. Relationships between vitreoretinal and refractive surgery. *Ophthalmology*. 2001;108:1663–1668.

56. Arevalo JF, Azar-Arevalo O. Retinal detachment in phakic eyes with anterior chamber intraocular lenses to correct severe myopia [letter]. *Am J Ophthalmol*. 1999;128:661–662.

57. Kwok AK, Young AL, Bhende P, Lam DS. Retinal detachment in phakic eyes with anterior chamber intraocular lenses to correct severe myopia [letter]. *Am J Ophthalmol*. 1999;128:395–396.

58. Melberg NS, Thomas MA. Nuclear sclerotic cataract after vitrectomy in patients younger than 50 years of age. *Ophthalmology.* 1995;102:1466–1471.

59. Blodi BA, Paluska SA. Cataract after vitrectomy in young patients. *Ophthalmology.* 1997;104:1092–1095.

60. Boyd BF. *Atlas of Refractive Surgery.* Panama: Highlights of Ophthalmology; 2001.

Please see the Pearls and Implantation Techniques for the Foldable Iris Fixated Phakic IOL video on the enclosed CD-ROM.

V

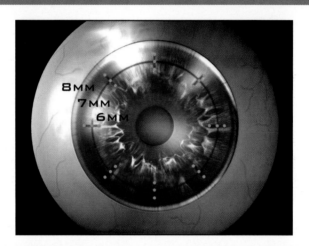

Miscellaneous

Chapter 31

CONDUCTIVE KERATOPLASTY AND POTENTIAL COMPLICATIONS

Roberto Pinelli, MD

Conductive keratoplasty (CK) with the ViewPoint System from Refractec, Inc (Irvine, California) is a nonlaser, radiofrequency-based procedure in which high frequency (350 KHz) energy is delivered into the stroma with a specially designed contact probe (Figure 31-1). The temperature and duration of the radiofrequency energy applied by the probe is optimal for collagen shrinkage without necrosis.

CK has been used primarily to treat low to moderate hyperopia[1-3] and to reduce the symptoms of presbyopia in presbyopic hyperopes (+1.00 to +2.25 D) or emmetropes through induction of mild myopia in the nondominant eye.[4] Other potential uses of the CK technique under investigation include treatment of over- or undercorrections following LASIK or other excimer laser procedures, enhancing outcomes of cataract surgery, and treating astigmatism.

COMPLICATIONS OF NEARVISION CK

The incidence and severity of complications from CK is very low, making for an excellent safety profile for the procedure.[5-12] Unlike most other corneal or lens-based surgeries, NearVision CK requires no ablation or incisions and does not invade the central cornea, cause flap-related complications, compromise the integrity or structure of the cornea, or cause dry eye or central haze.

As with any surgical procedure, of course, proper patient selection and education, a thorough preoperative examination, and appropriate postoperative care are important to the safety and success of the procedure. Complications may be avoided by ensuring that the patient has normal topography and adequate peripheral pachymetry (at least 560 µm) preoperatively. Proper surgical technique, including good centration and uniform, symmetrical placement of spots, is also important. The following are the most commonly encountered adverse events, along with pearls for prevention and/or resolution.

Induced Cylinder

Surgically induced astigmatism has been the most common adverse event following CK. However, it is much less common since the introduction of the LightTouch technique

Figure 31-1. Machine and instruments used in CK. (Image courtesy of Refractec, Inc.)

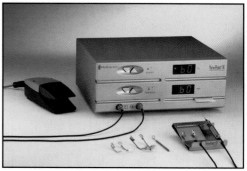

pioneered by Rick Milne. Using LightTouch, Milne and Durrie have reported no induced cylinder in 90% of patients, compared to 71% in the presbyopia clinical trial. The induction of > 1.00 D of cylinder has been reduced from 12% to 4% or less with the new LightTouch technique.

Cylinder can be assessed intraoperatively with the use of a ring light attachment to the operating microscope. Should any cylinder be detected during surgery (in the form of an oval or pear-shaped ring) or postoperatively, additional balancing spots can be placed on the axis of the minus cylinder, with one spot for each diopter of desired cylinder correction. Treatment spots should never overlap.

Relaxation of Effect

The initial over-response and subsequent relaxation of effect in the first few months following CK has been well documented. Even though the CK treatment is considered temporary, multiple follow-up studies demonstrate that the effects of the procedure are stable for 2 to 3 years or longer.

Presbyopia and hyperopia progress as we age. It is inevitable that, over time, patients will need additional CK treatment or a lens replacement to maintain the near visual acuity they desire as their presbyopia progresses.

Monovision Intolerance

Patients may be dissatisfied with the results of surgery if the difference between the 2 eyes is too great or if they experience difficulties in neuroadapting to their postoperative vision. Due to the blended vision effect of NearVision CK, however, anisometropia tends to be minimized, and patients experience far less difficulty with monovision or depth perception than they do with contact lens or LASIK-induced monovision.

Problems may be avoided by careful screening and counseling preoperatively to assess comfort with monovision, particularly if more than 1.00 D of effect is intended. Some patients with early difficulty may eventually adapt to their vision after CK within the first few months. In extreme cases, laser vision correction may be employed to "reverse" the procedure by returning to the full distance correction for both eyes.

If laser vision correction is needed after CK, surface ablation is recommended rather than LASIK. The creation of the LASIK flap severs the deep columns of treated collagen lamellae created by the CK procedure and could result in a sudden and unpredictable change in the patient's refraction. I do not use mitomycin-C (MMC) for post-CK laser vision correction cases.

Under- or Overcorrection

Ideally, surgeons should wait at least 6 months after NearVision CK before attempting enhancement, because the patient's vision may still be changing during that time. Undercorrected cases may simply be enhanced with additional rings of CK treatment.

Overcorrections are rare. To avoid overcorrections, the least number of CK spots possible should be performed. If a patient is on the borderline of 8 or 16 spots, for example, it may be wise to treat with 8 spots initially and enhance by adding another ring later, if necessary. Finally, surgeons using the LightTouch technique must use the appropriate nomogram for the number and placement of spots, as the standard pressure nomogram will yield significant overcorrections when less pressure is applied.

If an overcorrection does occur and the effect does not regress sufficiently within 3 to 6 months, it can be relatively easily resolved with surface laser vision correction. As noted above, creation of a lamellar flap is not recommended.

NEARVISION CK TO THE RESCUE: RESOLVING OTHER NIGHTMARES

Increasingly, practitioners are relying on conductive keratoplasty to resolve complications or unwanted refractive outcomes of other procedures, including IOL implantation, laser in situ keratomileusis (LASIK), and even penetrating keratoplasty. In the United States, these are all off-label uses of CK, although the manufacturer is pursuing US Food and Drug Administration (FDA) approval of some of these indications.

Postcataract/Intraocular Lens Enhancement

Patient expectations of visual quality and spectacle independence after intraocular lens (IOL) implantation have been on the rise in general, and especially with the advent of new IOL technologies. When surgeons implant a multifocal or accommodating IOL, an emmetropic outcome is critical to obtaining the best visual performance from the lens. When the refractive outcome is not as desired, it behooves surgeons to be able to offer enhancements that allow the patient to achieve their visual goals without an invasive IOL explant procedure.

I personally find CK to be an excellent modality for the correction of residual hyperopia or astigmatism or induced astigmatism after cataract surgery. It is stable and effective and may be healthier for the epithelium in older eyes than a LASIK enhancement would be.

As one example, I treated a 71-year-old male patient who had cataract surgery with a monofocal implant elsewhere. He presented at our institute with complaints of poor vision in the left eye. His uncorrected visual acuity (UCVA) was 20/50 in that eye; BSCVA was 20/30. The manifest refraction was +0.25 +1.5 x 70. Corneal topography (Figure 31-2) showed regular postcataract astigmatism in the left eye.

Given the patient's age and relatively thin corneas, we determined that LASIK was not appropriate and opted instead to place some CK spots to correct the cylinder. There were no astigmatic nomograms available at the time. I decided to place 2 spots at the 7-mm optical zone (Figure 31-3), one in each of the flat axes, which I had marked at the slit lamp. Six months following CK treatment, the patient's refraction is essentially plano and UCVA is 20/30, the same as his preoperative best-corrected acuity. The postoperative topography map shows no astigmatism remaining (Figure 31-4).

Of course, in addition to refining unwanted results after cataract surgery or refractive lensectomy, NearVision CK is also an effective tool to provide presbyopic pseudophakic patients with improved near vision.

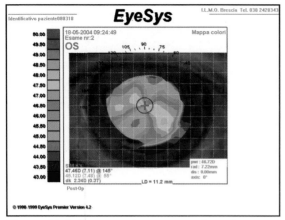

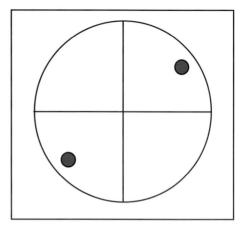

Figure 31-2. Preoperative topography of a post-cataract/IOL eye with astigmatism.

Figure 31-3. Placement of CK spots.

Figure 31-4. Postoperative topography shows resolution of cylinder.

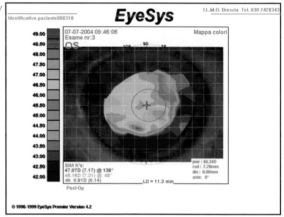

Post-LASIK or PRK Enhancement

Durrie and Stephen Pascucci have several times reported on results from their prospective study of conductive keratoplasty to treat presbyopia following LASIK or PRK. In their study, subjects went from wearing glasses for near 52% of the time preop to 10% postop, and reported dramatic improvements in ability to see at near and to perform common near tasks. They experienced little or no compromise in uncorrected binocular distance acuity. This is important because as the younger patients that we refractive surgeons have treated with the excimer laser become presbyopic, they are actively looking for a procedure that will allow them to remain spectacle independent.

Many of us are now routinely using CK for these normal post-LASIK enhancements. Pallikaris and Naoumidi in Greece have done some very interesting work with CK in eyes with more challenging LASIK complications. They have successfully treated patients with decentered ablations, striae or other topographic irregularities, and unwanted halos or ghosting.

One 47-year-old female patient they treated had LASIK for high myopia 9 months earlier and ended up overcorrected (+1.75 -1.00 x 10), with a decentered ablation.[11] Because so much tissue had already been ablated for the high myopia correction, further excimer laser ablation was undesirable. Instead, she was treated with 8 CK spots at the 7-mm optical zone

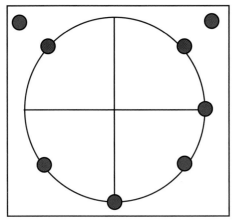

Figure 31-5. Following LASIK ablation over an incomplete flap, CK with the above spot pattern was successfully used to correct the patient's hyperopic shift and visual symptoms.

to correct the hyperopia and another 2 spots at the 8-mm optical zone opposite the decentered ablation area. One year after CK, her refraction was +0.50 -0.75 x 10. Placement of the 2 asymmetric spots successfully "pulled" the ablation zone closer to the center of the cornea, significantly improving her quality of vision.

I also have personal experience of treating aberrated post-LASIK eyes. A 33-year-old male patient of mine, for example, had LASIK in 2000. Preoperatively, his refraction was -3.75 -0.25 x 180, with UCVA of 20/100. During the procedure, the microkeratome stopped before finishing the pass, producing an incomplete flap. The ablation was performed anyway. The incomplete flap caused a hyperopic shift postoperatively, and the patient complained of halos, glare, and poor near vision. His postoperative UCVA was 20/33, with a refraction of +0.75 +0.25 x 180. I decided to perform NearVision CK to correct the hyperopic error and try to fix the visual symptoms. The treatment of 8 spots at the 7.0-mm optical zone and 2 balancing spots in the 8.0-mm optical zone (Figure 31-5) was successful. Following CK, the patient was seeing 20/20 and J2 uncorrected and said the halo and glare had disappeared.

Correction of Primary or Induced Astigmatism

Although we typically talk about the use of CK balancing spots to improve a result during or after NearVision CK surgery, they may also be utilized alone in the correction of primary astigmatism in emmetropes or to correct cylinder induced by another surgical procedure. CK does not appear to cause any coupling effect, so it is much less likely than incisional techniques for the correction of astigmatism to cause an unwanted hyperopic shift.

The amount of cylinder correction can be titrated for each case. To correct cylinder only, sequential spots should be applied at the 8.0-mm optical zone, beginning with the area of greatest elevation, or warmest colors on the topography map. Keratometry and autorefraction should be performed after placement of each spot to assess the effect. Note that an initial overcorrection of 50% to 75% is recommended, as the effect will relax somewhat in the postoperative period. More data are needed on the long-term stability and efficacy of this technique for the correction of astigmatism, but it is a very promising "rescue" indication for conductive keratoplasty.

Treatment of Keratoconus

Although not strictly a postrefractive surgery problem, keratoconus is an important exclusion for laser refractive surgery and can certainly be a "nightmare" to manage, for both patient and surgeon. Here again, CK may be useful. I treated a 34-year-old male patient who

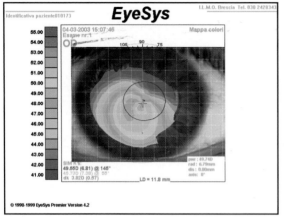

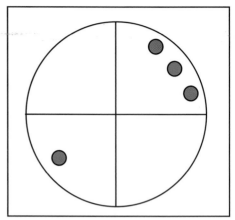

Figure 31-6. Preoperative topography in patient with pellucid marginal degeneration.

Figure 31-7. Placement of CK spots.

Figure 31-8. Postoperative topography shows the cone has moved toward the center of the cornea.

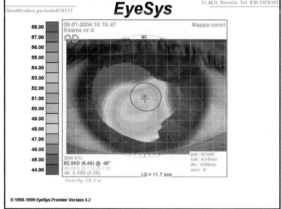

presented at the Institute seeking refractive surgery. BCVA was 20/40 in both eyes, UCVA was 20/400. His preoperative refraction was -0.25 -2.50 x 65 OD. Corneal topography revealed bilateral pellucid marginal degeneration (Figure 31-6). Central corneal thickness was 490 µm in each eye.

Obviously, LASIK or incisional procedures were inappropriate. However, we thought that placing asymmetrical CK spots in the flat zone in the superior area of the cornea might be able to move the cones centrally and improve the quality of vision. After discussion with the patient, we decided to proceed with CK one eye at a time. I placed 3 spots in the flat axis of the right eye and 1 additional spot on the opposite side to counterbalance the tension induced in the corneal tissue (Figure 31-7).

The results were very promising. UCVA improved from 20/400 to 20/50 in the treated eye. Six months postoperative, his refraction is -0.25 -0.75 x 90 and the cone has moved toward the center of the cornea (Figure 31-8). Importantly, we did not remove any tissue in this thinning cornea to achieve a better refractive result. The patient is very happy and has requested the same procedure on his other eye.

In retrospect, this treatment might have been even more effective in combination with a new treatment we have tested at the Institute, corneal collagen crosslinking with riboflavin. Custom-made riboflavin drops are applied to the cornea and then activated with ultraviolet light to increase collagen crosslinking and strengthen the cornea. Early results have shown this to be safe and effective at improving the quality of life of patients with keratoconus and other ectatic disorders.[12]

SUMMARY

Conductive keratoplasty is a nonlaser procedure for changing corneal curvature to treat presbyopia, low to moderate spherical hyperopia, and other refractive conditions. The US FDA multicenter study showed that CK was safe and effective for improving near vision in presbyopic patients, and the clinical results at our Institute have been similarly excellent.

KEY POINTS

1. Conductive Keratoplasty (CK) with the ViewPoint System from Refractec, Inc. (Irvine, California) is a non-laser, radiofrequency-based procedure in which high frequency (350 KHz) energy is delivered into the stroma with a specially designed contact probe.

2. NearVision CK requires no ablation or incisions, does not invade the central cornea, cause flap-related complications, compromise the integrity or structure of the cornea, or cause dry eye or central haze.

3. Surgically induced astigmatism has been the most common adverse event following CK. However, it is much less common since the introduction of the LightTouch technique pioneered by Rick Milne.

4. Presbyopia and hyperopia progress as we age. It is inevitable that, over time, patients will need additional CK treatment or a lens replacement to maintain the near visual acuity they desire as their presbyopia progresses.

5. CK is an excellent modality for the correction of residual hyperopia or astigmatism or induced astigmatism after cataract surgery. It is stable and effective and may be healthier for the epithelium in older eyes than a LASIK enhancement would be.

REFERENCES

1. McDonald MB, Davidorf J, Maloney RK, Manche EE, Hersh P. Conductive keratoplasty for the correction of low to moderate hyperopia: 1-year results on the first 54 eyes. *Ophthalmology.* 2002;109:637-649.

2. McDonald MB, Hersh PS, Manche EE, Maloney RK, Davidorf J, Sabry M. Conductive keratoplasty for the correction of low to moderate hyperopia: U.S. clinical trial 1-year results on 355 eyes. *Ophthalmology.* 2002; 109:1978-1989.

3. Asbell PA, Maloney RK, Davidorf J, Hersh P, McDonald M, Manche E; Conductive Keratoplasty Study Group. Conductive keratoplasty for the correction of hyperopia. *Trans Am Ophthalmol Soc.* 2001;99:79-84.

4. McDonald, MB, Durrie DS, Asbell PA, Maloney R, Nichamin L. Treatment of presbyopia with conductive keratoplasty: six-month results of the 1-year United States FDA clinical trial. *Cornea.* 2004;23:661-668.

5. Lin DY, Manche EE. Two-year results of conductive keratoplasty for the correction of low to moderate hyperopia. *J Cataract Refract Surg.* 2003;29(12):2339-2350.

6. Ehrlich JS, Manche EE. Long-term follow-up of conductive keratoplasty for correction of mild to moderate hyperopia. Presentation, 2006 American Society of Cataract and Refractive Surgery, Session 2K.

7. Stahl J, Durrie DS. Long-term results of conductive keratoplasty "blended vision" for presbyopia. Presented at: American Society of Cataract & Refractive Surgery; May 2, 2004; San Diego, Calif.

8. Pallikaris IG, Naoumidi TL, Astyrakakis NI. Long term results of conductive keratoplasty for low to moderate hyperopia. *J Cataract Refract Surg.* 2005;31(8):1520-1529.

9. Senft SH. Conductive keratoplasty to enhance multifocality after Array IOL implantation. Presentation at American Society of Cataract and Refractive Surgery; March 2006; San Francisco, Calif.

10. Neatrour, GP. Conductive keratoplasty after LASIK: Retrospective review. Presentation at American Society of Cataract and Refractive Surgery; March 2006; San Francisco, Calif.

11. Pinelli R, Pascucci SE, eds. *Conductive Keratoplasty: A Primer.* Thorofare, NJ: SLACK Incorporated; 2005.

12. Pinelli R. C3-riboflavin treatment for keratoconus and other ectatic disorders. Presentation at American Society of Cataract and Refractive Surgery; March 2006; San Francisco, Calif.

Chapter 32

Corneal Surgery for the Correction of Irregular Astigmatism After Corneal Refractive Surgery

Jose L. Güell, MD; Javier A. Gaytan Melicoff, MD; Felicidad Manero Vidal, MD; Merce Morral, MD; and Oscar Gris, MD

Introduction

The number of refractive surgeries has been increasing remarkably in the last few years. Of these procedures, the most popular is laser assisted in situ keratomileusis (LASIK). Logically, with the parallel increase in LASIK surgery, the incidence of complications has increased too. In a publication by Azar et al, the incidence of LASIK complications in series larger than 1000 cases has been analyzed. Flap complications are not that frequent: thinner than expected (0.3% to 0.75%), irregular (0.09% to 0.2%), buttonhole (0.2% to 0.56%), dislocation (1.1% to 2%), and incomplete (0.3% to 1.2%). Around 0% to 4.7% of the cases had lost their best spectacle-corrected visual acuity (BSCVA), regarding some authors. Flap folds or striae have been reported around 0.2 to 1.5 of incidence. Epithelial ingrowth is a little higher (1% to 2.2%) and presence of DLK is variable depending on the authors (0.2% to 3.2%). Infectious keratitis (0.1%), only reported by Stulting et al. Smaller series of cases have reported very similar data to the one mentioned before. On the other hand, optical complications now are more frequently diagnosed[1-7] and have been used as a reference when comparing it to other refractive procedures, as phakic IOL implantation.[8-10] Talking about late onset complications, the most important to follow and identify is progressive ectasia.[11-14]

Irregular Astigmatism

Irregular astigmatism is the final stage of several complications related to flap creation or laser ablation. It is the most frequent cause of loss of BSCVA. This could or could not be related to corneal scarring and opacification.

This kind of astigmatism is caused by folds or striae in the flap, decentered or irregular ablations, secondary ectasia, or recurrent epithelial ingrowth, with or without stromal melting. In some cases, the irregularity is the outcome of the final stage of DLK. Less important in the quantitative point of view is irregular astigmatism, which can result due to problems in other refractive procedures, like surface ablation (photorefractive keratectomy [PRK], laser epithelial keratomileusis [LASEK], Epi-LASIK, incisional keratotomy (radial keratotomy [RK],

Table 32-1
Surgical Approaches to Irregular Astigmatism

	Low	High
Stable	RGP CL	SALK±
	ICRS	Topography-guided ablation
	Topography-guided ablation	DALK/PKP/ICRS
Unstable	RGP CL	RGP CL
	PKP	PK
	DALK	DALK

Figure 32-1. Case of low irregular astigmatism corrected with a rigid gas permeable contact lens.

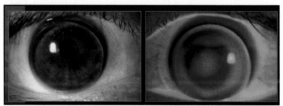

arcuate keratotomy [AK]), lamellar procedures (keratomileusis, intracorneal lenses, epikeratoplasty), and stromal techniques (LTK, CK).[15,16]

To evaluate visual capacity in a patient with irregular corneal astigmatism, it is necessary to adapt a gas permeable rigid contact lens. Although severe irregularities will not improve even with this technique, most of them will.

The clinical and surgical management of these patients will be dependant on the loss of BSCVA, and also if the refractive condition is stable after a follow-up period (Table 32-1).

In case of low irregular astigmatism (loss of 1 or 2 visual lines on Snellen's chart), we can correct it simply with a rigid gas permeable contact lens (Figure 32-1). Other good options are ICRS or topography-guided ablations: 2-step LASIK (topography-guided after flap creation) or transepithelial PRK.

Less frequent situations, like high stable irregular astigmatism, can be treated with microkeratome superficial anterior lamellar keratoplasty (SALK-mK) procedure, sometimes with additional topography-guided ablation. If the pachymetry is low, a SALK-mK with additional anterior lamella can be performed.

Other cases in this group can be treated with rigid contact lens, ICRS, lamellar keratoplasty, or penetrating keratoplasty (PKP).

High or low unstable irregular astigmatism can be corrected by ICRS, PK, or deep anterior lamellar keratoplasty (DALK), but never perform a SALK-mK to correct it because we need to make sure of future biomechanical stability (vertical incisions). Sometimes patients also respond well to rigid contact lens adaptation.

SURGICAL CORRECTION OF IRREGULAR ASTIGMATISM

Intracorneal Ring Segments

Our actual indications for the performance of this procedure are:
- Abnormal corneal topography because of congenital irregular astigmatism that contraindicates laser or incisional refractive surgery.

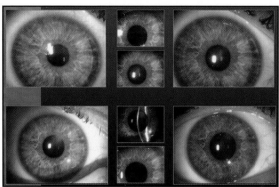

Figure 32-2. Postop pictures showing nightmares after SALK-mK. The top pictures show epithelial rejection and the bottom pictures show late stromal infiltrates. Resolution of both cases after topical treatment was observed.

- Mild keratoconus and other congenital ectasias. Ultraviolet (UV)/Riboflavin cross-linking should be considered in addition before performing DALK or PK.[15,16]
- Post-LASIK treatments to correct residual myopia with small optical zone and low pachymetry, decentered ablations, and secondary ectasia.

Reversibility is one of the most important advantages of this procedure; on the other hand, low predictability of the refractive outcome is an inconvenience, especially in postrefractive surgery patients.[17]

It is important to remember that the procedure should be done by experienced hands, considering central and peripheral pachymetry when performing the dissection tunnels. Controversy still exists in the localization of the incision and the position of the segments, but our technique (steepest meridian / lower U form)[17] has become successful in our patients. Refractive outcomes are not very constant, visual acuity and residual refraction are not always correlated, favoring the first, probably because of optical zone enlargement or the partial or total correction of residual irregular astigmatism.

Superficial Anterior Lamellar Keratoplasty

This procedure replaces the most anterior layers of the cornea, where the irregularity or opacity, secondary to a refractive procedure, is located. We employ the same technique as described by several authors:[18] using a microkeratome for receptor and donor corneas, the entire ocular globe, or a Moria anterior artificial chamber (Doylestown, Pa) (Figure 32-2).

This procedure has been a great tool in our experience. In cases of residual hyperopia and low pachymetry, we add refractively neutral extra lenticule. We also use it for corneal anterior irregularities, frequently associated with topography-guided ablations.

Recently, we are doing SALK-mK, exclusively in front of anterior opacities without irregularity (sometimes PTK can resolve it too, if very superficial), or corneal flap irregularity after lamellar surgery with regular residual stroma; the recommendation in this case is to simply remove the irregular flap with out a microkeratome use, to avoid the mirror image of superficial irregularity in the stroma when using the microkeratome in the recipient eye, with posterior placement of donor flap (microkeratome created). Some exceptional cases will resolve with simple removal of irregular flap without a substitute corneal cap.

Topography-Guided Ablation

This technique is used to regulate and smooth the anterior corneal curvature in a selective fashion. Most irregularities after laser refractive surgery will be corrected in this corneal layer. Other authors have suggested the use of wave front technology, viscoelastic substances and PALM (photo ablative laser modulation) to obtain the same purpose. Because of topography changes after flap creation,[19] we recommend performing a new manual dissection of the flap after SALK-mK or performing a 2-step LASIK or transepithelial PRK. We are actually working with the new topographically guided strategy with the MEL 80 (Carl Zeiss Meditec, Dublin, Calif) with excellent preliminary results.

Deep Anterior Lamellar Keratoplasty-Penetrating Keratoplasty

In this procedure, the goal is to substitute an abnormal, irregular, transparent or not, corneal tissue for a donor one, considering down to the deeper layers of the corneal stroma (DALK) (see Figure 14-8) or the whole thickness of the cornea (PK). The best indication for this technique is a high unstable irregular astigmatism.

CONCLUSIONS

The first thing to do is to diagnose and quantify irregular astigmatism, and the grade of corneal opacity and then decide on the mode of treatment. One should determine the potential maximum visual capacity in each case, after that we have to make sure of the stability of the problem, and frequently, it is necessary to wait several months. A few cases can get better (the physiological capacity of the cornea to remodel its surface is astonishing), and if it is not the case, we will have an objective idea about the stability or unstability of the topography-refraction-visual acuity and quality Also it is very important to evaluate our patients expectations, number of previous surgeries, contact lens tolerance and age among others. All these factors will influence in our therapeutic attitude. Finally, the most important factor to decide each particular treatment, will be the experience obtained by corneal surgeons in previous cases.

KEY POINTS

1. Irregular astigmatism is the final stage of several complications related to flap creation or laser ablation.
2. This kind of astigmatism is frequently caused by folds or striae in the flap, decentered or irregular ablations, secondary ectasia, recurrent epithelial ingrowth, with or without stromal melting.
3. To evaluate visual capacity in a patient with irregular corneal astigmatism, it is necessary to adapt a gas permeable rigid contact lens. Although severe irregularities will not improve even with this technique, most of them will.
4. High stable irregular astigmatism, can be treated with microkeratome Superficial Anterior Lamellar Keratoplasty (SALK-mK) procedure, sometimes with additional topography guided ablation.
5. High or low, unstable irregular astigmatism can be corrected by ICRS, PK or deep anterior lamellar keratoplasty (DALK).
6. Long-term follow up before any surgical decision is made is frequently needed.

REFERENCES

1. Perez-Santonja JJ, et al. Contrast sensitivity after laser in situ keratomileusis. *J Cataract Refract Surg.* 1998; 24(2):183-189.

2. Holladay JT, et al. Functional vision and corneal changes after laser in situ keratomileusis determined by contrast sensitivity, glare testing and corneal topography. *J.Cataract Refract Surg.* 1999;25(5):663-669.

3. McGhee CN, et al. Functional, psychological and satisfaction outcomes of laser in situ keratomileusis for high myopia. *J Cataract Refract Surg.* 2000;26(4):469-470.

4. Moreno-Barriuso E, et al. Ocular aberrations before and after myopic corneal refractive surgery: LASIK-induced changes measured with ray tracing. *Invest Ophthalmol Vis Sci.* 2001;42(6):1396-1403.

5. Malecaze F, Güell JL, et al. Abnormal activation in the visual cortex after corneal refractive surgery for myopia: demonstration by functional magnetic resonance imaging. *Ophthalmology.* 2001;108(12):2213-2218.

6. Marcos S, et al. Optical response to LASIK surgery for miopía from total and corneal aberration measurement. *Invest Ophthalmol Vis Sci.* 2001;42(13):3349-3356.

7. Oshika T, et al. Higher order wavefront aberrations of cornea and magnitude of refractive correction in laser in situ keratomileusis. *Ophthalmology.* 2002;109(6):1154-1158.

8. Malekaze F, Güell JL, et al. A randomised bilateral comparison of two techniques for treating moderately high myopia: laser in situ keratomileusis and Artisan phakic lens. *Ophthalmology.* 2002;109(9):1622-1630.

9. El Danasoury MA, El Maghraby A, et al. Comparison of iris-fixated Artisan lens implantation with excimer laser in situ keratomileusis in correcting myopia between –9.00 and –19.50 diopters: a randomized study. *Ophthalmology.* 2002;109(5):955-964.

10. Maroccos R, Vaz F, Marinho A, Güell JL, Lohmann CP. Glare and halos after "phakic IOL." Surgery for the correction of high myopia. *Ophthalmologe.* 2001;98(11):1055-1059.

11. Klein SR, Epstein RJ, et al. Corneal ectasia after laser in situ keratomileusis in patients without apparent preoperative risk factors. *Cornea.* 2006;25(4):388-403.

12. Abad JC. Idiopatic ectasia after LASIK. *J Refract Surg.* 2006;22(3):230.

13. Schallhorn SC, Amesbury EC, Tanzer DJ. Avoidance, recognition and management of LASIK complications. *Am J Ophthalmol.* 2006;141(4):733-739.

14. Binder PS, Lindstrom RL, Stulting RD, et al. Keratoconus and corneal ectasia after LASIK. *J Refract Surg.* 2005;21(6):749-752.

15. McCormick GJ, Porter J, et al. Higher-order aberrations in eyes with irregular corneas after laser refractive surgery. *Ophthalmology.* 2005;112(10):1699-1709.

16. Jabbur NS, Sakatani K, O'Brien TP. Survey of complications and recommendations for management in dissatisfied patients seeking a consultation after refractive surgery. *J Cataract Refract Surg.* 2004; 30(9):1867-1874.

17. Spoerl E, Seiler T. Techniques for stiffening the cornea. *J Refract Surg.* 1999;15(6):711-713.

18. Wollensak G, Wilsch M, et al. Collagen fiber diameter in the rabbit cornea after collagen crosslinking by riboflavin/UVA. *Cornea.* 2004;23(5):503-507.

19. Güell JL, Velasco F, et al. Intracorneal ring segments after laser in situ keratomileusis. *J Refract Surg.* 2004;20(4):349-355.

20. Calatayud M, Güell JL, et al. Tratamiento de las complicaciones de la cirugía refractiva mediante queratoplastia. *Microcirugía Ocular.* 2002;25(3):225-28.

21. Güell JL, Velasco F, Roberts C, et al. Corneal flap thickness and topography changes induced by flap creation during laser in situ keratomileusis. *J Cataract Refract Surg.* 2005;31(1):115-119.

22. Objective Optical Quality Comparison between penetrating keratoplasty and deep anterior lamellar keratoplasty. Presented at the Annual Meeting AAO; October 2004; New Orleans, La.

Chapter 33

INTRACORNEAL RINGS: KERARINGS AND INTACS

Jaime R. Martiz, MD; Carlos Manrique De Lara, MD, FACS; and Ramon Naranjo Tackman, MD

INTRODUCTION

Keratoconus disease is a bilateral, noninflammatory, progressive ectasia of the cornea that can result in severe vision loss and for a subset of patients requires corneal transplantation (penetrating keratoplasty [PK]). PK is undertaken to restore functional vision and until recently was the only option for these patients. Untreated keratoconus can lead to blindness in 10% of sufferers and is often debilitating for a larger percentage.

The objective is to return functional vision with contacts or glasses by using intracorneal rings (ICR) for keratoconus to normalize the shape of the bulging diseased cornea.[1-21] Appropriate candidates' vision has deteriorated to such a point that eyeglasses and contact lenses can no longer provide functional vision or cannot be tolerated throughout productive hours of the day due to excessive pain and irritation. As a result of limited options, ill-fitting contact lenses cause permanent scarring and central corneal opacities. Elimination of reliance on contact lenses or eyeglasses is achieved in a rare subset of patients with ICR for keratoconus. They are procedures whose objective is to restore the safe fitting and tolerance of contact lenses or functional vision with eyeglasses.

INCLUSION CRITERIA

Objectively defined selection criteria are similar to those currently used in PK for keratoconus. The subset of keratoconus patients to be treated are those:

- Who have experienced a progressive deterioration in their vision, such that they can no longer achieve adequate functional vision on a daily basis with their contact lenses or spectacles
- Who are 21 years of age or older
- Who have clear central corneas
- Who have a corneal thickness of 450 µm or greater at the proposed incision site
- Who have only PK as the remaining option to improve functional vision

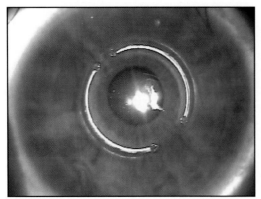

Figure 33-1. KeraRing intracorneal rings (Mediphacos, Brazil).

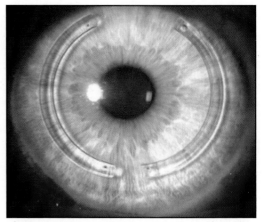

Figure 33-2. Intacs intracorneal rings (Addition Technology, Sunnyvale, Calif).

INTRACORNEAL RINGS SUPERIOR TO PENETRATING KERATOPLASTY

ICRs are a superior option to PK to return functional vision to contact lens-intolerant keratoconus sufferers because it is effective, less invasive, and significantly less risky. Potential complications associated with PK stem from the fact that it is an intraocular procedure as opposed to a corneal lamellar outpatient procedure. PK in keratoconus has a 17.9% rejection rate, and operative complications include expulsive hemorrhage and endophthalmitis in addition to inducement of cataract, glaucoma, corneal ulcer, neovascularization, induced astigmatism, unstable vision, and risk of viral transference. Following PK, the cornea is permanently weakened and constantly at risk of further trauma, a more likely occurrence in keratoconus sufferers because keratoconus is largely a young person's disease. Delaying a transplant as long as possible is in the best interest of patients since the average life expectancy of a transplant is roughly 20 years due to breakdown in the corneal endothelial cell layer, which has not been found to be an issue with intracorneal rings.

Significantly faster recovery is an additional benefit to keratoconus sufferers undergoing an ICR procedure instead of PK, resulting in only very limited time away from work and quicker resumption of normal activities, typically no more than 1 or 2 days.

KERARINGS AND INTACS

The KeraRing (Rockmed, Netherlands) has the following characteristics (Figure 33-1):
- Total diameter (external) of 6.2 mm
- Triangular section
- 600-μm base
- Variable thickness
- Two 160-degree segments
- One orifice in each extremity
- Made of CQ Acrylic

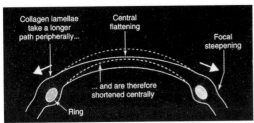

Figure 33-3. Barraquer and Blavatskaya postulates that an addition in the corneal periphery results in its flattening, and the ring diameter determines how much the cornea will be flattened.

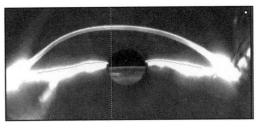

Figure 33-4. Normal anterior chamber depth. Pentacam, preop picture of keratoconus.

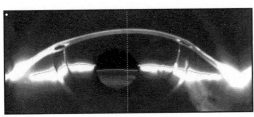

Figure 33-5. Anterior chamber depth after Intacs. Pentacam postop picture of Keratoconus. Notice the flattening of the cornea and decrease in the anterior chamber depth in response to the Intracorneal ring in the periphery.

Intacs (Addition Technology, Sunnyvale, Calif) have the following characteristics (Figure 33-2):
- Hexagonal cross-sectional
- Variable thickness
- Shape with 150-degree arc length
- 31-degree angulation
- One orifice in each extremity
- Clear polymethyl methacrylate (PMMA)

How the Intracorneal Rings Work

The corneal ring complies with Barraquer and Blavatskaya postulates. According to those, an addition in the corneal periphery results in its flattening, and the ring diameter determines how much the cornea will be flattened. Thus, the more tissue that is added (increasing ring thickness) and the smaller the diameter, the greater the myopia correction obtained (Figures 33-3 through 33-5).

Indications and Contraindications

The ICR implant is indicated in the following situations:
- Moderate to high myopias up to 11.00 D
- Keratoconus
- High irregular astigmatisms after cornea transplant
- Irregular astigmatisms after radial keratotomy
- Corneal ectasia after excimer laser

The ICR implant is not indicated in the following situations:
- Very advanced cones with curvature over 75.00 D and significant apical opacity
- Hydropsia
- Cases of high astigmatism after cornea transplant, the ring must not be implanted if the donor's cornea is very much decentralized
- Patients with intense atopia (these should be treated before the implant)
- Any ongoing infectious process, local or systemic

COMPLICATIONS

The incidence of complications after the learning curve is very low. The most significant complications in our sample were:
- *Infection*: Infection can occur in 2 cases—immediately after surgery or long after it, associated with the use of soft contact lenses. In the first case, the standard procedure consists of removing the anterior segment of the affected tunnel and applying intensive antibiotics therapy. There were 2 infection cases with tissue loss that compelled us to perform corneal transplant. In late infections, there may be a need to remove the segment, depending on the extension of the loss of corneal substance and on the seriousness of the infection. There was one case of infection caused by use of soft lenses. The infection was treated and the ring was kept in place.
- *Migration*: Usually keratoconus patients are atopic and report intense itching. Rubbing the eye may displace the segments, pushing them closer to the incisions and causing their extrusion.
- *Extrusion*: It can be caused by superficial implantation or segment migration. Its occurrence can be prevented with routine examination and removal of the segment before it gets exposed and later reimplanted. This complication occurred in 6 cases, corresponding to 3.0% of the total cases. In all of them, reimplantation was possible.
- *Decentralization*: The ring must be positioned at the cone base. Therefore, the centralization procedure must be executed, always considering the reflection. There was only 1 case of decentralization, and the procedure taken was to reposition the segments.
- *Halos and reflections*: Halos and reflections may be present in the first months, but they are seldom reported by patients. Whenever necessary, mild miotics can be prescribed. The incidence of patients complaining of halos and reflections is very low. Mostly, patients only report this phenomenon when asked about it.
- *Hypo- and hypercorrection*: These are relative complications if we considered that the main objective of the surgery is orthopedic and that the eventual visual correction should be made through conventional methods. Most of the cases are hypocorrected, when considering the spherical component. Astigmatisms in general are hypercorrected with an axis inversion.
- *Periannular opacity*: These are small white debris lying along the ring's internal face. They do not tend to grow and do not harm visual performance, being only anti-esthetical when submitted to biomicroscopic examination.

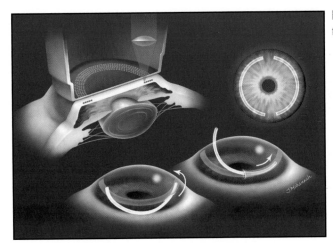

Figure 33-6. Creation of corneal tunnels for ICR using Intralase.

CREATION OF CORNEAL TUNNELS FOR INTRACORNEAL RINGS USING INTRALASE

ICR tunnels can be made with the femtosecond laser. Intrastromal tunnels (or rings) are an annular cut without a side cut at the desired depth. The annual cut is made at a predetermined inner radius from the corneal center and proceeds outward in a spiral fashion to a predetermined outer radius. This is followed by a small continuous entry cut along a radial direction that starts at the tunnel depth and progresses anteriorly to the corneal surface (Figure 33-6).

KEY POINTS

1. The objective is to return functional vision with contacts or glasses by using Intracorneal rings (ICR) for keratoconus to normalize shape of the bulging diseased cornea.
2. IntraCorneal rings are a superior option to PK to return functional vision to contact lens intolerant keratoconus sufferers because it is effective, less invasive and significantly less risky.
3. Significantly faster recovery is an additional benefit to keratoconus sufferers undergoing an ICR procedure instead of PK resulting in only very limited time away from work and quicker resumption of normal activities, typically no more than a day or two.
4. Infection can occur in two cases—immediately after surgery or long after it, associated to the use of soft contact lenses.
5. ICR tunnels can be made with the Femtosecond laser.

REFERENCES

1. Maurice DM. Nutritional aspects of corneal grafts and prosthesis. *Corneo- Plastic Surgery*. New York, NY: Pergamon Press; 1969:197.
2. Maurice DM. The cornea and sclera. In: Davison H, ed. *The Eye*. New York, NY: New York Academic Press; 1984:95.

3. Dohlman CM, Brown S. Treatment of corneal edema with a buried implant. *Trans Amer Acad Ophthal Otol.* 1966;70.

4. McCarey BE, Andrews DM. Refractive keratoplasty with intrastromal hydrogel lenticular implants. *Invest Ophthal Vis Sci.* 1981;21:107.

5. Burris TE, Ayer CT, Evensen DA, Davenport JM. Effects of Intrastromal corneal ring size and thickness on corneal flattening in human eyes. *Refract Corneal Surg.* 1994;7:45-50.

6. Barraquer JL. Cirurgia Refractiva de La Cornea Instituto Barraquer de America—Bogota, Tomo I, 1989

7. Barraquer JI. Modification of refraction by means of intracorneal inclusion. *Int Ophth Clin.* 1966;6:53.

8. Bock RH, Maumenee AE. Corneal fluid metabolism. *Arch Ophtalmol.* 1953;50:282.

9. Krwawicz T. New plastic operation for correcting refractive error of aphakic eyes by changing corneal curvature. Preliminary report. *Brint Ophthalmol.* 1961;45:59.

10. Schanzlin D, Verity SM. Intrastromal corneal ring. In: Elander R, Rich LF, Robin JB, eds. *Principles and Practice of Refractive Surgery.* Philadelphia, PA: WB Saunders; 1997:415-419.

11. Nose W, Neves RA, Burris TE, Schanzlin DJ, Belfort Jr R. Intrastromal corneal ring: 12 months sighted myopic eyes. *J Refract Surg.* 1996;12:20-28.

12. Flemming JF, Wan WL, Schanzlin D. The theory of corneal curvature change with the ICR. *CLAO J.* 1989;15(2):146-150.

13. Cunha PFA. Técnica Cirúrgica para Correção de Miopia com Implante de Anel Corneano Intraestromal, II Congresso Internacional da Sociedade Brasileira de Cirurgia Refrativa, São Paulo, 1994

14. Patel S, Marshall J, Fitzke III FW. Model for deriving the optical performance of the myopic eye corrected with intracorneal ring. *J Refract Surg.* 1985;11:248-252.

15. Belau PG, Dyer JA, Ogle KN, Henderson JW. Correction of ametropia with intracorneal lenses: An experimental study. *Arch Ophthalmol.* 1964;72:541.

16. Johnson R, Bhattacharyya G. *Statistics Principles and Methods.* New York, NY: John Wiley & Sons; 1986:578.

17. S.A.S. Institute Inc. *S.A.S. User's Guide: Statistics. Verrino.* 5th ed. Cary, NC: S.A.S. Institute; 1985.

18. Lovisolo C, et al. Intrastromal corneal ring segments in a patient with previous laser in situ keratomileusis. *J Refract Surg.* 2000;16(3).

19. Choyce P. Management of endothelial corneal dystropy with acrylic corneal inlays. *Br J Ophthalmol.* 1965;49:432.

20. Choyce P. The present status of intracorneal implants. *J Canad Ophth.* 1968;3:295.

21. Burris TE, Baker PC, Ayer CT, Loomas BE, Mathis L, Silvestrini T. Flattening of central corneal curvature with intrastromal corneal ring of increasing thickness: an eye bank eye study. *J Cataract Refract Surg.* 1993;19(Suppl):182-187.

Chapter 34

Refractive Surgery and Intraocular Pressure

Soosan Jacob, MS, FRCS, FERC, Dip NB and
Amar Agarwal, MS, FRCS, FRCOphth

Introduction

Even though optic disc and visual field are assuming increasingly important roles in the diagnosis of glaucoma, as of now estimating the baseline intraocular pressure (IOP) and target IOP are still extremely important in the management of glaucoma. Also, given the fact that great numbers of individuals are opting to go for refractive procedures for myopia, hyperopia, astigmatism, or even presbyopia, the number of individuals out of this patient population who would eventually develop glaucoma or ocular hypertension continues to increase. In this backdrop, it assumes enormous significance to understand the cause and effect relationship between IOP and refractive surgery. It is also important to understand the development, monitoring, and management of glaucoma in patients who have undergone refractive procedures as there come to play numerous confounding variables that affect the intraocular pressure readings in such a patient. The problem assumes great significance in the light of the fact that myopes who are the major category of patients undergoing refractive procedures are especially prone to develop glaucoma. Another interesting question that is raised is whether a patient with glaucoma is at increased risk of progression if he undergoes a refractive procedure.

Central Corneal Thickness and Intraocular Pressure

Central corneal thickness (CCT) was largely ignored in the armamentarium for diagnosis of glaucoma until the findings of the Ocular Hypertension Treatment Study (OHTS) showed that thinner corneas are an independent risk factor for progression to glaucoma. It is known that African Americans who are predisposed to glaucoma have thinner CCTs. Although Goldmann acknowledged the role of CCT on IOP measurements by applanation tonometry,[1] the real importance of this factor has come into play only in the recent past, mainly due to the popularity of refractive procedures that change the corneal pachymetry. Since IOP still plays a major role in glaucoma diagnosis and management, estimating the real IOP of the patient irrespective of his/her corneal thickness assumes great importance. The OHTS and other studies have shown that Goldmann's concept that the effect of pachymetry on IOP is

Figure 34-1. Cupping of the disc. (Reprinted with permission from Agarwal A. *Handbook of Ophthalmology.* Thorofare, NJ: SLACK Incorporated; 2006.)

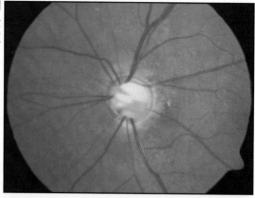

Figure 34-2. Optic nerve head scan on OCT showing a normal nerve head. The optic disc shows a characteristic contour on OCT. The NFL is thickest near the disc rim that is composed almost entirely of the NFL. The back-scattering decreases as the fibers turn to enter the optic disc, as they are no longer perpendicular to the light beam. The photoreceptor layer, retinal pigment epithelium (RPE), and choriocapillaris terminate at the lamina cribrosa.

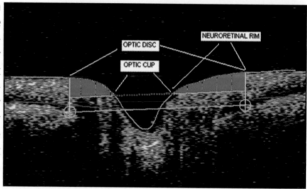

negligible in the normal range of corneal thickness is invalid. It has been shown that IOP can vary between ±4 to 5 mmHg within the normal pachymetry range.

Because laser assisted in situ keratomileusis (LASIK) procedures result in an alteration of the CCT, it is important to do a preoperative dilated, magnified stereoscopic disc evaluation in all patients (Figure 34-1) with documentation of the findings and, if indicated, to do an optic nerve head analysis (Figure 34-2), retinal nerve fiber layer analysis (Figure 34-3), and autoperimetry as baseline evaluation for purpose of comparing with in the future. It is also advisable to give the patient all these data as well for future use. While measuring IOP in post-LASIK patients, one can use correction factors, pay particular attention to other criteria for diagnosis of glaucoma, to take IOP measured from the peripheral nonablated areas of the cornea or use a Tono-Pen (Medtronic, Minneapolis, Minn).

INTRAOCULAR PRESSURE IN SURGICALLY ALTERED CORNEAS

IOP Changes Associated With Postmyopic LASIK/PRK Corneas

There has been an underestimation of the IOP following myopic LASIK and PRK.[2-4] A mean decrease of 1.9 to 3.8 mmHg in IOP measurements has been seen after LASIK.[5,6] Pneumotonometric readings were shown to be slightly less influenced by post-LASIK corneal changes than applanation tonometry.[6] A decrease in the central corneal thickness following myopic LASIK is postulated to be the main cause for obtaining false low IOP measurements after LASIK. The alteration in biomechanical strength that occurs due to the cut in the cornea in LASIK may be an additional cause for a further decrease in IOP after LASIK.

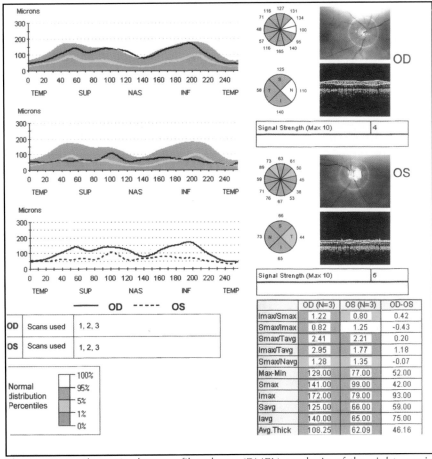

Figure 34-3. The retinal nerve fiber layer (RNFL) analysis of the right eye is within normal limits whereas the left eye shows marked loss of retinal nerve fibers predominantly in the superior and inferior quadrants and also mild loss in the temporal quadrant. There is loss of the double hump pattern in the plotting of the retinal nerve fibre layer of the left eye.

IOP Changes Associated With Posthyperopic and Astigmatic LASIK/PRK Corneas

Argento et al[7] first reported obtaining false high IOP measurements by Goldmann applanation tonometry after hyperopic LASIK. More recently, most studies have 8 to 11 reported false low IOP measurements after hyperopic and astigmatic LASIK. Flaws in the study design could have accounted for the results that Argento et al obtained.

IOP Changes Associated With Postconductive Keratoplasty Corneas

Though there is not expected to be any difference in the pre- and postoperative IOP measurements after conductive keratoplasty (CK), as this procedure has no effect on the corneal thickness, a postoperative IOP lower than preoperative was reported by Kymionis et al.[12] They have postulated that this could be due to an alteration in the biomechanical properties of the cornea, or secondary to an increased trabecular outflow, or due to an unknown effect of the thermal corneal stromal constriction. Further studies are required to verify the effect of CK on the measured IOP.

FACTORS AFFECTING INTRAOCULAR PRESSURE READINGS IN SURGICALLY ALTERED CORNEAS

The conventionally known factors that affect IOP readings are the corneal thickness, corneal curvature, presence of corneal edema, and to a smaller extent, scleral rigidity. Mark reported an increase in measured IOP of 0.34 mmHg with each additional diopter of corneal curvature.[13] Ehlers et al[14] reported the most accurate readings with the Goldmann tonometer to be at a corneal thickness of 520 μm and calculated an overestimation for thicker corneas or underestimation for thinner corneas by approximately 5 mmHg for every 70 μm of change in pachymetry. Whitacre et al[15] used a Perkins tonometer and proposed that applanation tonometry was most accurate between 540 and 550 μm. Real data relating pachymetry to the true IOP by intraocular cannulation studies are still awaited. It is also known that false high IOP values may be obtained in corneas with greater curvature and vice versa in less curved corneae. Similarly, an edematous cornea is associated with false low IOP readings.

These assumptions may not, however, apply to a surgically altered cornea. This is because other than the above-mentioned factors, other subsidiary factors also come into play such as the entire spectrum of corneal biomechanical properties, including corneal elasticity. Patel and Aslanides[16] concluded that a general softening of tissues following the natural healing process after PRK might affect ocular rigidity and IOP. Therefore, a correction factor based on postoperative pachymetry or curvature alone may not give the real IOP. As yet, no valid algorithm allows the calculation of the real IOP in these eyes.

In a study by Jarade et al,[11] a significant decrease of IOP measurement by Goldmann applanation tonometry was found following hyperopic and myopic LASIK, and the mean magnitude of IOP reading reduction was statistically similar in the hyperopic (2.37 ± 2.25 mmHg) and myopic (2.32 ± 2.89 mmHg) groups regardless of the nature of refractive surgery performed. After LASIK or PRK, the CCT decreases in the center in case of myopic LASIK and in the paracentral area in case of hyperopic LASIK. This results in a decrease in the ocular rigidity. The procedure may alter the elastic properties of the corneal collagen fibers.

Livecchi, Avalos, and Bores[17] suggested that changes in IOP could be the result of a persistent increase in drainage of the aqueous humor caused by the high pressure induced by suction. Another proposed factor that may affect the IOP measurements includes the peripheral cut in Bowman's layer, which may cause a change in the applanation properties of the residual cornea.[18,19] The size of the ablation zone may also affect IOP measurements.[20] Clinically undetectable fluid accumulation in the lamellar interface[21] and softening of the tissue due to epithelial and stromal edematization[3,20] or to topical steroids[22] are other factors that have been proposed.

Additionally, because glaucoma may develop decades after a refractive procedure, it is important to document the pre-LASIK/PRK IOP in order to closely follow patients at higher risk. IOP has to be adjusted for the corneal thickness. It is important to follow postrefractive patients closely if glaucoma risk is suspected. Against this background, practitioners should measure IOP 2 or 3 times in the immediate pre-LASIK period and then again 2 or 3 times after postoperative steroid drops are discontinued to establish a new baseline for the patient against which all measurements in the future can be compared.

ESTIMATION OF CENTRAL CORNEAL THICKNESS

Ultrasound pachymetry is reliable when used properly with the probe held perpendicular to the cornea. It is the most commonly used clinical means of measuring CCT. Other instruments that also measure CCT are the Orbscan (Bausch & Lomb, Rochester, NY) and the partial coherence inferometry (PCI), which are both noncontact optical systems. Rainer et al[23] have shown that CCT measured by ultrasound pachymetry was approximately 20 μm thicker than with the Orbscan or PCI. This may be due to the optical systems' lack of inclusion of the epithelium and endothelium. Garzozi et al[24] have reported measuring the IOP at the peripheral, unablated part of the cornea in the straight ahead gaze position with the Tono-Pen to be less affected as compared to conventional IOP-measuring techniques.

POTENTIAL EFFECTS OF THE PROCEDURE ON RETINAL NERVE FIBER LAYER THICKNESS AND VISUAL FIELD LOSS

The LASIK procedure as such may be expected to result in damage to the retinal ganglion cells and a decrease in the RNFL thickness. This is due to the extremely high levels that the IOP is raised to by the pressure applied during the suction head application and the microkeratome pass. The IOP is raised to a level more than 65 mmHg, sometimes up to 60 to 80 mmHg. Some studies[25-27] have shown a decrease in the RNFL thickness but in most of these, the RNFL analysis was done with the scanning laser polarimeter (SLP) with fixed corneal compensation and their results could also be due to a change in the corneal thickness and birefringerence induced by the LASIK procedure. Sony et al[28] have reported no significant changes in the RNFL thickness analysis using both the OCT as well as the scanning laser polarimeter with variable corneal compensation after LASIK.

THE GLAUCOMA PATIENT UNDERGOING LASIK

As LASIK gains more and more popularity and acceptance, there will be an increase in the number of already diagnosed glaucoma patients who want to undergo LASIK. It would be extremely inadvisable for any patient with moderate to advanced glaucoma to undergo LASIK, not only due to the well-documented problems in measuring IOP leading to problems in monitoring and appropriate management of the glaucomatous status, but also due to the potential for increasing glaucomatous nerve fiber loss and increasing visual field defects due to the transient, yet quite high, levels of IOP that occur during the LASIK procedure. It may, however, be considered in the mild forms of glaucoma in patients who have well controlled IOPs and absent to minimal stable field defects. LASIK might also be considered for the contact lens-wearing glaucoma patient needs filtering surgery. It would be inadvisable to do it in the presence of a pre-existing bleb for fear of damage to the bleb during suction ring application and the microkeratome pass.

In all these patients, a thorough baseline evaluation of the glaucoma status is mandatory before the LASIK procedure, including multiple measurements of diurnal IOP, leaving no room for doubt. It would also be advisable to use the dynamic contour tonometry, if available, to measure the IOP preoperatively as well as for postoperative follow-up of the patient. During the procedure, it is important to be careful to make the microkeratome pass as soon as possible after applying the suction ring and to then release the suction as early as possible. The other alternative in these patients is to do a surface ablation procedure such as a PRK. Presbyopes may also undergo CK. Postoperatively, one should be on the look out for

Figure 34-4. Proper placement of laser application in laser trabeculoplasty. This magnified cross section of the angle area shows a properly placed laser beam (L) being applied to the center of the posterior trabecular meshwork (P) or pigmented band. Notice the laser burns (B) centered on this pigmented band (P). If one were to divide the space between the scleral spur (S) and Schwalbe's line (A) in half (X), the laser burns (B) fall on the center of the pos-

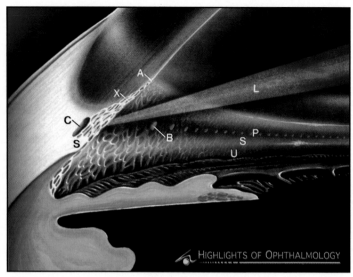

terior half (area between (X) and (S). The anterior half of the meshwork (area between (X) and (A)) is left untreated. Posterior to the scleral spur (S) is the uveal meshwork (U). Schlemm's canal (C). (Courtesy of Boyd BF, Luntz MH, Boyd S. *Innovations in the Glaucomas—Etiology, Diagnosis and Management*. Panama: Highlights of Ophthalmology; 2002.)

Figure 34-5. Trabeculectomy with fornix-based flap. Removing the trabecular window—surgeon's view. This is a surgeon's view of the final incision to remove the trabecular window. It also reveals the surgeon's view of the structures most important to proper trabeculectomy. The trabeculectomy flap that is being excised has been hinged backwards, exposing its deep surface to the surgeon's view. The Vannas

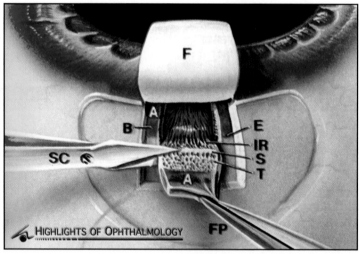

scissors (SC), make the final cut just in front of the scleral spur (S), on the trabecular tissue that is here being reflected back with forceps (FP). The scleral spur is localized externally (E) by the junction of white sclera and gray band (B). Scleral flap (F). Clear cornea (A). Iris (I). Iris root (IR). Trabeculum (T). (Courtesy of Boyd BF, Luntz MH, Boyd S. *Innovations in the Glaucomas—Etiology, Diagnosis and Management*. Panama: Highlights of Ophthalmology; 2002.)

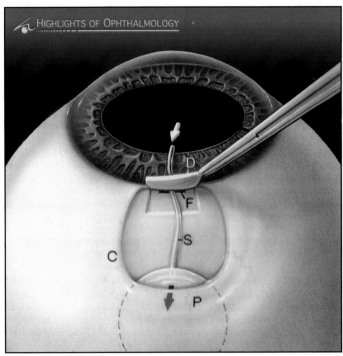

Figure 34-6. Seton implantation procedure. A fornix-based conjunctival flap (C) is raised and the methylmethacrylate baseplate (P) of the Seton is pushed under the conjunctival flap posteriorly and sutured to the scleral surface. The implant has a biconcave shape with the inferior surface shaped to fit the sclera. A small 3-mm square half thickness lamellar scleral flap (D) is raised just as in a trabeculectomy. An incision (F) is made into the anterior chamber under this scleral flap and the long silicone tube (S) of the Seton is placed into the anterior chamber (the end of the silicone tube can be seen in the anterior chamber near the tip of the white arrow). Next, the scleral flap (D) is sutured down around the tube (S) of the Seton. Finally, the conjunctiva is sutured back in place. Aqueous then drains from the anterior chamber (white arrow) down through the tube (S) to the baseplate (P) (black arrow), where a bleb forms. (Courtesy of Boyd BF, Luntz MH, Boyd S. *Innovations in the Glaucomas—Etiology, Diagnosis and Management*. Panama: Highlights of Ophthalmology; 2002.)

steroid-induced glaucoma. It is important to use either the OCT or the SLP with variable corneal compensation for analysis of the RNFL after LASIK in patients with or suspected to have glaucoma.

If glaucoma is present, one can manage these patients with medication, argon laser trabeculoplasty (Figure 34-4), trabeculectomy (Figure 34-5), nonpenetrating procedures, etc. In very bad cases, a Seton operation (Figure 34-6) can be done.

RECENT ADVANCES

Numerous studies have demonstrated that the Goldmann applanation tonometer is affected more by refractive surgery than other types of applanation tonometers, such as the handheld Tono-Pen or air tonometers.[6,22,29,30] The dynamic contour tonometer (DCT) measures IOP independent of the CCT. It is based on contour matching. It is not based on the applanation principle and is, therefore, not largely affected by the corneal structural properties. It has a concave tip that approximates the corneal surface contour when intraocular and extraocular pressures are equal (eg, as if the eye were submerged in a pressurized water bath). This tip matches the radius of the central cornea and provides for a constant appositional force and contact area. It has a piezoresistive pressure sensor that samples, digitizes, and computes pressure readings by a microprosessor-based control unit. In cadaver eyes, the DCT measured IOP closer to actual values than either Goldmann applanation or pneumotonometry.[31] In a study by Kaufmann et al,[32] the DCT readings tended to be 1.6 mmHg higher than Goldmann Tonometer (GAT) readings. This is in good agreement with a recently published study that states that IOP readings made by applanation tonometry were 1.2 mmHg lower than true IOP measured manometrically in human eyes in vivo.[33]

KEY POINTS

1. Given the fact that great numbers of individuals are opting to go for refractive procedures for myopia, hyperopia, astigmatism, or even presbyopia, the number of individuals out of this patient population who would eventually develop glaucoma or ocular hypertension continues to increase. In this backdrop, it assumes enormous significance to understand the cause and effect relationships between intraocular pressure and refractive surgery.

2. There has been seen to be an underestimation of the IOP following myopic LASIK and PRK. Most studies have reported false low IOP measurements after hyperopic and astigmatic LASIK. Postoperative IOP lower than pre-operative has been reported following conductive keratoplasty.

3. Other than the decreased central corneal thickness (CCT), other factors such as alterations in the entire spectrum of corneal biomechanical properties including corneal elasticity also contribute to false IOP readings after refractive surgery. Therefore, a correction factor based on post-operative pachymetry or curvature alone may not give the real IOP.

4. Other factors which have been proposed to result in postoperative changes in IOP include a persistent increase in drainage of the aqueous humor caused by the high pressure induced by suction, the peripheral cut in Bowman's layer, which may cause a change in the applanation properties of the residual cornea, the size of the ablation zone, clinically undetectable fluid accumulation in the lamellar interface and softening of the tissue due to epithelial and stromal edematization or to topical steroids.

5. No significant changes in the RNFL thickness analysis after LASIK have been reported using both the optical coherence tomography (OCT) as well as the scanning laser polarimeter with variable corneal compensation.

6. Preoperative multiple measurements of the diurnal IOP, dilated, magnified stereoscopic disc evaluation, reliable baseline fields, and preoperative pachymetry data with documentation of the findings is essential in all patients.

7. The dynamic contour tonometer is not based on the applanation principle and is, therefore, not largely affected by the corneal structural properties.

REFERENCES

1. Goldmann H, Schmidt T. Applanation tonometry [in German]. *Ophthalmologica*. 1957;134:221-242.

2. Faucher A, Gregoire J, Blondeau P. Accuracy of Goldmann tonometry after refractive surgery. *J Cataract Refract Surg*. 1997;23:832-838.

3. Gimeno JA, Alonso L, Aguilar L, et al. Influence of refraction on tonometric readings after photorefractive keratectomy and laser assisted in situ keratomileusis. *Cornea*. 2000;19:512-516.

4. Mardelli PG, Piebenga LW, Whitacre MM, Siegmund KD. The effect of excimer laser photorefractive keratectomy on intraocular pressure measurements using the Goldmann applanation tonometer. *Ophthalmology*. 1997;104:195-198.

5. Fournier AV, Podtetenev M, Lemire J, et al. Intraocular pressure change measured by Goldmann tonometry reading after corneal refractive surgery. *J Cataract Refract Surg.* 1998;23:905-910.

6. Zadok D, Tran DB, Twa M, et al. Pneumatonometry versus Goldmann tonometry after laser in situ keratomileusis for myopia. *J Cataract Refract Surg.* 1999;25:1344-1348.

7. Argento C, Cosentino MJ, Moussalli MA. Intraocular pressure measurement following hyperopic LASIK. *J Cataract Refract Surg.* 1998;24:145.

8. Alonso-Munoz L, Lleo-Perez A, Rahhal MS, Sanchis-Gimeno JA. Assessment of applanation tonometry after hyperopic laser in situ keratomileusis. *Cornea.* 2002;21:156-160.

9. Zadok D, Raifkup F, Landao D, Frucht-Pery J. Intraocular pressure after LASIK for hyperopia. *Ophthalmology.* 2002;109:1659-1661.

10. Wang X, Shen J, McCulley JP, et al. Intraocular pressure measurement after hyperopic LASIK. *CLAO J.* 2002;28:136-139.

11. Jarade EF, MD, Abi Nader FC, Tabbara KF. Intraocular pressure measurement after hyperopic and myopic LASIK. *J Refract Surg.* 2005;21:408-410.

12. Kymionis GD, Naoumidi TL, Aslanides IM, et al. Intraocular pressure measurements after conductive keratoplasty. *J Refract Surg.* 2005;21:171-175.

13. Mark HH. Corneal curvature in applanation tonometry. *Am J Ophthalmol.* 1973;76:223-224.

14. Ehlers N, Bramsen T, Sperling S. Applanation tonometry and central corneal thickness. *Acta Ophthalmol (Copenh).* 1975;53:34-43.

15. Whitacre MM, Stein RA, Hassanein K. The effect of corneal thickness on applanantion tonometry. *Am J Ophtahlmol.* 1993;115:592-596.

16. Patel S, Aslanides IM. Main causes of reduced intraocular pressure after excimer laser photorefractive keratectomy. *J Refract Surg.* 1996;12:673-674.

17. Livecchi J, Avalos G, Bores L. Presented at: Annual meeting of the American Cataract and Refractive Surgery Society; 1999; Seattle, Wash.

18. Emara B, Probst LE, Tingey DP, et al. Correlation of intraocular pressure and central corneal thickness in normal myopic eyes and after laser in situ keratomileusis. *J Cataract Refract Surg.* 1998;24:1320–1325.

19. Mills RP. If intraocular pressure measurement is only an estimate then what? *Ophthalmology.* 2000; 107:1807–1808.

20. Montes-Mico R, Charman WN. Intraocular pressure after excimer laser myopic refractive surgery. *Ophthalmic Physiol Opt.* 2001;21:228–235.

21. Rosa N, Cennamo G. Goldmann applanation tonometry after PRK and LASIK. *Cornea.* 2001;20:905–906.

22. Garzozi HJ, Chung HS, Lang Y, Kagemann L, Harris A. Intraocular pressure and photorefractive keratectomy: a comparison of three different tonometers. *Cornea.* 2001;20:33–36.

23. Rainer G, Findl O, Petternel V, et al. Central corneal thickness with partial coherence Interferometry, ultrasound, and the Orbscan system. *Ophthalmology.* 2004;111:875-879.

24. Garzozi H.J, Kagemann LE, Harris A. Letter to the editor. *J Refract Surg.* 2002;18:89-90.

25. Nevyas JY, Nevyas HJ, Nevyas-Wallace A. Change in retinal nerve fiber layer thickness after laser in situ keratomileusis. *J Cataract Refract Surg.* 2002;28:2123-2128.

26. Roberts TV, Lawless MA, Rogers CM, Sutton GL, Domniz Y. The effect of laser-assisted in situ keratomileusis on retinal nerve fiber layer measurements obtained with scanning laser polarimetry. *J Glaucoma.* 2002;11:173-176.

27. Hollo G, Nagy ZZ, Vargha P, Suveges I. Influence of post-LASIK corneal healing on scanning laser polarimetric measurement of the retinal nerve fibre layer thickness. *Br J Ophthalmol.* 2002;86:627-631.

28. Sony P, Sihota R, Sharma N et al. Influence of LASIK on retinal nerve fiber layer thickness. Letter to the Editor. *J Refract Surg.* 2005;21.

29. Levy Y, Zadok D, Glovinsky Y, Krakowski D, Nemet P. Tonopen versus Goldmann tonometry after excimer laser photorefractive keratectomy. *J Cataract Refract Surg.* 1999;25:486–491.

30. Duch S, Serra A, Castanera J, Abos R, Quintana M. Tonometry after laser in situ keratomileusis treatment. *J Glaucoma.* 2001;10:261–265.

31. Kniestedt C, Nee M, Stamper RL. Dynamic contour tonometry: a comparative study on human cadaver eyes. *Arch Ophthalmol.* 2004;122:1287-1293.

32. Kaufmann C, Bachmann LM, Thiel1 MA. Intraocular pressure measurements using dynamic contour tonometry after laser in situ keratomileusis. *Invest Ophthalmol Vis Sci.* 2003;44:3790–3794.

33. Feltgen N, Leifert D, Funk J. Correlation between central corneal thickness, applanation tonometry, and direct intracameral IOP readings. *Br J Ophthalmol.* 2001;85:85–87.

Chapter 35

DRY EYE AND REFRACTIVE SURGERY

Ahmad M. Fahmy, OD and David R. Hardten, MD

INTRODUCTION/EPIDEMIOLOGY

In order to develop and implement the most appropriate treatment plan for the post-refractive surgery dry eye patient, a good understanding of pathogenesis of chronic dry eye is the key. The pre- and postoperative evaluation and treatment of the refractive surgery patient with dry eye should be approached with a similar strategy used in treating chronically dry eyes. Comparing the physiologic changes postoperatively to eyes without prior surgery can help us better understand and anticipate iatrogenic pathology or exacerbation of existing pathology. Patients suffering from ocular irritation caused by tear film instability are very difficult to manage successfully. An estimated 10 million people in the United States comprise this group of patients suffering from dry eye syndromes.[1] Chronic dry eye is much more prevalent in females than males, and more advanced in postmenopausal women. Patients developing chronic dry eye after laser in situ keratomileusis (LASIK) are also more likely to be female, as demonstrated by a more frequent appearance of corneal punctate epitheliopathy after LASIK.

DEFINITION AND CLASSIFICATION

Dry eye researchers have historically struggled to produce a concise definition and classification of dry eye conditions. As defined by the National Eye Institute (NEI), dry eye, or keratoconjunctivitis sicca, is a "disorder of the tear film due to tear deficiency or excessive evaporation that causes damage to the intrapalpebral ocular surface and is associated with symptoms of discomfort."[6] This classification of dry eye is further delineated into patients with aqueous tear deficiency and those with increased evaporative loss. Deficient aqueous production is a hallmark finding in patients with Sjögren's syndrome and other autoimmune diseases. Evaporative loss can be exacerbated by meibomian gland disease or other surface abnormalities such as excessive exposure or evaporation due to lid abnormalities. Other terms often used for this constellation of symptoms are *dysfunctional tear syndrome* or *ocular surface disease*.

Table 35-1
Pertinent Medical History

Systemic Conditions	Medications	Symptoms
Acne rosacea	Antidepressants	Foreign body sensation
Ocular cicatricial pemphigoid	Antihistamines	Redness
Sjögren's syndrome	Antihypertensives	Fluctuation of vision
Stevens-Johnson syndrome		Contact lens intolerance
Rheumatoid arthritis		
Sarcoidosis		
Environmental allergies		
Neurological pathology		
Menopause		
Systemic lupus erythematosus		

PATIENT SELECTION AND EDUCATION

Patients interested in decreasing their dependence on contact lenses by undergoing refractive surgery who also report dry eye symptoms should be approached carefully. Patient education regarding postoperative visual acuity fluctuation and irritation should be performed due to the typical increased dryness, especially in the early phase of recovery. For most patients, increased dryness after LASIK is tolerable and not visually significant. Therefore, chronic dry eye is not a definite contraindication to refractive surgery. However, patients with ocular surface disease prior to refractive surgery should be treated aggressively and counseled regarding the likelihood of exacerbation of symptoms postoperatively. Systemic pathology and medications used by the patient can contribute to a dry ocular surface (Table 35-1). The most common symptoms are chronic irritation and uncomfortable foreign body sensation.

Just as it is important to identify systemic causes of dry eye, there are many clinical findings that can help the careful clinician identify ocular surface pathology (Table 35-2). Improving surface lubrication and if present, controlling a concomitant inflammatory component such as blepharitis will improve objective and subjective success postoperatively. Postrefractive surgery patients with a markedly compromised tear film due to a combined mechanism etiology can experience significant fluctuations in visual acuity. Most patients report this fluctuation improves just after a blink or instillation of artificial tears. It has been reported that the surface regularity index (SRI) does not significantly change just after instillation of artificial tears in healthy, nonoperative eyes.[4] It is reasonable to attribute some visual acuity fluctuation to poor tear spread over the newly contoured central depression in myopic LASIK cases and the resultant increased dioptric power of the precorneal tear film. Intermittent blur after blinking and irritation are bothersome symptoms that can disappoint refractive surgery patients as the expectations of visual outcome continue to increase with progressive improvements in refractive surgery technology. With improved surgical technique and increased experience of the surgeon, LASIK may still be the procedure of choice for mild to moderate levels of myopia in healthy eyes, as well as those with mild to moderate dry eye.[5]

Table 35-2
Preoperative Clinical Evaluation

Ocular Surface	*Systemic*
Tear meniscus/Schirmer's	Rhinophyma
Tear break up time	Dental and gum disease (Sjögren's)
Punctate epithelial keratopathy	
Palpebral fissure	
Exposure/ectropion	
Meibomian gland inspissation	
Conjunctival tylosis	
Conjunctival pleating	
Eyelid collarette formation and telangectasia	

Table 35-3
Significant Factors Affecting Chronic Dry Eye and Regression

Female
Smoker
Moderate to high refractive error/ablation depth
Decreased corneal sensation
Ocular surface disease
Subjective reports of dry eye symptoms
Dry working environment
Prolonged computer use

It is important to carefully look for evaporative as well as inflammatory causes of dry eye, as many patients will present with both a tear production deficiency and an evaporative component (Table 35-3). In a survey conducted in 2001, members of the American Society of Cataract and Refractive Surgeons, the most common "complication" of LASIK as dry eye.[6] Once chronic dry eye has been identified and treated aggressively, evidence shows that regression after LASIK is also reduced.[7] It is always best to proceed with refractive surgery after a smooth, well-lubricated ocular surface has been achieved. In other procedures, such as conductive keratoplasty (Figure 35-1), one should also carefully evaluate the ocular surface.

POST-LASIK TEAR PRODUCTION, CLEARANCE, AND SENSITIVITY

The ocular surface and the lacrimal gland work together as a functional unit to stimulate lacrimal tear production. Sensory nerves in the corneal epithelium and stroma trigger the blink mechanism to spread tears uniformly and clear tears from the ocular surface by pumping used tears into the nasolacrimal ducts. Eyelid inflammation, surgical severing of corneal

Figure 35-1. Conductive keratoplasty. (Image courtesy of Refractec, Inc.)

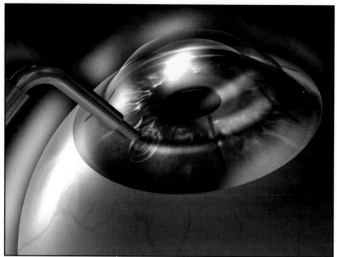

nerves, and laser ablation results in disruption of this important feedback loop, obstructing neural sensory input to the lacrimal gland. As a result, tear production, clearance, and ocular surface sensitivity to touch, including the conjunctiva, decrease. It has been reported that depressed conjunctival sensation postoperatively is caused by placement of the microkeratome suction ring on perilimbal conjunctival nerves.[5] On the question of clearance, it has been suggested that a decreased blink rate caused by corneal denervation and the resultant increased tear film evaporation are important altered tear dynamic factors postoperatively.[5] Decreased tear clearance exacerbates dry eye conditions, as pooling of inflammatory constituents damage the ocular surface. Precorneal tear film dysfunction may be more prominent in eyes that have undergone procedures prior to LASIK, such as photorefractive keratectomy (PRK) and radial keratotomy (RK), as the irregular corneal surface limits sustained, even corneal lubrication.[5]

NEUROTROPHIC EPITHELIOPATHY

A temporarily neutrophic cornea results from creation of the flap during LASIK.[8] Nerve bundles course through the corneal tissue to carry neural input through the stroma and the epithelium centrally. This corneal denervation effect is more prominent in higher refractive corrections and deeper ablations for myopic, as well as hyperopic cases. Disruption of corneal innervation induces anesthesia and hyposthesia that result in significant punctate epithelial erosions. Ablation results in depression of corneal sensation of surface dryness and results in decreased feedback and stimulation of the lacrimal gland, putting in motion a cycle of events adversely affecting ocular lubrication. The incidence of symptomatic neurotrophic epitheliopathy has been reported to be approximately 4% at 1 to 3 months.[8]

Most patients present early postoperatively without discomfort when the clinical presentation of epithelial erosion is significant due to early hyposthesia. Many notice the blur in vision, but not discomfort. It has been demonstrated that the number of stromal nerve fiber bundles decreases by nearly 90% early after LASIK.[9] The regeneration of these nerve fiber bundles takes place slowly. At 1 year postoperatively, some reports show that the number of nerve fiber bundles remains less than 50% of that just prior to LASIK, although most studies demonstrate corneal sensation returns back to normal preoperative levels at approximately the 6 month period.[5,8] Nasally hinged flaps tend to sever less of these nerve fiber bundles and therefore dry eye symptoms postoperatively may be less when creating a nasally-hinged flap during LASIK.[9] Enhancement may cause a return of symptoms and clinical evidence of neutrophic epitheliopathy because lifting the flap once again interrupts reinnervation. Patients after PRK have been thought not to develop a clinically significant degree of epithelial neuropathy, even though corneal sensation is reduced for approximately 3 months postoperatively. Yet in our experience, PRK can still be associated with relatively long periods of epitheliopathy in some patients.

REGRESSION

Sustained dysfunction of the precorneal tear film after LASIK exacerbated by the wound healing response has been reported to contribute significantly to regression of the refractive result. Albietz and colleagues demonstrated an incidence of 27% myopic regression in chronic dry eye patients after LASIK compared to 7% without chronic dry eye in a group of 565 eyes studied retrospectively.[7]

There are several proposed mechanisms of regression. One proposed by Albeitz and colleagues involves epithelial hyperplasia due to increased release of epidermal growth factor. It is reasonable to consider that repeated mechanical trauma during blinking of the dry ocular surface postoperatively increases the release of epidermal growth factor, leading to epithelial hyperplasia and regression.[7]

A second reasonable mechanism to consider involves keratocyte apoptosis. It has been suggested that dry eye after LASIK is related to apoptosis of stromal keratocytes induced by inflammatory cytokines. Autoimmune disorders direct cytotoxic reactions in which antibodies and lymphocytes damage surrounding tissue. The most common inflammatory disorder encountered is blepharitis, but as discussed earlier, many patients suffer from a variety of autoimmune conditions that cause similar inflammatory cellular damage.

When antibodies to specific cells affix to their corresponding antigen and activate complement on their cell surface to accomplish cytolysis, they are referred to as cytotoxic antibodies. When the cells are foreign, cytolysis is protective; when the cells are self, autoimmune disease occurs. Cells containing mediators are activated by stimuli other than an antigen-antibody union on their surface. Neural, chemical, and physical stimuli also induce mediator release, initiating symptoms that resemble allergic reactions, even though no allergen exposure has taken place. Even in the case of the perfectly healthy postoperative eye, during the wound healing inflammatory cascade, infiltration of the ocular surface with T-cells causes tissue damage that leads to apoptosis of stromal keratocytes, underscoring the importance of anti-inflammatory medical treatment.

TREATMENT

Tear Film Supplements

There has been a significant increase in our understanding of the pathogenesis of dry eye syndrome and how to successfully treat it. Traditionally, a very common treatment of dry eyes has been supplementing the tear film with artificial tears. Although artificial tear film supplements in solution and ointment form provide immediate lubrication of the ocular surface and patient comfort, it has been shown that use of artificial tear solutions preserved with benzalkonium chloride (BAK) causes significant epithelial toxicity.[1] Nonpreserved formulations provide the added benefit of avoiding increased irritation and are indicated for patients that are increasingly symptomatic shortly after using preserved formulations. Precorneal tear film supplements can alleviate symptoms temporarily and provide an excellent additional treatment, but patients typically achieve long-term relief by addressing the inflammatory component along with decreased tear production. Chronic inflammation of the ocular surface exacerbates early dissipation of the precorneal tear film.

In addition to replenishing the tear film, the addition of nutrients and fatty acid-enriched formulations containing eicosapentaenoic acid (EPA) has also been proven to be very helpful in decreasing inflammation, stimulating aqueous tear production, and augmenting the tear film oil layer.[19,21]

Oral administration of essential fatty acids that contain sufficient amounts of gamma-linolenic-acid (GLA) stimulate the natural production of anti-inflammatory series one prostaglandins (PGE1).[20] These prostaglandins reduce ocular surface inflammation and reduce the inflammatory process associated with meibomitis. The nutrient cofactors vitamin A, vitamin C, vitamin B_6, and magnesium act to facilitate this conversion and are functionally disrupted by alcohol, aging, smoking, elevated cholesterol levels, and other environmental factors.[21] Vitamin E also plays an anti-inflammatory role by stabilizing the essential fatty acids and preventing oxidation. It also works to inhibit cyclooxygenase-2 (COX-2) enzyme activity that promotes the inflammatory response.[22] Vitamin C also enhances the production of immunoglobulin E (IgE) concentrates in tears, which is the first line of basophil and mast cell defense against invading pathogens and allergens that frequently exacerbate dry eye symptoms.[23] These nutrient cofactors also work to modulate goblet cell production.

Autologous Serum

Another approach aimed at prolonging surface lubrication is the addition of topically applied autologous serum that incorporates growth factors naturally present in the tear film.[2] Autologous serum application has been proven to significantly decrease staining and improve symptoms of ocular surface dysfunction associated with dry eye. This has been especially observed in patients with Sjörgen's syndrome.[11] Although patients subjectively report autologous serum eye drops are superior to artificial tears in relieving signs and symptoms of dry eye disease, it is not widely used due to limitations, including required special preparation and increased risk of infection.[11]

Eyelid Hygiene

In staphylococcal blepharitis (Figure 35-2), inspissation of the meibomian glands may lead to early evaporation of the tear film and the classic punctate keratopathy that is consistent with symptomatic dry eye. The most effective treatment aimed at improving meibomian gland function and the oily contribution to the tear film is the application of warm compresses to both the upper and lower eyelid, followed by eyelid massage with warm water and a mild soap. During the application of warm compresses, we find it helpful to use heat-absorbing substances rather than repeatedly reheating a clean face towel. We typically advise patients to perform the warm compresses and lid hygiene routine for approximately 5 to 10 minutes twice a day. If the severity of blepharitis is marked, we recommend more sessions (4 times) each day. It is also important to remind the patient to be careful not to use a high concentration of soap that may irritate the eye and break down the tear film further. Meibomitis is significantly improved with diligent application of warm compresses and massage in most patients.

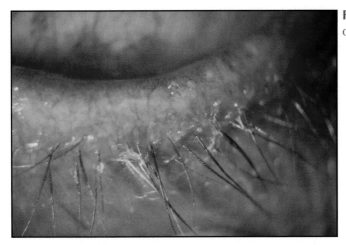

Figure 35-2. Blepharitis. (Courtesy of Guillermo Simon-Castellvi.)

Ocular Rosacea

The addition of doxycycline to the treatment regimen may be indicated in many patients with rosacea. Tetracycline (and its derivates) has decreased bacterial lipase activity in vitro.[12] Interestingly, in addition to its bacteriostatic effect, its proposed anti-inflammatory effects play a significant role in reducing meibomitis. The acceptance of anti-inflammatory aspects of doxycycline and other antibodies was advocated by gastrointestinal disease experts who pondered why antibiotics helped many patients with Crohn's disease despite no clinical evidence of infection. Studies suggest that the clinical anti-inflammatory effect of doxycycline is due in part to its antioxidant effects.[13] Free fatty acid concentrations in the meibum from acne rosacea patients have been shown to decrease with oral minocycline treatment. Adding 100 mg of doxycycline po twice a day reduces meibomitis. This dosage is titrated according to severity and tolerance. Patients using doxycycline should be counseled regarding birth control and possible photosensitivity, nausea, and vaginal candidiasis.

Eyelid involvement can also be limited by topically treating the periocular skin and scalp of rosacea patients. Metronidazole (0.75% topical gel) application twice a day and ketoconazole (2.0% shampoo diluted as a lather) once a day are common treatments. With oral and topical skin treatment, 70% to 80% of rosacea patients reported significant improvements in facial redness, papules, pustules, and telangiectasia.[12] In our practice, we typically instruct the patient to avoid applying the metronidazole topical gel close to the eyelid margin, drawing a clear distinction between an eyelid ointment to be applied to the lid margin and a topical gel that is to be applied to the skin around the eye. The brand name version of metronidazole (Noritate [Dermik, Berwyn, Pa]) is tolerated directly on the lids by many patients who find this helpful in controlling ocular rosacea symptoms. Rosacea patients are also advised to avoid sunlight because it is the single-most common factor triggering exacerbation of rosacea.

Cyclosporine A

In addition to using warm compresses and lid massage, using eyedrops that have an anti-inflammatory effect can improve tear film quality. It has been shown that 0.05% cyclosporine A (CsA) (Restasis, Allergan, Irvine, California), an immunomodulator, significantly decreases the concentration of the inflammatory cytokine interleukin-6 (IL-6) in the conjunctival epithelium of moderate to severe dry eye patients.[14] This decrease in IL-6 concentration was not different from baseline at the 3-month interval; however, showed a significant decrease from baseline at 6 months. When adding topical ophthalmic cyclosporine emulsion to the chronic dry eye treatment, the clinician should remind the patient that immediate results are not expected, and consistency in compliance past the 3-month interval is important, although many patients still obtain symptomatic relief with Restasis sooner. We now routinely start patients on topical CsA 1 to 2 months preoperatively when dry eye symptoms or signs are present. This regimen is continued for up to 6 months postoperatively. This may help to speed the recovery of vision in the early postoperative period when patients are most symptomatic.

Corticosteroids

When a symptomatic patient presents with significant dry eyes, blepharitis, and conjunctival inflammation that is not improved sufficiently with lid hygiene and artificial tear supplements, it may be helpful to use an anti-inflammatory medication such as lotoprednol etabonate 0.2% or 0.5% and CsA in combination. Studies demonstrate that dry eye patients treated with lotoprednol etabonate showed statistically significant improvement in signs and symptoms, especially those presenting with advanced dry eye and corneal staining. A combined approach could limit further inflammatory damage to the ocular surface by adding a site-specific corticosteroid while CsA begins to deplete cytokine concentrations. As the inflammation and symptoms improve, the regimen can be altered by tapering lotoprednol etabonate while continuing to use CsA for prophylactically.

Nonsteroidal Anti-Inflammatory Drugs

Nonsteroidal anti-inflammatory drugs are used to treat mild to moderate pain and relieve inflammation and swelling associated with rheumatoid arthritis. They inhibit prostaglandin synthesis and has been proven to be effective as an added treatment in patients with chronic dry eye symptoms exacerbated by autoimmune inflammation.

Allergies

If there is an allergic component to the ocular inflammation, targeting the allergic cascade with anti-allergy medications is essential. We typically use olopatadine hydrochloride 0.1% (Patanol [Alcon, Ft. Worth, Tex]) and epinastine hydrochloride 0.05% (Elestat [Allergan, Irvine, Calif]) twice a day to limit allergic conjunctival inflammation. Patients suffering from chronic environmental allergies will often times be already taking a systemic antiallergy medication such as cetrizine hydrochloride (Zyrtec [Pfizer, New York, NY]).

Although its exact mechanism of action has not been identified, an immunomodulator: tacrolimus also was shown to inhibit T-cell activation.[15,16] Pimecrolimus 1% cream and tacrolimus 0.03% or 1.0% ointment (Fujisawa Healthcare, Deerfield, Ill) used in the treatment of a common allergic condition affecting the skin have also been shown to be especially effective in treating steroid-induced rosacea.

Investigational Treatments

Rebamipide 1.0% and 2.0% ophthalmic suspension (Otsuka Maryland Research Institute, Rockville, Md) currently in a phase 3 investigational study is a quinolinone derivative. The oral form was developed and marketed as a new therapy for gastric ulcers. It causes mucin to cover the internal surface of the stomach, providing a protective coating. It is the increased mucus-producing effect of rebamipide that is spurring the investigation into its use as a promising dry eye treatment.

Punctal Occlusion

Conservation of the tear film by punctual occlusion is one of the most useful treatments available for dry eye patients. Having the option of placing punctal plugs in either the lower eyelid or the upper eyelid or both enables the clinician to titrate the amount of tear film conservation needed precisely. While the main therapeutic mechanism of punctual occlusion is simply increasing retention of the tear film, doing so may exacerbate ocular surface dysfunction if inflammatory blepharitis is a factor. Since punctal occlusion also decreases tear clearance by limiting outflow, keeping inflammatory mediators on the ocular surface longer can worsen the condition. In contrast to punctal cautery, reversible occlusion offers needed flexibility as tear production volume fluctuates over time. Cautery is generally a more permanent solution, although we sometimes see cauterized punctae reopen spontaneously. Punctal occlusion has been reported to improve Schirmer's test scores, reduce punctate staining, and, therefore, patient comfort.[10]

Temporary collagen punctal occlusion lasting approximately 4 to 7 days can be used to ascertain if punctal occlusion is effective. If improvement is noted clinically or subjectively, then permanent silicone punctal plugs are implanted. Silicone punctal plugs are permanent in that they do not dissolve; however, they can be removed.

Smart Plug (Medennium, Irvine, Calif), is a temperature-sensitive punctal occlusive device. It is made from a thermodynamic acrylic polymer. At room temperature, the device is a thin rigid rod 10.0 mm long and 0.4 mm in diameter. As it is inserted into the puncta, it begins to shorten and expand, forming a soft, gel-like glue that conforms to fit the punctal space. Unlike traditional plugs, no part of the Smart Plug lies above the surface of the eyelid after insertion, offering added comfort to patients.

Tarsorrhaphy

Conservation of the tear film can also be accomplished by limiting exposure and evaporation. In severe cases in which other treatments have not been successful, this can be achieved surgically. In the case of the patient who has developed severe epitheliopathy, persistent nonhealing epithelial defects, or sterile corneal ulceration, tarsorrhaphy is indicated. As with punctal occlusion, this can be done permanently or temporarily. Tarsorrhaphy has been proven to be very effective in healing the compromised cornea after chronic corneal tissue damage from dry eye.[1,2]

Hormone Therapy

Several studies strongly suggest that the low incidence of Sjögren's syndrome in males is due to the protective effects of androgenic hormones such as testosterone, and that patients suffering from Sjörgen's syndrome are significantly androgen deficient.[17,18] Repeatable findings have demonstrated that the meibomian gland is an androgen target organ that becomes dysfunctional with androgen deficiency and that androgens regulate lipid production of sebaceous glands throughout the body. Acinar cells in sebaceous glands respond to these androgens by producing proteins that increase both the synthesis and secretion of lipids that, in turn, contribute to tear film stability. Androgens also act to attenuate autoimmune reactions, whereas estrogens tend to contribute to many autoimmune disorders. The immunosuppressive effects of androgens are due in part to the stimulation of TGF-ß, a potent immunomodulator and anti-inflammatory cytokine.[17]

Summary

Dry eye is a very important issue to be considered in patients contemplating refractive surgery and during the postoperative management of refractive surgery patients. Postsurgical management is very similar to management in patients without refractive surgery, including careful attention to concomitant lid abnormalities, lid hygiene, artificial tear replacement, and medical therapy such as cyclosporine. In most patients, there is a temporary exacerbation of symptoms and signs for 3 to 6 months with eventual return to the preoperative state. By implementing these controlling measures, most patients can actually be more comfortable with their eyes in the long run than they were in their contact lenses.

Key Points

1. As defined by the National Eye Institute (NEI), dry eye, or keratoconjunctivitis sicca is a "disorder of the tear film due to tear deficiency or excessive evaporation that causes damage to the intrapalpebral ocular surface and is associated with symptoms of discomfort."

2. For most patients, increased dryness after LASIK is tolerable and not visually significant. Therefore chronic dry eye is not a definite contraindication to refractive surgery. However, patients with ocular surface disease prior to refractive surgery should be treated aggressively and counseled regarding the likelihood of exacerbation of symptoms postoperatively.

3. Improving surface lubrication and if present, controlling a concomitant inflammatory component such as blepharitis will improve objective and subjective success postoperatively.

4. Postrefractive surgery patients with a markedly compromised tear film due to a combined mechanism etiology can experience significant fluctuations in visual acuity.

5. Sensory nerves in the corneal epithelium and stroma trigger the blink mechanism to spread tears uniformly, and clear tears from the ocular surface by pumping used tears into the nasolacrimal ducts. Eyelid inflammation, surgical severing of corneal nerves and laser ablation results in disruption of this important feedback loop, obstructing neural sensory input to the lacrimal gland.

6. It is well documented that a temporarily neutrophic cornea results from creation of the flap during laser in situ keratomileusis (LASIK).

7. Sustained dysfunction of the precorneal tear film after LASIK exacerbated by the wound healing response has been reported to contribute significantly to regression of the refractive result.

References

1. Krachmer JH, Mannis MJ, Holland JE. *Dry Eye. Cornea: Fundamentals, Diagnosis, and Management.* 2nd ed. London, UK: Elsevier Mosby; 2005:521-540.

2. Alm AA, Anderson DR, Berson EL. The lacrimal apparatus. In: Hart WM, ed. *Adler's Physiology of the Eye: Clinical Application.* 9th ed. London, UK: Mosby Yearbook; 1992:18-27.

3. Spalton, DJ, Hitchings, RA, Hunter PA. The cornea. *Atlas of Clinical Ophthalmology.* 2nd ed. London, UK: Mosby;1994: 6.2-6.30.

4. Nichols KK, Mitchell LG, Zadnik K. Repeatability of clinical measurements of dry eye. *Cornea.* 2004;23:272-285.

5. Battat L, Marci A, Dursun D, et al. Effects of laser in situ keratomileusis on tear production, clearance, and the ocular surface. *Ophthalmology.* 2001;108:1230-1235.

6. Solomon KD, Holzer MP, Sandoval HP. Refractive surgery survey 2001. *J Cataract Refract Surg.* 2002; 28:346-355.

7. Albietz JM, Lenton LM, McLennan SG. Chronic dry eye and regression after laser in situ keratomileusis for myopia. *J Cataract Refract Surg.* 2004; 30:675-684.

8. Wilson SE. Laser in situ keratomileusis-induced (Presumed) neurotrophic epitheliopathy. *Ophthalmology.* 2001;108:1082-1087.

9. Toda I, Asano-Kato N, Komai-Hori Y, et al. Laser-assisted in situ keratomileusis for patients with dry eye. *Arch Ophthalmol.* 2002;120:1024-1028.

10. Yen MT, Pflugfelder SC, Feuer WJ. The effect of punctal occlusion on tear production, tear clearance, and ocular surface sensation in normal subjects. *Am J Ophthalmol.* 2001;131:314-323.

11. Poon CA, Geerling G, Dart JK. Autologous serum eyedrops for dry eyes and epithelial defects: clinical and in vitro toxicity studies. *Br J Ophthalmol.* 2001;85:1188-1197.

12. Stone DU, Chodosh J. Oral tetracycline for ocular rosacea: an evidence-based review of the literature. *Cornea.* 2004;23:106-109.

13. D'Agostino P, Arocoleo F, Barbera C, et al. Tetracycline inhibits the nitric oxide synthase activity induced by endotoxin in cultured murine macrophages. *Euro J Pharmacol.* 1998;346:283-290.

14. Sall K, Stevenson DO, Mundorf TK, et al. Two multicenter, randomized studies of the efficacy and safety of cyclosporine ophthalmic emulsion in moderate to severe dry eye disease. *Ophthalmology.* 2000;107:631-639.

15. Ashcroft DM, Dimmock P, Garside R, et al. Efficacy and tolerability of topical pimecrolimus and tacrolimus in the treatment of atopic dermatitis: meta-analysis of randomized controlled trials. *BMJ.* doi:10.1136/bmj.38376.439653.D3.

16. Nghiem P, Pearson G, Langley RG. Tacrolimus and pimecrolimus: from clever prokaryotes to inhibiting calcineurin and treating atopic dermatitis. *J Am Acad Dermatol.* 2002;46:228-241.

17. Schaumberg DA, Buring JE, Sullivan DA, et al. Hormone replacement therapy and dry eye syndrome. *JAMA.* 2001;286:2114-2119.

18. Sullivan DA, Wickam LA, Rocha EM, et al. Androgens and dry eye in Sjögren's syndrome. *Annals New York Academy of Sciences.* 1999; 876:312-324.

19. Barham JB, Edens MB, Fonteh AN, et al. Addition of eicosapentaenoic acid to gamma-linolenic acid-supplemented diets prevents serum arachadonic acid accumulation in humans. *J Nut.* 2000;130(8):1925-1931.

20. Barabino S, Ronaldo M, Camicione P. Systemic linoleic and γ-linolenic acid therapy in dry eye syndrome with an inflammatory component. *Cornea.* 2003;22(2):97-101.

21. Wu D, Meydani M, Leka LS, et al. Effect of dietary supplementation with black currant seed oil on the immune response of healthy elderly subjects. *Am J Clin Nutr.* 1999;70:536-543.

22. Fujikawa A, Gong H, Amemiya T, et al. Vitamin E prevents changes in the cornea and conjunctiva due to vitamin A deficiency. *Graefe's Arch Clin Exp Ophthalmol.* 2003;241:287-297.

23. McEven AR, Blewell SA. The inhibition of mast cell activation by neutrophil lactoferrin: uptake by mast cells and interaction with tryptase, chymase and gathepsin G. *Biochem Pharmacol.* 2003;65(6):1007-1015.

POSTREFRACTIVE SURGICAL FITTING OF CONTACT LENSES

Kenneth Daniels, OD, FAAO

INTRODUCTION

Any surgical intervention will often leave the cornea contours irregular or the patient with a visual difficulty that cannot be properly addressed with spectacles. Contact lens fitting for keratoplasty, aphakia, and refractive surgery will vary dramatically from standard rigid or soft lens-fitting concepts.[1-21] Corneas altered by either incisional or lamellar refractive surgery techniques are more challenging to fit with contact lenses than nonsurgically altered eyes. These types of fits require numerous lens trials and chair time to rectify the induced visual distortions created by the surgical intervention. The basic concept is to allow the contact lens to act as a new primary refracting surface prior to the entry into the surgically altered cornea and through the entry pupil of the human optical system. Despite the continuing success of refractive surgery, contact lenses will be required after surgery in some patients with postoperative regression, irregular astigmatism, or surface irregularities to optimize their postoperative vision.

The primary goal in these types of fits is to adequately center the lens over the visual axis without compromising the corneal physiology or inducing further change to the corneal structure and optics. The greatest difficulty involved with these fits is proportional to the amount of distortion and irregularity of the corneal topography and the visual demands of the patient. Additionally, the motivation of these patients is dramatically different than the traditional contact lens patients. These patients expected to have got rid of contact lenses, instead they require them to see due to a postoperative complication. Therefore, the approach is to find materials that will allow for a continuous wear scenario to give the option to the patient to achieve vision without the inconvenience of daily lens maintenance. Table 36-1 shows the potential adverse reactions or side effects of refractive surgery.

PHYSIOLOGICAL ALTERATION OF THE POSTREFRACTIVE SURGERY CORNEA AND THE EFFECTS OF POSTOPERATIVE CONTACT LENS RELATIONS

When the cornea is surgically changed, and prior to a contact lens fit postoperatively, not only does the anatomy change but also the physiology and the supportive tissue and

Table 36-1

Potential Adverse Reactions or
Side Effects of Refractive Surgery

Visual Complications With Refractive Surgery	Ocular Health Complications With Refractive Surgery
Intentional undercorrection	Neovascularization
Unplanned overcorrection	Inclusion cysts or plugs
Multifocal effect	Hudson stahli line
Induced astigmatism	Epithelial basement membrane dystrophy
Fluctuation of vision	Recurrent corneal erosion
Difficulty in scoptopic (dim) lighting conditions	Bacterial keratitis—ulceration
	Corneal perforation
Disability glare	Traumatic cataract
Induced anisometropia	Endophthalmitis
Monocular diplopia	Incisional—junctional leukoma
Loss of depth perception	Diffuse lamellar keratopathy
Ghosting and contrast difficulties	Microkeratome—juncture anomalies

glands. Photorefractive keratectomy (PRK) and laser assisted in situ keratomileusis (LASIK) patients have induced neurological deficits in the feedback loop pertaining in lid, blink, and tear function. In LASIK or laser assisted subepithelial keratectomy (LASEK), the corneal epithelium remains relatively intact leading to a lesser duration of recovery. If the corneal epithelium and the tear production appear intact, yet a contact lens is required, the fit can proceed in the short course. However, if the lid and tear production demonstrate a deficit, then the issues at hand need to be treated prior to a contact lens fitting. LASIK-induced neuron-trophic epitheliopathy[1,2] results in a form of superficial punctate keratopathy with dry eye symptoms that may require up to 6 months of intensive therapy with artificial tears before contact lenses can be successfully fitted.

Tear function and postlaser refractive surgery can be dramatically attenuated due to the denervation of the sub-basal neurons. Much like when corneal hypoxia occurs under stressed conditions, such as with continuous wear contact lenses, the neurological feedback loop is altered. In a laser procedure, the ablation of the stromal tissue creates similar changes to the sensitivity of the neurons and disrupts the same feedback loop as described in Figures 36-1 and 36-2. There is a significant loss of neurons 50% immediately postoperatively and creates a sensitivity of approximately 80% over a 5-year period.[3]

Contact lens fitting is extremely difficult in postoperative patients due to the unusual variance in anatomy, and a further challenge is posed with patients who have dry eyes. Therefore, special care should be given to the tear deficiency problem with appropriate treatment prior to lens fitting. Paradoxically, and anecdotally, patients who experienced dry eye problems preoperatively have fewer dry eye complaints postoperatively than patients who never described dry eye in their preoperative evaluations. Since many of these patients had worn contact lenses prior to surgery, they have already experienced contact lens induced dry eye (CLIDE)[4-6] and, therefore, find no great differences pre- and postoperatively.

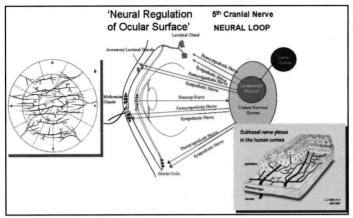

Figure 36-1. Innervation of contributory structures.

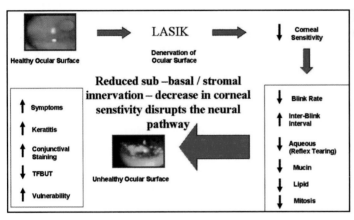

Figure 36-2. Effect of surgical denervation of the cornea.

Traditionally, to enhance healing and encourage neuronal sensitivity, it is suggested to utilize short- (10 day) or long-term (60 day) collagen punctal occlusion E1-E4 (all puncta)[7,8] accompanied by antioxidant electrolyte balanced or gel-like drops such as Systane (Alcon, Ft. Worth, Tex) or Endura (Allergan, Irvine, Calif) qid for a minimum of 30 days.[9]

USE OF SOFT AND BANDAGE THERAPUETIC CONTACT LENSES FOLLOWING REFRACTIVE SURGERY

Soft lenses after RK, PRK, LASIK, and LASEK have been met with varying degrees of success and sometimes catastrophes due to associated complications. Thinner disposable lenses may yield comfort, convenience, and adequate visual acuity due to the resultant draping effect, whereas the use of thicker conventional lenses may lead to vaulting and ultimate buckling over the flattened central cornea, resulting in visual fluctuation.

The use of higher water, hyperpermeable contact lenses is preferred to reduce hypoxia and chances of vascularization. Extended or continuous wear itself is contraindicated due to the potential for hypoxia and hypercapnia that may initiate vascularization along the incision lines and junctural edges. The risk is greater with incisional procedures. However, the advent of new silicone polymers for extended wear hold promise for these patients, as the risks of hypoxic complications should be greatly minimized.

Table 36-2
Uses for Therapeutic Contact Lenses

Provides the traumatized cornea with a mechanical barrier against the shearing forces of the lids

Amplifies drug delivery to the anterior segment

Possibly heightens lubrication therapy, since the lens acts as a reservoir for continuous sustained hydration

Provides a mechanical splinting effect

Avoids prescribing ointments thus reducing visual disturbances to the patient

Therapeutic lenses include collagen-based shields, soft hydrophilic, and silicone hydrogel contact lenses. Collagen corneal shield are made of a natural protein involved in the support and protection of vital structures. Drugs can be instilled, absorbed, and dissoluted via the collagen shield in various rates of 6, 12, 24, 48, and 72 hours and even 1 week.

Perioperatively, pain management utilizing soft contact lenses have been used effectively for pain management during healing of epithelial defects following PRK or LASIK in the immediate postoperative recovery stage. With the exception of therapeutic bandage use, it is best to avoid contact lens use in most cases during the initial postoperative month due to the potential hypoxic effects that may influence healing and disrupt the flap during the process of inserting and removing. However, it has been reported that a plus power soft lens worn overnight may promote regression in cases of significant overcorrection of myopia.

Soft hydrophilic contact lenses are utilized to reduce discomfort from corneal epithelial defects and to protect the cornea from drying or mechanical trauma while promoting a healing response to a corneal wound, post-PRK or for the splint of radial keratometric incisional gaps. The uses of therapeutic contact lenses are shown in Table 36-2.

FLAP SLIPPAGE

Flap slippage is not a catastrophic event; it is an "inconvenience." Treatment requires patient reassurance and refloat with interface stromal bed cleansing using sterile balanced salt solution (BSS) and the readministration of the proper fluoroquinolone antibiotic with steroid accompanied by the application of a bandage contact lens with punctal occlusion (Figure 36-3).

CONTACT LENS-ASSISTED PHARMACOLOGICALLY INDUCED KERATO STEEPENING

Contact lens-assisted pharmacologically induced kerato steepening (CLAPIKS) is a process to correct residual hyperopia, myopia, and possibly astigmatism after refractive surgery with the use of extended wear contact lenses and the nonsteroidal anti-inflammatory drug (NSAID) Acular (ketorolac tromethamine [Allergan, Irvine, Calif]). This is an off-label use of the eye drops. CLAPIKS has shown to be effective on patients who have been overcorrected by 0.50 to 3.00 D of hyperopia following refractive surgery. There is some concern

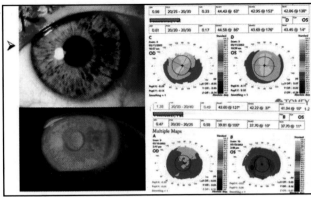

Figure 36-3. Flap slippage with sutures and bandage silicone hydrogel contact lens.

about NSAIDs side effects of corneal melting post-LASIK, LASEK, or PRK. Patients with collagen diseases or other corneal melt problems should not be treated with this technique. Acular is thought to encourage epithelial cell thickening, reducing the thickness by several microns.[10]

The process usually takes several weeks of continued contact lens fitting and use of the drug before significant refractive change is achieved. If the patient demonstrates a hyperopic overcorrection on the first day postoperative visit, do nothing. This is expected, however, monitor carefully for the persistence of the overcorrection. If at 1 week there is significant hyperopia demonstrating 1.50 D or greater, the patient should be fit with a contact lens to induce corneal steepening in conjunction with Acular or an NSAID qid. The patient should be told that this process is a slow "fine-tuning" that takes approximately 8 to 10 weeks.

The lens curve should be selected 8.3 mm (preferred) to 8.6 mm using a silicone hydrogel allowing for continuous use. Remember, the lens should be sparingly removed, one due to the psychology of the patient, and secondly to avoid disturbance to the re-epithelization process or annealing of the flap. The only drawback of dosing the Acular with the lens in place, is the possible deposit of the drug in and on the lens leading to clouding. The patient can be given a 6-pack supply of lenses and allowed to carefully change lenses on a weekly basis.

The patient should be seen at 1 week, 3 weeks, 5 weeks, and so forth until the stabilization of the refraction into an acceptable low plus range or plano. It is unlikely that the patient will reverse into a myopic posture. Once the manifest has shown stability, it is best to maintain the lens for approximately 2 additional weeks as a retainer while continuing the Acular qid for the same period. Once the lens is discontinued, the Acular can be continued under standard label indications for ocular allergy if deemed necessary (Figure 36-4).

POSTREFRACTIVE SURGICAL GAS PERMEABLE AND ALTERNATIVE CONTACT LENS OPTIONS

Radial keratotomy (RK), conductive keratoplasty (CK), and Laser in situ keratomileusis (LASIK) are the most predominant refractive surgical methods known to induce visual aberrations. Results are promising in correcting low to moderate myopia using custom wavefront guided laser, yet many visually induced complications still occur. These complications include decentration of the ablated area leading to monocular diplopia and a nocturnal halo due to a multifocal effect of the corneal surface overlying the entrance pupil, ghosting, halos, loss of contrast, and induced irregular astigmatism. Even though the aim of corneal refractive surgery is to correct myopia by inducing a flattened central cornea, unfortunately, large optical

Figure 36-4. Topographies demonstrate the pre- and postoperative topographies and the subtle effects of the CLAPKIS procedure.

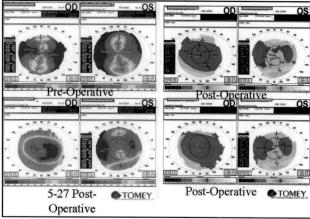

aberrations have been reported in eyes following surgery which suggests the need for a longitudinal study which documents the change in aberrations before and after surgery.[11,12]

In general, to address the visual concerns postoperatively, large-diameter tetra-curve RGP lenses, approximating a mean diameter of 11.85 (SD 0.16) mm, are more beneficial than contact lenses with a standard geometry which do not appear to be useful due to excessive movement and inadequate centration.[13] Contact lenses with large diameters, in combination with a back optic zone radius resting at least 0.2 mm on the periphery of the refractive ablation zone, will facilitate a contact lens fitting that will restore best corrected visual acuity (BCVA) in LASIK patients with a multifocal corneal aberration. GP lenses are seen as more successful, and sometimes the only alternative, for patients with surgically induced irregular astigmatism.[14] Even though there is no one unique fitting parameter for postoperative corneas, the argument of vaulting the ablated or treatment area with RGP lenses is acceptable in around 50% of the cases.[15]

The general concept of fitting gas permeable lenses postsurgically is to select an initial trial lens central posterior curve based upon the presurgical topography or keratometry.[16] In the simplest words, the fitter is making the assumption that he or she is using a similar technique as if they had been fitting the preoperative eye. Using this concept, the lens design will vault the central treatment zone, balance on the edge of the zone and become tangent to the midperipheral cornea.

STANDARD GAS PERMEABLE DESIGNS—LARGE DIAMETERS

Hyperpermeable rigid gas permeable lenses are usually the lenses of choice particularly after RK. If the central flattening is not excessive, standard RGP designs, spherical or aspherical, can be utilized but may require modification of optic zone and lens diameters. For more severe central flattening, special lenses with a lens periphery steeper than traditional gas permeable fitting will allow for a tangential relation between the lens and the peripheral cornea (reverse geometric designs) are preferred. If post-LASIK, the microkeratome cuts can result in more abrupt junctions necessitating reverse geometry lenses for better centration. Common diameters are 9.0 to 10.5 mm, with an optic zone generally 1.5 to 4.0 mm smaller. The optic zones should vault the ablation zone to allow for adequate pupillary coverage in dim illumination.

A large lens diameter of approximately 10 to 11 mm, intralimbal or macroLens design, will facilitate a more optimal lens centration, comfort, and acuity. These lenses will incorporate a large optic zone, approximately 1.5 to 2 mm less than the overall lens diameter to allow for balance over the corneal cap. Optionally, on larger diameter lenses, one could consider fenestrated lenses if air bubbles become trapped under the lens and/or tears accumulate and pool as a result of poor tear exchange.

In a more standard GP fitting approach, the preoperative On K fit would allow for lid attachment or lid interaction but will create edge lift, an increased inferior pooling, central clearance, and superior bearing. The base curve selection would be the average of the keratometric readings. For example, a 44/46 at 90 average would be 45.00 D or 7.5 mm base curve. An averaged base curve will approximate a midperipheral touch with central vaulting. Midperipheral touch is necessary to support the lens on the minimally altered midperipheral corneal tissue.

The diameter of the lens will approximate the standard 8.8 mm to 9.6 mm. The optic zone will minimally vary from traditional designs other than being slightly larger than the corneal cap and allow the edge of the optic zone to balance on the midperipheral cornea. The fluorescein pattern will demonstrate a significant central apical clearance, midperipheral touch, and low axial edge clearance. There may also be an exhibition of touch over the incisional lines if used for post-RK. This fit, is more appropriate for the smaller diameter cornea with the ability and tolerance for the lens to position superiorly on the cornea and is considered more appropriate with post-RK fitting.

A central vault technique requires the use the preoperative averaged keratometric measures with a larger optic zone diameter (ie, 7.8 to 8.2 mm) and subsequently a larger diameter lens.[17] The larger optic zone should be mathematically at least 2 times greater than surgical optical zone if post-RK and 1.0 to 2 mm larger the corneal cap if post-LASIK or LASEK. This will allow the optic zone to "vault" the treatment zone and balance the mass of the lens midperipheral cornea. For example, an RK surgical optical zone is 3.5 mm making the optic zone of the lens approximately 7 mm or greater. If post-laser, the optic zone should be at least 2 mm or greater than the treatment zone such that with a 6-mm ablation zone the optic zone of the lens should be no less than 8 mm and preferably larger. The overall lens diameter should be large enough to allow for a lid interaction without creating excessive superior bearing or inferior lift (ie, 9.4 to 10 mm). Peripheral curves (ie, tricurve design or aspheric hyperbolic) should be employed to allow for back surface of the lens to contour the anterior peripheral cornea.

If the lens decenters superiorly, slightly steepen the base curve, increase the optic zone diameter or lens diameter can be employed. If the lens and optic zone diameters are adjusted, 0.2 mm steps are recommended with only 0.1 mm steps in base curve adjustments. An alternative is to add base down prisms. If prism is added, one-half to third-fourths prism diopters should be used as the initial trial increasing in one-half prism diopter steps as needed, bearing in mind that truncation is not necessary.

If the lens decenters inferiorly, it is necessary to increase the lid interaction. To increase the lid interaction, one may increase the lens diameter and subsequently flatten the base curve appropriately. Conversely, the lens diameter and center thickness may be decreased to reduce the weight of the lens and allow it to position more superiorly. Otherwise, consider a myoflange design that will increase the peripheral bulk of the lens and encourage lid grab.

REVERSE GEOMETRIC DESIGNS

A second method is to utilize the philosophy of orthokeratology by fitting a lens flatter to enhance the flattened effect of the surgery if the patient is undercorrected.[18,19] This method works well on 1) corneas with abrupt contour changes around the surgical optical zone which lead to lens decentration; 2) Asymmetrical, surgically altered corneal peripheries such as post-RK and CK; and 3) history of low preoperative corneal eccentricity (e=0.3), which implies a spherical periphery cornea.[20] After corneal ablating or incisional procedures, a large disparity may exist between the peripheral cornea that will be complemented better with a specialty lens design called "reverse geometry" or "pseudo-orhtokeratology design." Specialty RGP designs such as reverse geometry use ultra large diameter and hyper Dk RGP polymers. These are used to limit the harsh bearing effect on areas at the mid to far periphery of a spherical lens.

In contrast to a reverse geometric or orthokeratological design for the myopic LASIK, a hyperopic LASIK patient benefit with a "pseudokeratoconic design." Smaller optic zones complemented with a steeper base curve and a smaller difference in peripherals curves as compared to the central curve. Keratoconic lens designs, such as the Rose K (Blanchard Labs, Manchester, NH), Dyna Z Cone (Lens Dynamics, Golden, Colo), or a FDACL (First Definite Apical Clearance—from CLEK study) would be appropriate.

PIGGYBACK LENS FITTING

Piggyback lens fitting is a method that utilizes a soft lens carrier for a "best fit" gas permeable lens. The soft lens acts as a "cushion" and "protective barrier" between the GP lens and the corneal surface. The soft lens supports the GP in fostering better centration without excess bearing onto the corneal surface. It is most often used for patients with keratoconic or pellucid degenerations, corneal dystrophies, or in higher cylindrical patients to allow for lens stabilization. When applying a piggyback system to posthyperopic LASIK or CK, the method is simple. A daily disposable or silicone hydrogel lens of maximum refractive power is first fit. Based on the residual visual needs of the patient, particularly glare and halos, the GP is fit based on a conventional fitting nomogram with the luxury of potential fitting to the slightly flatter side if necessary. This would be done if the fitter wants to expand the central visual optical region.

Hybrid designs are considered "pseudopiggybacks" in which the gas permeable material is infused as a single piece lens with a soft lens skirt. The concept of fitting these lenses, even though they are more specific to high cylindrical and keratoconic fits, is similar to a scleral type lens design. A base curve selection of the postoperative RK or LASIK is to utilize the preoperative data. The lens will vault the central cornea and balance the infused GP material juxtaposed to the surgical area. The soft lens creates a "suspension bridge" type lift of the GP lens so that there is no bearing onto the cornea. The soft skirt allows for the support of the GP lens but also added comfort to the patient. The vaulting will create a significant plus power tear lens effect and subsequently the need for a higher minus lens power sometimes approximating the pre-surgical refraction. The major concern is that the vault is inefficient and that a central air pocket forbidding the fit. The Softperm (Ciba Vision, Duluth, Ga) has a limited skirt curve selection, however the Synergeyes (Carlsbad, Calif) generally has two to three skirt curve selections. The adjustment in the skirt curve will be able to lift the GP lens to increase the vault or be decreased as needed.

COSMETIC LENSES TO CONTROL GLARE

Glare problems, particularly after RS, can occur. Simple miosis can solve the concern accomplished by pharmocological intervention or artificial pupil soft contact lenses. Dapiprazole HCl 0.5% is an alpha-adrenergic blocking agent indicated for reversing pharmacological midriasis, generally used postdilated examination, can also constrict the pupil to the size smaller than the surgical optic zone in conjunction with the contact lens.

Generally used postdilated examination, this drop can also constrict the pupil to a size smaller than the optical zone. However, it stings upon instillation and causes temporary redness. Low dosed pilocarpine 0.25% is an optimal therapuetic miotic agent. However, even though it may cause accommodative spasm and increase the risk of retinal detachment, at a low dose it is extremely unlikely. Brimonidine tartrate 0.2%, used as an ocular hypotensive, also has a miotic effect with generally favorable patient tolerance.[21]

Soft contact lenses are available with an artificial pupil that can be made smaller than the optical zone. These lenses sometimes vault over the ablation zone. In such cases, neutralize the tear lens by adding minus power in the contact lens. You can also use the contact lenses to correct residual refractive error or deliberately overminus.

DISCLOSURES

The author is not a paid consultant for any manufacturer but does own common stock in Johnson and Johnson (Vistakon), Coopervision, and Bausch & Lomb. The author does participate on research projects for many of the contact lens and medical device companies and is on the advisor panel for Coopervision, Optical Connection, Hydrogel, and the Sarnoff Corporation.

KEY POINTS

1. Corneas altered by either incisional or lamellar refractive surgery techniques are more challenging to fit with contact lenses than nonsurgically altered eyes. The primary goal in these type of fits is to adequately center the lens over the visual axis without compromising the corneal physiology or inducing further change to the corneal structure and optics.

2. Tear function, post laser refractive surgery, can be dramatically attenuated due to the denervation of the sub-basal neurons.

3. Soft-hydrophilic contact lenses are utilized to reduce discomfort from corneal epithelial defects and to protect the cornea from drying or mechanical trauma while promoting a healing response to a corneal wound, post-PRK, or for the splint of radial keratometric incisional gaps .

4. The general concept of fitting gas permeable postsurgically is to select an initial trial lens central posterior curve based upon the presurgical topography or keratometry.

5. Contact Lens Assisted Pharmacologically Induced Kerato Steepening (CLAPIKS) is a process to correct residual hyperopia, myopia, and possibly astigmatism after refractive surgery with the use of extended wear contact lenses and the nonsteroidal anti-inflammatory drug (NSAID) Acular (ketorolac tromethamine [Allergan, Irvine, Calif]).

6. Piggyback lens fitting is a method that utilizes a soft lens carrier for a "best fit" gas permeable lens. The soft lens acts as a "cushion" and "protective barrier" between the GP lens and the corneal surface. The soft lens supports the GP in fostering better centration without excess bearing onto the corneal surface.

7. Soft contact lenses are available with an artificial pupil that can be made smaller than the optical zone. This can solve the problem of glare.

References

1. Wilson SE. Laser in situ keratomileusis-induced (presumed) neurotrophic epitheliopathy. *Ophthalmology.* 2001;108:1082-1087.

2. Breil P, Frisch L, Dick HB. Diagnosis and therapy of LASIK-induced neurotrophic epitheliopathy. *Ophthalmologe.* 2002;99:53-57.

3. Probst L. Refractive surgery research: the cutting edge. *Review of Ophthalmology.* Available online at: http://www.revophth.com/index.asp?page=1_730.htm. Accessed August 30, 2006.

4. Foulks GN. What is dry eye and what does it mean to the contact lens wearer? Continuous wear contact lens symposium for the new millennium: 2002. *JCLAO.* 2003;29(1 suppl).

5. Daniels KM, et al. *Comparative Analysis of Dry Eye Symtoptomolgy and Disposable Contact Lenses. Corporate Sponsored Research Grant, Coopervision, Inc.* Pennsylvania College of Optometry, Unpublished report; 1997.

6. Lee M, Symthe J, Bergenske P, Caroline, P. Comparison of symptomatic dryness and overall comfort of two continuous wear modalities. Poster presentation from: American Academy of Optometry; December, 2003, CITY, STATE?

7. Albietz JM, Lenton LM. Management of the ocular surface and tear film before, during, and after laser in situ keratomileusis. *J Refract Surg.* 2004;20:62-71.

8. Albietz JM, Lenton LM, McLennan SG, et al. A comparison of the effect of refresh plus and bion tears on dry eye symptoms and ocular surface health in myopic LASIK patients. *CLAO J.* 2002;28:96-100.

9. Trespalacios R, Davis R. Early Intervention for Post-LASIK Trouble. Available online at: http://www.ophmanagement.com/article.aspx?article=86558. Accessed August 31, 2006.

10. MacDonald JE, Mertins A. CLAPIKS. Available online at: http://www.usaeyes.org/faq/subjects/CLAPIKS.pdf. Accessed August 31, 2006.

11. Oshika T, Klyce SD, Applegate RA, Howland HC, El Danasoury MA. Comparison of corneal wavefront aberrations after photorefractive keratectomy and laser in situ keratomileusis. *Am J Ophthalmol.* 1999;127:1-7.

12. Hong X, Thibos LN. Longitudinal evaluation of optical aberrations following laser in situ keratomileusis (LASIK) surgery. *J Refract Surg.* 2000;16(5):S647-650.

13. Eggink FA, Beekhuis WH, Nuijts RM. Rigid gas-permeable contact lens fitting in LASIK patients for the correction of multifocal corneas. *Graefes Arch Clin Exp Ophthalmol.* 2001;239(5):361-366.

14. Alio JL, Belda JI, Artola A, Garcia-Lledo M, Osman A. Contact lens fitting to correct irregular astigmatism after corneal refractive surgery. *J Cataract Refract Surg.* 2002 Oct;28(10):1750-1757.

15. Astin CL, Gatry DS, McG-Steele AD. Contact lens fitting after photorefractive keratectomy. *Br J Ophthalmol.* 1996;80:597-603.

16. Shivitz IA, et al. Contact lenses in the treatment of patients with overcorrected radial keratotomy. *Ophthalmology.* 1987;94(8):899-903.

17. Moore CF Expert opinion: gas permeable lenses are most successful in post-RK patients. *Contact Lens Spectrum.* 1988; December:25.

18. Aquavella JV, Shovlin JP, DePaolis MD. Contact lenses and refractive surgery. *Problems of Optometry.* 1990; 2(4):685-693.

19. Martin R, Rodriguez G. Reverse geometry contact lens fitting after corneal refractive surgery. *J Refract Surg.* 2005;21(6).

20. Szczotka LB. Fitting the irregular cornea. Available online at: http://www.clspectrum.com/article.aspx?article=&loc=archive\2003\May\0503033.htm. Accessed August 31, 2006.

21. McDonald JE, Kotb AM, Decker BB. Effect of brimonidine tartrate ophthalmic solution 0.2% on pupil size in normal eyes under different luminance conditions. *J Cataract Refract Surg.* 2001;27:560-564.

INDEX

aberrometers, 121–123
  problems with, 218–219
aberrometry, 122, 172
  problems with, 216–217
  wavefront, 121, 123, 125, 128
ablation
  decentered, 119–120
    in axial and elevation maps, 214
    case presentation of, 120, 122–129
    management of, 121–124
    surgical treatment of, 122
    topographic, 121
    wavefront aberrations and, 121
  diameter of, in iatrogenic keratectasia, 132
  in diffuse lamellar keratitis, 148
  eye tracking for accuracy in, 37
  topography-guided, in irregular astigmatism correction, 341–342
  wavefront-guided customized
    in early refractive outcomes, 203–204
    for postoperative glare and halos, 195
accommodation, 27–28, 207
acetazolamide, 48
Acrysof ReStor multifocal intraocular lens, 302–303
agentamicin, post-LASEK, 69
air pump, in phakonit procedure, 249
alcohol leakage, in LASEK surgery, 68
allergic dry eye, 368
Alphagan, for night vision problems, 194

amblyopia, after pediatric cataract surgery, 269
ametropia, intraocular lens power formulas for, 242

anesthesia, in phakonit procedure, 245
anterior chamber
  gas bubbles in, 198
  inflammatory reaction in, 255
anterior chamber depth (ACD)
  Orbscan determining, 10
  postoperative, 237–238
anterior float, 3-D, 13, 20
anterior segment
  dynamic evaluation of, 27–28
  new imaging techniques for, 25–33
  static measurement of, 26–27
antibiotics, postoperative, 45, 60, 262
antidesiccation chamber, 108
antihypertensive, topical ocular, for post-LASIK keratectasia, 135
anti-inflammatory agents, for corneal haze prevention, 45, 47–48
aphakia, versus pseudophakia, 268–269
apoptosis, in post-LASEK haze, 76–77
Array IOLs, 293
Artisan IOL implantation techniques, 317–318
ASCRS White Paper, 157–158, 160
astigmatism
  dystrophic, 174
  with epithelial ingrowth, 166
  in iatrogenic keratectasia, 133
  induced, correction of, 335
  irregular, 213
    axial maps of, 125–126
    classifications of, 175
    clinical causes of, 218
    correction of after refractive surgery, 339–342
    with Crystalens implant, 298

definition of, 171
etiology of, 172–175
examination for, 171–172
grading of, 174
indexes used to describe, 215
misreading curvature maps in identifying, 216
S/P keratorefractive surgery for, 218–227
surgical approaches to, 340
treatment of, 176–182
macroirregular and microirregular, 175–176
myopia and, customized LASIK for, 230–231
paraxial optics to correct, 3
surgically induced, 331–332
with-the-rule, 18
autologous serum, for dry eye, 366
automated corneal shaper (ACS), 106, 107, 115
autorefraction, 207, 218
axial length, 238–241
inaccurate measurement of, 237
interocular difference in and refractive shift, 268
axial maps
of decentered ablation with dry eye, 128
in hyperopic LASIK treatment, 219
of irregular astigmatism, 125–126, 223, 224
in keratoconus, 119–120
azithromycin, for post-LASIK keratitis, 159

back-scattered reflection, versus specular reflection, 4–5
band scale filter, normal, 7, 13, 19
beam and camera calibration, 6
best-corrected visual acuity (BCVA), loss of, 61, 150
best spectacle-corrected visual acuity (BSCVA), 80, 93

biometry
accurate, 237
causes of unexpected outcomes in, 237–238
in measuring axial length, 238–241
blepharitis, 367
brimonidine tartrate, 48, 194
buttonholes, 110–114

cannulas, contaminated, 11
capsular contraction syndrome, 298
capsular phimosis, 252, 297
capsule opacification, 190, 191
posterior, 296, 303
capsulorrhexis, creating perfect, 296–297
Carl Zeiss Meditec Stratus, 25–33
cataract surgery
capsule opacification after, 190
corneal topography in, 8–10
pediatric, refractive shift after, 265–273
phakonit techniques in, 245–263
cataracts
extracapsular extraction of, 255–256
with phakic IOLs, 322
unilateral versus bilateral, 267–268
central islands, post-PRK, 62
central opacity, post-LASEK, 74
Chandelier illumination, 258, 260
children
IOL power calculation in, 270
refractive shift cataract surgery in, 265–273
choroidal neovascularization, 284–286
clarithromycin, 159
coherence laser interferometry, partial, 238–239
collagen crosslinking with riboflavin (C3-R treatment), 136–137, 139
collagen punctal occlusion, 369
combination immersion A/B-scan, 240
Compeed, for skin blister, 69–70
confocal microscopy, post-LASIK, 159
connective tissue diseases, preoperative assessment of, 57
contact lenses
alternative options for, 377–378
bandage, after laser surgery, 91
to control glare, 380–381
gas permeable, postrefractive, 377–379
for irregular astigmatism, 176
piggyback, fitting of, 380
postoperative pain with, 70–71
postrefractive surgical fitting of, 373–381
reverse geometric designs of, 379–380
rigid gas permeable, postoperative, 135, 195
soft, eye color-changing, 195
soft and bandage therapeutic, 375–376
therapeutic uses for, 376
contrast, reduced, 188, 189

cornea
    biomechanics in healing response of, 204
    cloudy with edema of, 100
    decompensation of, 252
    edema of, 31, 308
    endothelial injury to, 252, 253, 321
    gas bubbles in, 198
    hydration of in refractive outcomes, 203
    perforation of, 115–116
    phakonit-related complications of, 252–254
    post-LASIK sensitivity of, 363–364
    post-PRK infection of, 60
    posterior changes of in refractive surgery,
        17–22
    qualitative imaging of, 29–30
    recurrent erosion syndromes of, 115
    scarring of, post-PTK, 99–100
    surface irregularities of, 213–214
        nonlaser surgery for, 180–182
    surgical denervation of, 375
    transparency of after laser surgery, 92–93
    ulcers of, 60, 156
corneal bed
    irregular, 113–114
    residual thickness of, 131–132, 139
corneal curvature
    anterior, analysis of, 3, 14–15
    keratometric measures of, 4
    mapping of, 10
        with BSCVA, 220
        in irregular astigmatism, 216, 222
        misinterpretation of, 213–214
    in posterior corneal elevation, 20, 21
corneal dystrophy, 98–99
corneal erosion, post-PTK recurrence of, 62,
    97–98, 101
corneal irregularity measurement (CIM),
    215
corneal thickness
    in anterior keratoconus, 12
    central
        estimation of, 355
        intraocular pressure and, 351–352
    in iatrogenic keratectasia, 133
corneal topography
    anterior segment, future of, 30–33
    for cataract surgery, 8–10
    complications of, 213–227
    iatrogenic keratectasia and, 133–134
    irregular astigmatism pattern in, 171–172

    posterior, 18
    pre-existing posterior abnormalities of,
        18–20
    pre-LASIK, 17, 139
    problems of, 213–216
corneal tunnels, for intracorneal rings using
    Intralase, 349
corneoscleral melting, Mitomycin-C and,
    94–95
corticosteroids
    for corneal haze, 80
    for dry eye, 368
    postoperative, side effects of, 59
cryotherapy, for epithelial ingrowth, 167, 169
Crystalens, 294, 295–299
crystalline lens
    OCT evaluation of, 27–28
    pseudophakic artificial, 28–29
custom-CAP procedure, 221
Custom-Corneal Ablation Pattern, 122–123
cycloplegia, 207, 298
cycloplegics, for corneal decompensation,
    252
cyclosporine A, 367–368

dandelion keratectasia, 132
dapiprazole, 194
decentration
    causes of, 128
    diffuse lamellar keratitis and, 129
    evaluation of, 128
    inferotemporal, 125
    with intracorneal rings, 348
    with phakic IOLs, 323
    post-PRK, 62, 232–233
    with ReZoom implants, 301–302
    topographic, 121
defocus errors, inadequate correction of, 3–4
Descemet's membrane damage, 253
Desmarres sharp blade, 90
dexamethasone, postoperative, 45, 47–48, 69
diclofenac, post-LASEK, 69
diffraction, 185
diplopia, with decentered excimer ablation,
    128
dispersion, 185
    dry eye
    aggressive treatment of, 126–127
    chronic and regressive, factors affecting,
        363

decentered ablation and, 128
definition and classification of, 361
epidemiology of, 361
with epithelial ingrowth, 165
medical history of, 362
patient selection and education on, 362–363
post-LASIK treatment for, 365–366
postoperative, 192
with presbyopic correcting IOLs, 295
refractive surgery and, 361–370

ectasia
clinical presentation of, 133
diagnosis of, 134–135
iatrogenic post-LASIK, 131–139
pathogenesis of, 131
predisposing factors in, 131–133
topography in, 133–134
treatment of, 135–137
ELASHY technique, 177–178
electromagnetic radiation, 185
elevation, 10
in anterior keratoconus, 11
in decentered ablation, 124
in irregular astigmatism, 172
in LASIK candidates, 14
mapping
with BSCVA, 220
for corneal irregularities, 219
in irregular astigmatism, 223
in keratoconus, 119–120
measurement of, 4
in microns, 20
posterior, 18–21
diagnostic criteria in, 21
iatrogenic keratectasia and, 134
intraocular lens calculation and, 21–22
Orbscan analysis of, 7–9
posterior abnormalities in, 18–20
topographic analysis in, 18
emmetropia, 271, 301
emulsification technique, complications related to, 251–252
endophthalmitis
differential diagnosis of, 309
with phakic IOLs, 324–325
with phakonit techniques, 262–263
toxic anterior segment syndrome and, 307
endotoxins

balanced salt solution and, 310
in detergent and ultrasonic bath, 310
in diffuse lamellar keratitis, 147, 151
in instrument contamination, 311
Epi-LASIK, 82, 85–86
histological findings and, 82
irregular astigmatism after, 172
postoperative period in, 83–85
technique in, 83
epikeratome, Centurion SES, 83, 85
epithelial cell dehiscence, minimizing, 151
epithelial fistulas, 166
epithelial reference markings, 108
epithelial scraping, 167
epithelial sheets
alcohol-assisted separation of, 85–86
mechanically separated, 82–83
replacement of, 83
epithelium
defects in, 114–115
delayed healing of, 60–61
hyperplastic layer thickness and haze, 49
ingrowth of, 163, 169
classification of, 164
complications of, 166
follow-up of, 166
forms of, 166
histopathology of, 163
prevention of, 168
recent advances in, 169
removal of, 167, 168
risk factors for, 164–165
signs of, 166
symptoms of, 165
treatment of, 167–168
intraoperative management of, 67–68
phakonit-related injury to, 253
post-LASEK regrowth of, 75
post-LASEK thinning of, 72–74
postoperative healing of, 58
removal of, 90
excimer laser surgery, 176–180
eye
acoustic shock waves through, 280
tracking of, 37
eyelid hygiene, 366

FAVIT technique, complications of, 256–259
Ferrara Rings, 136
flap melting, 166

flaps
    complications of, 105–116
    development of, 105
    epithelial defects on, 114–115
    folds and wrinkles in, 113
    incomplete, 109–110
    LASIK
        complications of, 105–116
        intraoperative complications in creating, 197–200
        postoperative complications in creating, 200–201
        thickness of, 32
    lifting of in LASIK enhancement, 206
    post-LASEK
        inclusions under, 74
        tears in, 68, 71, 72
    slippage of, 376, 377
    thickness of in iatrogenic keratectasia, 133
    thin, 110–114
    unliftable, 198–199
fluorometholone, 59
fluoroquinolones, 159
Fourier analysis, 172, 173
free cap, 105–106
    complications of, 108–109
    management of, 106–108
fundoscopy, 56

gamma-linolenic acid (GLA), 366
gas bubbles, 198, 199
geometric bending measures, 4
geometric optics, 3–4
ghosting, 128
glare
    computer simulation of, 186
    cosmetic lenses to control, 380–381
    daytime and dim-light, 186
    post-LASIK, 190–195
    pupil size and, 187–189
    in refractive surgery, 37–38
glaucoma
    angle-closure, 31
    intraocular pressure changes in, 354
    LASIK and, 355–357
    OCT imaging in, 30
    preoperative assessment for, 56
    in refractive shift in pediatric cataract surgery, 269
Goldmann applanation tonometer, 357–358

Haigis formula, 241, 242
halos, 186
    after refractive surgery, 37–38
    colored, causes of, 188
    computer simulation of, 187, 189
    with intracorneal rings, 348
    management of, 38
    post-LASIK, 190–195
    post-PRK, 61
    pupil size and, 187–189
    with ReZoom implants, 300–301
Hartmann-Shack technology, 122–123, 219
haze, 52
    case study of, 45–51
    causes and definitions of, 43–44
    diffuse, 63, 252
    with epithelial ingrowth, 165
    grading of, 44
    Mitomycin-C for, 89, 90–95
    onset of, 44
    post-LASEK, 76–77
    with post-PRK regression, 64–65
    prophylaxis and treatment of, 45, 47–48, 94
    stromal, 44, 64, 76–77
hemorrhage, expulsive, 255
Hoffer-Q formula, 241, 242
Holladay IOL formulas, 241, 242
hormone therapy, 369
hydrocarbons, 147
hydrodissection, 246
hyperopia, 218
    after pediatric cataract surgery, 270
    after radial keratotomy, 232
    customized LASIK for, 229–230
hyperopic enhancements, 205
hyperopic regression, 232
hyperosmotics, 252

image exploitation software, prototype of, 27
imaging techniques, anterior segment, 25–33
infections
    with intracorneal rings, 348
    irregular astigmatism after, 175
    in phakonit procedures, 253
    post-LASIK, 155–169
infrared wavelengths, in optical coherence, 25–26
Intacs, 153

characteristics of, 347
diffuse lamellar keratitis and, 150
irregular astigmatism with, 172
for post-LASIK keratectasia, 135–136
intracorneal rings
  complications of, 348–349
  corneal tunnels for, 349
  function of, 347
  inclusion criteria for, 345
  indications and contraindications to, 347–348
  in irregular astigmatism correction, 340–341
  types of, 346–347
  versus penetrating keratoplasty, 346
Intralase, complications with, 197–201, 349
intraocular lens (IOL) drop, with phakonit procedures, 257–258
intraocular lens (IOL) power
  calculation methods for in children, 270
  formulas for, 237–242, 243
  inaccurate measurement of, 237–238
  posterior corneal elevation effects on, 21–22
  size and in refractive shift in pediatric cataract surgery, 269
intraocular lenses (IOLs)
  decentration of, 256
  dislocated, 261
    removal of, 260
  extrusion of with phakonit procedures, 257
  3M diffractive multifocal, 293
  NearVision, 333–334
  opacification of, 256
  phakic, 36–37
    angle-supported, 315–316
    classification of, 315
    complications of, 320–325
    foldable posterior, 319, 320
    inserting, 29, 316
    iris-supported, 316–319
    LASIK after, 231
    myopia after, 230
    recent advances in, 325
    repositioning/removal of, 323
    retinal breaks and detachment with, 282
    types of, 315–320
    versus refractive surgery, 36–37
  piggyback, 28, 271–272

posterior chamber phakic, 319–320
presbyopic correcting, 293–305
intraocular pressure (IOP)
  central corneal thickness and, 351–352
  increased, with phakic IOLs, 322–323
  in surgically altered corneas, 352–354
intrastromal corneal rings, 38–39, 135–136
IOLMaster, 238–239, 242
irido-corneal angle, 31
iris injury, in phakonit procedures, 254
irrigating solution, contaminated, 310

K reading, 21–22
keloid formation, preoperative assessment of, 57
KeraRings, 346–347
keratectasia
  iatrogenic
    clinical presentation of, 133
    diagnosis of, 134–135
    pathogenesis of, 131
    predisposing factors in, 131–133
    topography in, 133–134
    treatment of, 135–137
  post-LASIK, 18–19
    prevention of, 138–139
keratectomy
  automated lamellar, 177–178
  irregular bed in, 113–114
  loss of suction in, 113, 114
  photorefractive (PRK)
    after other surgical procedures, 57–58
    case study of corneal haze in, 45–50
    complications of, 55–65
    contact lens fitting after, 373–374
    corneal haze after, 43, 44–45
    for decentered ablation, 122
    decentration after, 232–233
    intraocular pressure changes with, 352–354

    irregular astigmatism after, 172, 339–340
    LASIK for hyperopic regression after, 232
    Mitomycin-C prophylaxis in, 45
    NearVision contact keratoplasty in, 334–335
    postoperative management in, 58–59
    preoperative assessment in, 46, 55–57
    results of, 46–47

retinal breaks and detachment after, 276
risk-benefit assessment of, 57
risk factors for infection after, 155
vitreoretinal complications of, 275–287
phototherapeutic (PTK)
complications of, 97–102
corneal dystrophies after, 98–99
corneal scarring in, 99–100
for epithelial ingrowth, 167
Mitomycin-C with, 49–50
outcomes of, 50–51
recurrent erosion after, 97–98
keratitis
diffuse lamellar (DLK), 124, 143, 153–154
corneal features of, 143–144
delayed onset, 149
diagnosis of, 144–145
differential diagnosis of, 149
etiology of, 146–148
Hatsis classification of, 145–146
Intacs intralase, 150
late onset, 149–150
ocular features of, 144
pathogenesis of, 144
postoperative, 127, 190–191, 200–201
prevention of, 150–152
topographical decentration and, 129
treatment of, 152–153, 190–191
fungal, 156, 158–159
herpetic, 175, 253
in phakonit procedures, 253
post-LASIK
clinical signs and symptoms of, 156–157
complications of, 157
epidemiology of, 156
histopathology and microbiology of, 157
prevention of, 158
risk factors for, 155
treatment of, 158–159
postoperative, 200
sicca, 57
viral, 150
kerato steepening, contact lens-assisted pharmacologically induced, 376–377
keratoconus
anterior, Orbscan analysis of, 11–15
anterior-to-posterior curvature in, 20
axial and elevation maps in, 119–120
contact keratoplasty for, 335–337
criteria for intracorneal rings for, 345

early, detection of, 19
general quad map in, 9
irregular astigmatism in, 174
preoperative assessment of, 56
producing glare, 191
keratoglobus, irregular astigmatism in, 174
keratometers, 3, 4–5
keratometric mean curvature, 12
keratometry
inaccuracy of, 21
irregular astigmatism pattern in, 171–172
mean toric (MTK), 215
simulated (SimK), 4, 213, 215
keratomileusis, sutureless technique for, 105
keratopathy
band-shaped, phototherapeutic keratectomy for, 101
central toxic, 150, 153
in phakonit procedures, 252, 253
punctate, in diffuse lamellar keratitis, 145
keratoplasty
automated anterior lamellar, for irregular astigmatism, 180–181
automated lamellar, 180–181
conductive, 364
intraocular pressure changes in, 353–354
LASIK after for low hyperopia and presbyopia, 229–230
potential complications of, 331–337
contact, 333–334
deep anterior lamellar (DALK)
for irregular astigmatism, 181
in irregular astigmatism correction, 342
for post-LASIK keratectasia, 137, 138
NearVision conductive
complications of, 331–333
in resolving other complications, 333–337
penetrating
versus intracorneal rings, 346
irregular astigmatism and, 172, 181–182, 342
myopia and astigmatism after, 230–231
photorefractive keratectomy after, 57–58
for post-LASIK keratectasia, 137, 139
reinfection with hypopyon after, 159
for post-LASIK keratectasia, 137–139
superficial anterior lamellar, 341

keratorefractive surgery, for irregular astigmatism, 218–227
keratotomy
   arcuate, irregular astigmatism after, 172
   radial
      irregular astigmatism after, 172, 215,
         339–340
      LASIK for hyperopia after, 232
      photorefractive keratectomy after, 57–58
ketoconazole, 367
Klebsiella pneumonia, 310

LASEK, 81
   complications of, 67
      intraoperative, 67–68
      long-term, 75–78
      postoperative, 69–75
   drawbacks of, 81, 86
   irregular astigmatism after, 172
   for refractive shift after pediatric cataract
      surgery, 272
laser ablation
   depth of in iatrogenic keratectasia, 133
   for epithelial ingrowth, 167
   Mitomycin-C use in, 89–95
   night glare and halos after, 37–38
   pupil size and, 38
laser Nd-YAG capsulotomy, 190
laser programming, accuracy of, 208
LASIK, 81
   accurate refraction after, 207–208
   avoiding difficulties in, 207
   complications of, 86, 208, 275
   contact lens fitting after, 373–374
   contraindications for, 55
   cornea-sparing, 137
   corneal perforation in, 115–116
   customized, after previous refractive sur-
      gery, 229–233
   diffuse lamellar keratitis after, 146
   early refractive outcomes of, factors in,
      203–204
   enhancement techniques in, 205–206
   epithelial ingrowth after, 163–169
   femtosecond laser-assisted, 222–224
   flap complications after, 105–116
   free cap in, 106–109
   in glaucoma patient, 355–357
   iatrogenic ectasia after, 131–139
   inadequate suctioning in, 111

incomplete flap in, 109–110
infections after
   clinical signs and symptoms of, 156–157
   complications of, 157
   epidemiology of, 156
   histopathology and microbiology of,
      157
   prevention of, 158
   risk factors for, 155
   treatment of, 158–159
intraocular pressure changes with, 352–354
irregular astigmatism after, 172, 222–224,
   339–340
long-term stability and regression after,
   204–205
macular holes after, 282–284
NearVision contact keratoplasty after,
   334–335
neurotrophic epitheliopathy after, 364–365
patient counseling and selection for, 207
photorefractive keratectomy after, 57–58
postoperative infections in, 155–159
predictability factors of, 203–204
preoperative topographic analysis for, 13–
   15
rational advertising of, 207
recurrent erosion syndromes after, 115
retinal breaks and detachment after, 276–
   279
retinal conditions of, 278
submacular lacquer cracks and hemorrhage and choroidal neovascularization after, 284–286
thin glass and buttonholes in, 110–114
under- or overcorrection management
   after, 205
vitreoretinal complications of, 275–287
latanoprost, 48
light
   colored halos around, 188
   physics of, 185
   transient postoperative sensitivity to, 200
LightTouch technique, 331–332

macular detachment, stage 4 macular hole
   with, 283
macular edema, cystoid, 324
macular hole, after refractive surgery, 282–
   284
map colors conventions, 6

masking solutions, for irregular astigmatism, 177–178
Merocel microsponge, 90
metronidazole, 367
microkeratome
  corneal perforation by, 115–116
  in diffuse lamellar keratitis, 151
  malfunction of, 110, 112
  in post-LASIK keratectasia prevention, 139
  producing incomplete flap, 109–110
microphakonit, 249–250
MIRLEX (microincisional refractive lens exchange)
  air pump for, 249
  Chandelier illumination in, 258
  complications with nucleus manipulation for, 251–252
  conversion to extracapsular cataract extraction, 255–256
  corneal complications with, 252–253
  expulsive hemorrhage and, 255
  history of, 245
  IOA problems in, 256–258
  iris injury and, 254
  microphakonit techniques for, 249–250
  phakonit techniques for, 245–249
  vitreous loss and, 254–255
  wide-angle viewing in, 259–263
  wound construction in, 251
Mitomycin-C
  actions of, 90
  with contact keratoplasty, 332
  for corneal haze, 45, 48, 49–50
  for epithelial ingrowth, 167
  in LASEK surgery, 68
  in laser refractive surgery, 89–95
  PRK/PTK outcomes with, 49–51
  prophylactic, 94
  safety issues with, 94–95
  side effects and complications of, 93
modulated transfer functions (MTF), 219
monovision intolerance, after NearVision CK, 332
multicoated glasses, 192–193
Mycobacterium, post-LASIK, 156, 157, 159, 160
myopia
  accurate refraction in, 207
  after pediatric cataract surgery, 272
  astigmatism and, 230–231

customized LASIK for, 230
Epi-LASIK treatment of, 86
in iatrogenic keratectasia, 133
overcorrection of, 205
preoperative assessment of, 56
myopic refraction shift, factors affecting, 265–270

near infrared femtosecond laser
  intraoperative complications in, 197–200
  postoperative complications in, 200–201
near-work, excessive, 269–270
neuroadaptation, 300, 304
neurotrophic epitheliopathy, 364–365
night driving, yellow glasses for, 193
night glare, 37–38
night vision, 189, 193–194
nomograms, personalized, 205
nondissected islands, 199–200
nonsteroidal anti-inflammatory drugs (NSAIDs)
  for dry eye, 368
  postoperative, 58, 60
nucleus
  dislocation of with phakonit procedures, 256–257
  dropped, 257–258
  manipulation of, complications related to, 251–252

ocular hypertension, postoperative, 59
ocular rosacea, postoperative, 367
ocular surface slicing, 6
ofloxacin, post-LASEK, 69
ointment, intraocular, contaminated, 311
opaque bubble layer (OBL), 198, 199
optical coherence tomography (OCT)
  anterior chamber, 26, 28
  anterior segment, 29–33
  in under- or overcorrection management, 205
optical slit scan, 17–18
optical zone size, 35–36
Orbscan analysis
  in anterior keratoconus, 11–15
  clinical applications of, 7–10
  of corneal topography, 17–18
  imaging in, 6
  of normal eye, 6–7
  for post-LASIK keratectasia prevention, 138–139

of posterior corneal changes, 21–22
slit-beam and back-scattered reflection in, 3–4
understanding, 3–10
Orbscan II, 4
overcorrection
with contact keratoplasty, 333
with intracorneal rings, 348
post-LASEK, 75–76
post-LASIK, 205
post-PRK, 64

pachymetry, 20–21, 32
pain
with epithelial ingrowth, 165
postoperative, 59–60, 69–70, 77
paraxial optics, 3
patient selection
for LASIK surgery, 207
for refractive surgery, 362–363
pellucid marginal degeneration, 174
periannular opacity, 348
phacoemulsification, 248
phakonit
anesthesia in, 245
complications of, 251–254
converting to extracapsular cataract extraction, 255–256
with cut sleeve, 248–249
hydrodissection in, 246
incision in, 246
versus microphakonit, 251
rhexis forceps in, 246
techniques of, 247–248
wide-angle viewing systems in, 259–262
wound construction in, 251
photoablatable lenticular modulator (PALM) technique, 177
pigmentary dispersion syndromes, 322
pilocarpine, 194
placido disc systems, 3, 4, 56
pneumotonometry, 357–358
point spread function (PSF), 219, 225
polymerase chain reaction testing, 159
polymorphonuclear neutrophils (PMNs), 144, 152
posterior float, 3-D, 13, 20
posterior segment lesions, 286
prednisolone, 47–48, 152
premacular subhyaloid hemorrhage, 284

presbyopia
correcting implants for, 293–305
customized LASIK for, 229–230
post-PRK, 64
prostaglandins, 366
pseudodendrites, post-PRK, 61
pseudophakia, 268–269, 271–272
pseudosands, 153
pterygium, 100
punctal occlusion, 369
pupil constriction, 193–194
pupil size
in glare and halos, 187–189
glare and halos and, 37–38
laser ablation and, 38
measurement of, 35–36
preoperative measurement of, 189
pupillary ovalization, 322–323
pupillometers, binocular and monocular infrared, 36
pupillometry, accurate, 187–189

quad maps, 6–7, 10
in keratoconus, 9, 11–13
in posterior corneal elevation, 8, 9, 19

ray-tracing, 3–4, 172
rebamipide, 368
reflection, 185, 348
refraction measurements, 207–208, 220
refractive errors
correction of, 192–193, 269–270
hereditary, 267
multicoated glasses to correct, 192–193
preoperative assessment of, 55–56
residual, 321
refractive lensectomy, 282
refractive shift, after pediatric cataract surgery, 265–273
factors affecting, 265–270
prevention of, 270–271
treatment of, 271–273
refractive surgery
aberrations reducing quality of, 185
accuracy in, 35
complications of, 186–195
contact lens fitting after, 373–381
corneal dryness treatment after, 192
corneal topography problems in, 213–216
customized LASIK after, 229–233

dry eye and, 361–370

glare and halos after, 185–195

intraocular pressure and, 351–358

for irregular astigmatism, 218–227

irregular astigmatism correction after, 339–342

macular holes after, 282–284

mechanisms of retinal breaks and detachments after, 279–281

Mitomycin-C use in, 89–95

optical zone size and, 36

posterior corneal changes in, 17–22

posterior segment lesions after, 286

postoperative healing period after, 191–192

potential adverse and side effects of, 374

preoperative clinical evaluation for, 363

presbyopic correcting, 293–305

pupil size and, 35–39

recent advances in, 357–358

retinal nerve fiber layer thickness and visual field loss and, 355

submacular lacquer cracks and hemorrhage and choroidal neovascularization after, 284–286

toxic anterior segment syndrome after, 307–313

vitreoretinal complications associated with, 275–287

ReStor implant, 302–304

retinal breaks/detachment

after phakic IOL and refractive lensectomy, 282

after refractive surgery, mechanisms of, 279–281

distribution of, 279

with phakic IOLs, 323–324

with photorefractive keratectomy, 276

post-LASIK, 276–279, 281–282

pre-LASIK, 281–282

subtotal inferotemporal, 277

retinal holes, location and types of, 57

retinal nerve fiber layer thickness, 353, 355

retinoscopy, irregular astigmatism pattern in, 171–172

ReZoom implant, 299–301

rhexis forceps, 246

S/P keratorefractive surgery, 218–227

salt solution, balanced, 310

Sands of Sahara Syndrome. *See* diffuse lamellar keratitis

Scheimpflug imaging, 25, 123–124

Schwind ESIRIS, 204

segment migration, 348

Seidel, aberrations of, 185

septic infiltrations, post-LASEK, 71–72

Seton implantation procedure, 357

shape factor (SF), 213, 215

silicone-coated gloves, 148–149

slit-lamp examination

of anterior segment, 25

of corneal scars, 99

for diffuse lamellar keratitis, 144

slit-scan imaging, 3, 225

Smart Plug, 369

Snellen letter, 219, 226

specular reflection, versus back-scattered reflection, 4–5

SRK/T formula, 241, 242

Staphylococcal Aureo toxin, post-LASEK, 72

Staphylococcus aureus, 158, 307

starbursts, 186

steep cornea, 112

sterile corneal ulceration, 253

sterile glove contamination, 148–149

sterile infiltrates, post-PRK, 60

sterilization, short cycle, 311

sterilizer steam impurities, 311

steroids

for diffuse lamellar keratitis, 152

long-term topical use of, 192

postoperative, 58, 59

for toxic anterior segment syndrome, 309

Streptococcus, post-LASIK keratitis, 156, 157

stromal apoptosis, post-LASEK, 76–77

stromal melting, 166, 253

stromal surface, irregular, 92

stromal tissue, residual, 48–49

submacular hemorrhage, 284–286

submacular lacquer cracks, 284–286

suction loss, 113, 197

suction ring, 111, 113

sunglasses, polarizing and multicoated, 193

surface asymmetry index (SAI), 213, 215

surgical instruments, contaminated, 311

tarsorrhaphy, 369

tear film
   post-LASIK dysfunction of, 365
   supplements, 365–366
tear production, post-LASIK, 363–364
temporal globe, post-LASIK retinal breaks in, 277–279
temporal vitreous base, 280
testosterone, for dry eyes, 369
thermal insult, in diffuse lamellar keratitis, 148, 151
thermokeratoplasty, laser, 172
Thornton ring, 119
TOPOLINK procedure, 178–179
toxic anterior segment syndrome (TASS), 313
   clinical features of, 308–309
   conditions implicated in, 310
   definition of, 307
   differential diagnosis of, 309
   etiology of, 309–311
   outbreak investigation of, 311–312
   treatment of, 312
toxic endothelial cell destruction syndrome (TECDS), 308
toxic insult, in diffuse lamellar keratitis, 147, 151
trabeculectomy, postoperative, 31
trabeculoplasty, 356
trauma
   in diffuse lamellar keratitis, 147–148, 149–150
   irregular astigmatism and, 174
tropicamide, 69
two-dimensional topographic machines, 3

ultrasonography
   A-scan technology, 239–241
   of anterior segment, 25–26
   applanation A-scan, 241
   in axial length measurement, 239–241
   B-scan technology, 240
   immersion A-scan, 239–240
   in under- and overcorrection management, 205
uncorrected visual acuity (UCVA), 84, 85
undercorrection
   with contact keratoplasty, 333
   with intracorneal rings, 348
   postoperative, 63, 75–76, 205
UV exposure, in corneal haze, 44
uveitis, with phakic IOLs, 322

vascular occlusion, after refractive surgery, 286
Vexol, for postoperative ocular hypertension, 59
videokeratography
   computerized, 21–22, 56
   Fourier analysis of, 173
   showing corneal irregularity, 99–100
   showing regular cornea, 101
Visante optical coherence tomography, 32–33
   for anterior segment imaging, 25–26
   in under- or overcorrection management, 205
vision loss, with epithelial ingrowth, 166
visual acuity
   loss of, with epithelial ingrowth, 165
   in refractive shift in pediatric cataract surgery, 269
visual axis opacification, 269
visual field loss, refractive surgery effect on, 355
visual rehabilitation, after Epi-LASIK, 84–85
vitrectomy, 254–255
vitreoretinal complications, 275–287
vitreoretinopathy, post-LASIK proliferative, 278
vitreous
   collecting specimens of, 262–263
   loss of, 254–255, 303
vitritis, in toxic anterior segment syndrome, 309

wavefront
   in irregular astigmatism evaluation, 172, 219, 223
   in irregular astigmatism screening, 179–180
   problems with, 217
wavefront-guided lenses, customized, 193
wavefront-oriented excimer laser, for irregular astigmatism, 179–180
wide-angle viewing system
   contact, 261–262
   noncontact, 259–261
wound construction, in phakonit, 251
YAG laser, for complications of Crystalens implant, 298–299

Zernicke polynomials, 216, 219
zonal ablations, for irregular astigmatism, 176–177

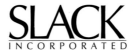

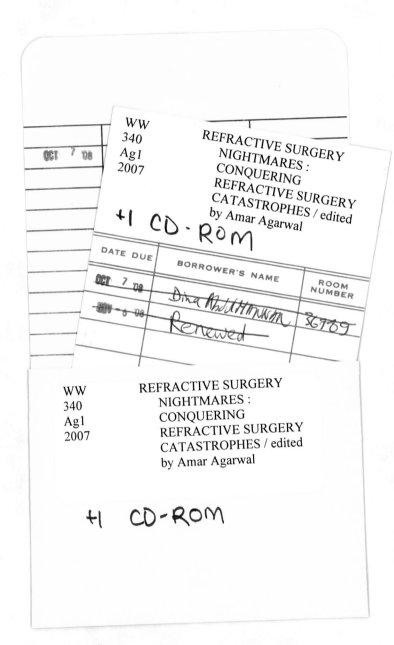

WW
340
Ag1
2007

REFRACTIVE SURGERY
NIGHTMARES :
CONQUERING
REFRACTIVE SURGERY
CATASTROPHES / edited
by Amar Agarwal

+1 CD-ROM

WW
340
Ag1
2007

REFRACTIVE SURGERY
NIGHTMARES :
CONQUERING
REFRACTIVE SURGERY
CATASTROPHES / edited
by Amar Agarwal

+1 CD-ROM

Earthquakes